Knee Surgery using Computer Assisted Surgery and Robotics

Fabio Catani • Stefano Zaffagnini
Editors

Knee Surgery using Computer Assisted Surgery and Robotics

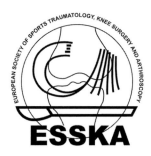
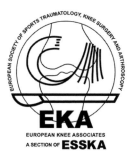
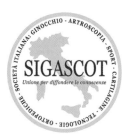

Editors
Fabio Catani
Department of Orthopaedic Surgery
University of Modena
Modena
Italy

Stefano Zaffagnini
Clinica Ortopedica Traumatologica III
Istituti Ortopedico Rizzoli
Bologna
Italy

Project Coordinator
Julie Agel
Department of Orthopedic Surgery
University of Minnesota
Minneapolis
USA

ISBN 978-3-642-31429-2   ISBN 978-3-642-31430-8   (eBook)
DOI 10.1007/978-3-642-31430-8
Springer Heidelberg New York Dordrecht London

Library of Congress Control Number: 2012954676

Foreword I

We are what we do, especially what we do to improve who we are!

The success of a surgery depends on an accurate and irreproachable technique. The awareness of surgical risks and complications is one of the most important purposes inside the operating room.

Currently we follow the trend to prevent human error and we need more than surgery carried out exclusively by human hand. Nevertheless, we must not forget the irreplaceable part of surgeons' knowledge and experience regarding the decision process.

This volume of *Knee Surgery* using *Computer Assisted Surgery and Robotics* shows very clearly the advantages of this tool and its usefulness in the near future. Moreover it includes a thorough range of opinions from outstanding surgeons.

The future is exciting and enthusiastic and we must continue to define what is best for our patients and profit from the newest technologies.

I am absolutely certain that this book will have a key role in education in this field.

João Espregueira-Mendes
ESSKA President

Foreword II

The computer world entered our life many years ago affecting the relation we have with time, space, distance or communication. The computer systems have also reached the field of surgery and particularly orthopedic surgery probably later than in other areas such as aeronautics or three-dimensional manufacturing. Nevertheless, it is now a reality to use any form of three-dimensional assistance to perform a knee arthroplasty. This may occur either at the time of planning the surgery, designing personalized tools, choosing the appropriate orientation of cutting guide, or performing the bone cuts using robotic surgery.

We are living in a world of permanent evaluation and the computer science technology brings in the operating room the possibility to check every step of the surgery when performing a uni-/bicompartmental or total knee arthroplasty. This relates to the location decided for the placement of the tibial and femoral cutting guides which was the first attempt to provide the surgeon with three-dimensional information while performing a knee arthroplasty. Then the orthopedic surgeon had the possibility to evaluate soft tissue tension and patellar tracking. Finally the kinematics data became available during surgery aiding the surgeon to address range of motion, femoro-tibial translation during flexion, and stability. The exact position of the implants is also provided as well as the overall lower limb axis.

After the first generation use of computer assisted surgery, some limitations and concerns appeared in the orthopedic literature world. The first one was related to time consumption for the registration process and the potential morbidity linked with rigid bodies. The second one focused on the precision of the information given to the computer at the time of registration since this impacts directly the quality of the data provided to the surgeon by the computer. The third one was related to the potential differences between the exact position of the guide as given by the computer and the actual precision of the bone cut performed by the surgeon. These last aspects led to the development of robotic or micro-robotic surgery in order to reduce this conflict, and the future evolutions in that field are probably unlimited.

At the end of the day the critical question is to define which surgical factors will influence significantly both functional and long term results of knee arthroplasty in terms of implant position, limb alignment or soft tissue tension. There is no doubt that any form of computer assisted surgery will play a key role for achieving these roles in their second generation of use when all the concerns and limitations have been addressed. The virtual imaging process provided by computer assisted surgery has also the potential to take a place of choice in the education of young orthopedic surgeons in order to plan and simulate the surgery while evaluating the kinematic consequences of the knee arthroplasty. The aim of this book is to provide the knee surgeon with the updated information related to computer assisted surgery and robotics and its application for the treatment of sportive and degenerative knee pathologies.

Jean-Noel Argenson

Foreword III

It has been always difficult to determine the real aims of Computer Assisted Surgery (CAS). During past years, several debates about the importance of this method in knee surgery, in particular in prosthetic knee surgery, have arisen.

The accuracy of surgery, the reduction of the invasiveness, and the possibility to monitor intraoperative parameters have been always claimed as among the biggest advantages of CAS. However, its role in younger surgeons' education has also to be considered essential.

Recently, its usefulness in pre- and intra-operative evaluation of ligament laxity has been investigated, thus making CAS an excellent tool also in the choice of surgical indication and type of treatment.

CAS and robotics with their several applications may represent for surgeons a strong incentive to improve the surgical technique, the research and the analysis of results. I am certain that this book will be also a new opportunity for young surgeons to learn the basis of these methods.

Paolo Adravanti
SIGASCOT President

Contents

Introduction

1

Fabio Catani and Stefano Zaffagnini

The idea to write a book on the use of computer-assisted surgery and robotics in orthopedic surgery can appear not up to date due to the low impact that this technology has had in the everyday practice for most orthopedic surgeons. AAOS recently made a survey of the use of CAS and found that only 7 % of the orthopedic surgeons use CAS for TKA.

However, we believe that this technology has been underestimated in its surgical application and clinical outcome impact because of the limited understanding of the anatomical and technical features of the technology and the complexity of the procedure implemented in the joint arthroplasty surgical technique. The purpose of this book is to give the clinical and surgical rationale for applying the use of CAS and robotics in treating patients affected by knee instability, knee osteoarthritis, and patello-femoral disease. This difficult task has been fulfilled by the contribution of the expertise of clinicians, engineers, and surgeons that have had effective benefit in their scientific and clinical work.

Computer-assisted surgery (CAS) and robotics have been introduced many years ago for joint replacement (hip and knee) with the aim to improve the accuracy in prosthesis components alignment. The technology was appealing but the learning curve of the orthopedic surgeons was quite steep. CAS introduced more costs, more materials to be sterilized and longer time for the surgeon in performing joint replacement, meaning increasing time of surgery and increasing hospital costs. The learning curve was difficult for many surgeons because of the understanding of the geometrical principles that the technology utilizes to correctly align the prosthetic components. Active and passive systems demonstrated advantages and disadvantages. Moreover, each company dedicated the CAS technology to their own prosthetic devices. All these factors limited the use of CAS, particularly for surgeons with little knowledge of joint replacement surgery.

Literature data comparing CAS with standard joint replacement technique demonstrated statistically significant differences in prosthesis component alignment particularly for the femur, less for the tibia. The strongest advantage was the reduction in patients' outliers. No literature data showed better clinical results using CAS with standard or minimally invasive surgery (MIS). Intraoperative osteoarthritis deformity kinematics assessment and soft tissue kinematics and balancing have not been enough studied; in fact no peer review data have been published on these topics.

F. Catani (✉)
Department of Orthopaedic Surgery,
University of Modena and Reggio Emilia,
Via del Pozzo 71, Modena 41125, Italy
e-mail: catani.fabio@unimore.it

S. Zaffagnini
Clinica Ortopedica e Traumatologica III,
Istituto Ortopedico Rizzoli,
via di Barbiano 1-10, Bologna 40136, Italy

Laboratorio di Biomeccanica e Innovazione Tecnologica,
Istituto Ortopedico Rizzoli,
via di Barbiano 1-10, Bologna 40136, Italy
e-mail: stefano.zaffagnini@unibo.it

F. Catani, S. Zaffagnini (eds.), *Knee Surgery using Computer Assisted Surgery and Robotics*,
DOI 10.1007/978-3-642-31430-8_1, © ESSKA 2013

The use of CAS or robotics in clinical practice is in the order of 8–10 % of all TKR and probably less than 2–3 % in THR. Only high-volume joint replacement surgeons working in teaching hospital are using CAS or robotics technology. We believe that CAS and robotics improve the accuracy of joint replacement surgery and for those who were using these technologies for many years enabled them to teach orthopedic surgeons, residents, and fellows to be more accurate and aware about the surgical mistakes we perform during surgery. The most important advantage, in fact, using CAS and robotic technology is the understanding of the mistakes that we face during surgery and also the kinematic relationship between OA deformity and soft tissue behavior. One of the most important results for many surgeons using CAS and robotics has been to perform less soft tissue releases to correctly balance the knee.

We strongly believe that CAS and robotics should be improved for the next generation of surgical techniques and, no less important, in teaching how to perform an excellent joint replacement and to improve patients' satisfaction and clinical outcomes.

To obtain patient satisfaction and lower limb high functional performance, we need to develop the new generation of digital surgery that will allow the surgeon to use less bulky instrumentation, to be less invasive, decrease tissue morbidity, and reach higher implant technique accuracy. A strong clinical research effort should be made to improve the current technologies in order to quantify the relationship between intra-operative measurement (prosthesis component alignment and soft tissue release) and patient clinical outcomes. An augmented virtual reality could allow us to foresee the effect of each surgical step and should permit a less invasive and time-consuming procedure.

All the applications for improvement of total knee arthroplasty are described: soft tissue balancing, alignment correction, functional performance of implanted prosthesis, as well as the application for unicompartmental prosthesis and bicompartmental procedure.

Navigation of patellar tracking and component and revision total knee are described as the latest applications. Tibial osteotomy and computer-assisted surgery of ligament reconstructions is described as well as the possibility to perform a kinematic evaluation of the knee in order to restore as much as possible the native knee pathway.

The availability of the state of the art of each surgical technique will allow the reader to have the possibility to judge his own thinking and surgical practice. This process in improving the surgeon knowledge in performing a more quantitative surgery could end up with new ideas and technical applications.

Only a full awareness of the CAS and robotics technology can widen our professional horizon and allow the surgeon to develop effective surgical improvements for the next surgical technology generation.

Accuracy of Computer-Assisted Surgery

2

Alberto Leardini, Claudio Belvedere, Andrea Ensini,
Vincenza Dedda, and Sandro Giannini

2.1 Introduction

2.1.1 Definitions

Computer-assisted surgery was introduced to improve the performance of surgical interventions with electronic instruments and software. In total knee arthroplasty (TKA) surgical navigation was primarily exploited and introduced, essentially for improving the accuracy of implant positioning [4]. The main advancement pursued is an 'augmented reality' in the operating theatre, made up of a number of digital cameras and trackers attached to the bones and to the standard instrumentation. Information such as optimal resection planes and targeted limb alignment is displayed to the surgeon during the operation before performing bone preparation, also according to a surgeon's specific preference (posterior slope, femur flexion, bone resections, varus/valgus, joint line, etc.). This tracking of bones and instruments is usually obtained by means of a stereophotogrammetric system made of digital cameras and emitting or reflective markers. Another series of navigation systems for TKA are based on electromagnetic tracking devices, not the topic of this present chapter, for which specific information can be found elsewhere [34, 74]. In general, surgical navigation systems are meant to enhance the final positioning of the implant (accuracy), as well as the visibility in inaccessible areas (security), and the prediction of the effects of the surgical actions (control).

It is fundamental to clarify the meaning of a series of relevant terms in this discipline and very recurrent in this present chapter, for which confusion may exit. Navigation systems are meant to track rigid objects in the three-dimensional space (see Fig. 2.1), i.e. to measure their position and orientation (hereinafter referred to as 'pose'). This pose therefore is usually expressed, in this three-dimensional space, in terms of three position coordinates and three orientation angles, with six values at each time instant, i.e. six degrees of freedom. These degrees of freedom are traced by the navigation system trackers, via the technical reference

A. Leardini, Ph.D. (✉) • C. Belvedere, Ph.D. • V. Dedda
Movement Analysis Laboratory,
Istituto Ortopedico Rizzoli, via di Barbiano 1/10,
Bologna, 40136, Italy
e-mail: alberto.leardini@ior.it;
claudio.belvedere@ior.it; vincenza.dedda@ior.it

A. Ensini, M.D.
Department of Orthopedic Surgery,
Istituto Ortopedico Rizzoli, University of Bologna,
via di Barbiano 1/10, Bologna, 40136, Italy
e-mail: andrea.ensini@ior.it

S. Giannini, M.D.
Department of Orthopedic Surgery,
Istituto Ortopedico Rizzoli, University of Bologna,
via di Barbiano 1/10, Bologna, 40136, Italy

Movement Analysis Laboratory,
Istituto Ortopedico Rizzoli, via di Barbiano 1/10,
Bologna, 40136, Italy
e-mail: sandro.giannini@ior.it

F. Catani, S. Zaffagnini (eds.), *Knee Surgery using Computer Assisted Surgery and Robotics*,
DOI 10.1007/978-3-642-31430-8_2, © ESSKA 2013

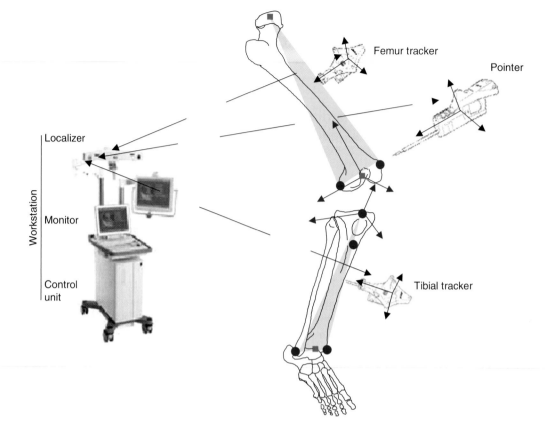

Fig. 2.1 Diagram showing the main instruments and references in a knee navigation system. The main workstation is made of the control unit with the computing power, a monitor for control, and graphical restitution to the surgeon and the localiser with the digital cameras to track motion of the trackers. These are implanted into the bones, and an additional one can point anatomical landmarks (*blue circles*) from which anatomical reference frames (*blue co-ordinate systems*) are defined. Each tracker/ pointer has its own technical reference frame (*black co-ordinate systems*) tracked in space by the localiser. Joint centres (*red squares*) are estimated in a number of ways and serve for the anatomical reference frames and mechanical axes. The pointer serves also to digitise clouds of points on the surfaces, for spatial registration, bone morphing, and other geometrical calculations

frames, which in themselves do not bring any anatomic value. These references are then rearranged with anatomical meanings, i.e. set in relation to the anatomy of the tracked bones, after the so-called anatomical survey to determine the anatomical reference frames. In the fields of science, engineering, industry, and statistics, accuracy of a measurement system is the degree of closeness of the obtained measurements to the corresponding actual true value. Precision of a measurement system, also called reproducibility or repeatability, is the degree to which repeated measurements under unchanged conditions show the same results. In the context of scientific methods therefore, the two words imply very different concepts. To emphasise and contextualise the contrast, a navigation system can be very precise if repeated measurements of the same quantity are very similar but not accurate if these are far away from the corresponding real value; in this case a systematic error is affecting the measures. Resolution, or sensibility, is the smallest change in the quantity that produces a response in the measurement. This is another important concept in navigated surgery: if the display shows bone thickness in millimetres with only integer numbers and no decimal figures (as in the snapshots in Fig. 2.3a, b), the overall resolution is 1 mm, irrespective to the nominal accuracy of the system. In other words, it is the minimum appreciable change of the information provided by the system.

2.1.2   State of the Art

The original surgical techniques for TKA were designed with basic knowledge of functional anatomy and biomechanics, utilising only mechanical tools and instruments, and relying on visual inspection by the surgeon. The accuracy with which orthopaedic surgeons can figure out visually lower limb alignment has been questioned [65]. In the early 1990s, easy access to computer-based motion tracking with the relevant user-friendly interfaces contributed to the development of a number of surgical navigation systems. These are now able to support the surgeon in many of the surgical decisions, such as the level and inclinations of osteotomy planes for both the femoral and the tibial components, component size selection, and also ligament release. The feasibility and value for the navigation-based control of these procedures have been established in many studies, largely for standard TKA, but recently for partial knee replacement [41, 62, 82, 85], and in osteoarthritic knees with severe extra-articular deformity [20, 81], where traditional instrumentation cannot be utilised. Recently, the patella seems to be traceable in TKA [8, 10], with considerable potential benefits for femoral and tibial component implantation.

It has been recognised that an accurate reconstruction of leg alignment offers the best opportunity for achieving good long-term results in TKA [4, 6, 13]. The extent to which the misalignment obtained with the conventional techniques was shown compared to that measured by navigation technology [9, 42, 77]. A large number of issues in TKA, such as early loosening, patellofemoral disorders, and uneven wear of the polyethylene liner, which all result in limitation of function and ultimately failure of the prosthesis are also associated with the optimal final alignment of the implant [13], for which computer-aided surgery, and in particular surgical navigation, provides significant facilitations. With this technology, the surgeon can

now plan the correct surgery, define bone cuts according to standard or preferred personal criteria, check the exact execution of these cuts, and adjust them to better match the surgical goals. It is now established that navigation can generate precise, accurate, and reproducible alignments [4, 5, 13, 20, 51, 62, 79, 86]. Rather than simply better mean results in component positioning, what has been shown is a considerable improvement of the rate of good alignments, usually at ±3° from the optimal final position [7, 23, 33, 51]. Evidence has also been provided that navigation surgery produces at least a tighter spread of deviations from neutral alignment of the coronal mechanical axis than conventional surgical techniques with intramedullary and extramedullary guides [7]. Surgical navigation also allows for careful intraoperative inspection of the kinematics before and after surgery, both at the tibiofemoral [18, 46] and patellofemoral joints [10]. Better restoration of the joint line has also been claimed [32, 63]. The value in obtaining more standardised surgical procedures and possibly more consistent outcomes [62], in assessing intraoperatively the natural and prosthetic range of knee motion [3, 68], and in performing less invasive surgeries [12, 40] has also been pointed out. Finally, intraoperative evaluations by navigation systems of anteroposterior knee joint laxity and relevant reliability have been discussed [46], but these are beyond our present scopes.

2.1.3   Limitations

Surgical navigation has been developed to achieve more accurate postoperative leg alignment through more precise and reproducible bone resections and more cautious ligament balancing [1, 19]. No long-term clinical studies have provided evidence of lower revision rates, and no difference in functional results was claimed at 2 years follow-up [33, 73]. Little clinical advantage of navigated over conventional surgical techniques in primary TKA has been claimed at early follow-ups [24]. Revision rates should be assessed carefully for a long time after surgery, by comparing groups of patients operated with and without this technique, and the possible advantage in patient outcomes of correct implant alignment should be assessed at mid and long terms. Many studies have provided large evidence that implant alignment is significantly improved compared with that achieved by conventional surgery, either with intramedullary or extramedullary guides. This has been shown by using radiography [13, 53, 62, 66, 79, 86] and computed tomography [13, 52]. It has been pointed out that radiographic and navigation-based measurements of limb alignment do not correlate [86], likely accounted for by the inherent limitations of the former technique, i.e. very qualitative and with subjective references.

The improvement in accuracy of prosthesis component implantation with navigation comes with additional costs. The technology in itself has a considerable cost, though the initial investment and maintenance over time can be shared among surgeons and spread over a large number of operations. Perhaps the most concerning general expense for the hospital is the increased operative time, reported to be from 0 [5] to 30 % [13] longer than any standard TKA, with both extramedullary and intramedullary guides. Learning curves can be another issue, the operative time reported to be significantly longer for a novice surgeon in navigation in the first 20 cases [72]; his final 20 cases had no difference, and all 50 cases in that study achieved the same results as the experienced surgeon in terms of post-implant mechanical alignment in the coronal and sagittal planes after operation and in mean Oxford score, mechanical axis and range of movement at 6 weeks and 1 year post-surgery. This study therefore showed that the learning curve for navigated TKA is approximately 20 cases and that a beginner can reproduce the results of an expert from the outset. The fact that residents implanting their initial TKA using navigation can perform as accurately as experienced consultants have been reinforced recently, though these operations can take longer [64]. It has been claimed that experience in navigation surgery can even reduce significantly the surgical time [49]. But much of the additional costs for this technology would be paid off over the social health-care service by the considerable reduction

of the TKA revisions, achieved possibly with a more accurate surgery, for which navigation can contribute enormously [57, 71].

2.1.4 Inaccuracies and Possible Errors

The surgical navigation systems are based on optoelectronic cameras; define surgical targets according to different surgical goals; rely on rigid fixations of trackers on bones and surgical instruments; are subject to deterioration of the instrumentation also because of the special surgical conditions and of sterilisation; require manual definition of axes and calibration of landmarks; imply anatomical, functional, and mathematical conventions; ought to communicate with the surgeon through a visual or numerical interface; and even have to monitor surgical actions which cannot be controlled, i.e. final standard impaction of the tibial and femoral components following all necessary bone resections and cement. The latter procedure in itself definitely results in alignment deviation between bone resection and final implant positioning, which the navigation system can monitor [19]. All these processes involve necessarily potential errors, i.e. unexpected and unknown deviations from what is planned and what can be performed and achieved. The necessary full knowledge of these errors is possible only with a profound understanding of all these processes, but this has been achieved only limitedly in this community so far. This present chapter contributes to this knowledge by looking at the literature and also by providing a consistent set of relevant results from experiments explicitly designed and performed for this purpose by these authors.

2.2 Sources of Error

Various and potentially very critical are the sources of error in conventional TKA in itself, which have also been quantified by surgical navigation systems [9, 42, 77]. The final accuracy is certainly affected by the different anatomical references and therefore targets. Even when these references and targets are fully determined in a navigation system, a number of inaccuracies may arise, as discussed below.

2.2.1 Instrumental and Technical Errors

The original source of possible inaccuracy is associated with the motion capture system in itself. Motion tracking of human bone segments by means of stereophotogrammetry is a largely studied discipline [17, 26, 30, 45]. Differently from surgical navigation research areas, many of the relevant definitions, options, and algorithms have been investigated and discussed within the relevant communities internationally. This thorough exercise has resulted in large and important evidence, reported in the literature; therefore, these issues are more known in the area of human motion and clinical gait analysis than in surgical navigation.

In surgical navigation, trackers are rigidly fixed to bone segments by standard Steinmann pins or equivalents; the classical soft tissue artefact [45] is overcome, but instrumental error still applies [26]. As for the instrumentation in itself, the current systems include pre-calibrated and rigidly connected camera arrays integrated into a suitable mobile unit. These can be moved around the space during acquisition of position data. A large series of studies in human motion analysis apply to surgical navigation for the correct definition of the necessary coordinate reference frames. The technical reference frames are those associated to the trackers, which hold a number of markers which can be active, i.e. light emitting diodes (LED) usually infrared, or passive, i.e. little balls reflecting this light emitted from LEDs around the cameras. In both cases, calculation is necessary by the navigation software to define the technical frames from the 3D positions of the relevant markers [17]. These procedures are not simple mathematical connections between markers but frequently take into account the full cluster of markers with an optimisation process [26]. The accuracy of the pose estimation for the relevant technical reference frame depends on the number, quality, visibility, and configuration of these markers, the larger the number of markers and the larger their relative distance, the better the accuracy is a correct tracking of bones and surgical instruments implies complete rigidity between these and the relevant tracker, for the technical frame to represent reliably segment pose throughout the operation. The most critical source of systematic error in this respect is a displacement of the tracker with respect to the segment, for any reason during the operation. This does affect severely the calculations of the system and would impair, if not realised, the final surgical result. Causes for this displacement are related to the mechanical loosening of the tracker fixation to the bony structure, due to either mechanical overload of the assembly or loosening of the fixation device. For this reason a number of navigation systems require digitising, from time to time during operation, both trackers and segments in reference points, for the relative position to be figured out and the possible displacement identified, i.e. integrity check. In this case the surgical procedure must restart from the beginning.

Little evidence of these issues has been reported explicitly for surgical navigation systems. These systems imply clusters of markers for rigid body tracking and also pointer probes utilised to indicate landmarks, axes, etc. For these probes, in addition to the accuracy in their pose estimation, the manufacturing and calibration of the instrument in itself may affect the final accuracy in defining these landmarks and axes. A recent study [48] has assessed in vitro with phantoms the reliability of the most elemental and critical measurements in navigation for TKA, i.e. angles and distances. The accuracy in locating single points, distances, and angles was found to be respectively about 0.6 mm (from 0.2 to 0.9 mm), 0.4 mm (from 0.001 to 1.3 mm) and 0.4° (from 0.06° to 0.69°). These demonstrate the superiority of the navigation systems to goniometres [3] and even to tomography [84]. These figures were claimed to be more than enough for TKA, but, as mentioned in that paper [48] and discussed here, the instrument in itself is only the original and smallest part of the overall error in navigation surgery. Another study had assessed the accuracy of image-free navigation system in phantom legs in which normal or abnormal mechanical axes are imposed [61] and claimed similarly good accuracy for position and orientation, but this was associated with the overall surgical navigation procedure. Because a phantom leg was used and hip and knee joints were simulated, this should be considered merely an analysis of the instrumental error, being the anatomical variability and relevant inaccuracy in landmarking not dealt with. It should also be pointed out that the reported good accuracy is typical in optimal conditions, i.e. perfect visibility, appropriate orientation, and vicinity of the cameras to the trackers, which may not always be achievable within a normal operating theatre.

2.2.2 Anatomical Calibrations and Survey

The procedure for the identification of the anatomical reference planes necessary to define and to target surgical goals, i.e. also called referencing [4], can be based on CT or fluoroscopy, i.e. the image-based navigation systems, or on landmark calibration, i.e. the image-free or imageless navigation systems. Imaging the patient is invasive, expensive, and time consuming; the image-free are therefore the most frequent, though the final anatomical reference frames differ considerably among the systems, which makes the comparison of results impractical. These are based on different clusters of anatomical landmarks, joint centres, and axes; even in case of similar primary references, the corresponding anatomical frames can be defined according to different criteria and conventions. The extent to which these definitions can be critical for the final results has been pointed out in human movement science [28, 30]. Even in the absence of the skin interposition between the bony landmark and the digitiser [28], large errors can be observed. Every navigation system has defined its own references also because the relevant TKA has its own design criteria and features, which may imply, for example, the identification of special mediolateral axes as target for the flexion axis of the femoral component. In the few image-based navigation systems, these landmarks are identified manually, but can be calculated automatically; in the many non-image-based systems, the landmarks have to be defined by visual

inspection within the standard surgical field and therefore must be easily identifiable. Reference axes can be defined from landmarks (the farther apart these are the better), can be indicated directly by the surgeon via instrumented pointers, or can be the combination, i.e. midway, of these two. Particularly in case of calibration of large relevant areas of the cartilage and bone surfaces, the system is enabled to work out the most appropriate size of the prosthetic components.

In surgical navigation for TKA, there is little evidence explicitly on this matter, likely because of the variety of systems and the complexity of the anatomy at the knee and the surrounding structures, as discussed for surgical navigation [38] as well as for traditional TKA [37].

The variability in individual digitisation was found to vary from 2 to 5 mm in standard deviation for certain landmarks, with ranges of 15–25 mm across surgeons [59]. Inter- and intra-surgeon errors in calibrating selected anatomical landmarks were investigated in vitro [88, 89]. In 100 repetitions of the same survey by a single surgeon [88], the maximum error in the transepicondylar axis was $8.2°$, whereas the maximum combined errors in the mechanical axis of the lower limb were only $1.3°$ in the coronal plane and $4.2°$ in the sagittal plane, the larger error of the former axis being accounted likely to the vicinity of the two landmarks. Once divided over the two bones [89], the maximum error in the femoral mechanical axis was $0.7°$ in the coronal and $1.4°$ in the sagittal planes; in the tibial mechanical axis these were respectively $1.3°$ in the coronal and $2.0°$ in the sagittal plane. Another study has evaluated, in sawbones, the effect of known incorrect landmarking onto final bone alignments [14], reporting significant deviations of the tibial bone cuts in the coronal plane: lateral displacements of the tibial plateau centre of 5, 10, and 15 mm caused mean differences of $1.3°$, $2.2°$, and $2.6°$ to valgus of the tibial coronal cut, respectively; corresponding medial displacements caused mean differences of $0.3°$, $1.4°$, and $2.2°$ to varus.

The reliability of the target for tibial component rotation, a critical issue in TKA [25], was assessed explicitly on 40 tibias by looking at seven possible reference frames as determined by

34 different anatomical landmarks [58]. High variability was found between these anatomical reference frames particularly those widely used in TKA, i.e. based on the transmalleolar axis and via the posterior condylar axis, 9.3° standard deviations for both. Large variability was observed for those based on the tibial tuberosity and the anterior condyles, respectively 6.1° and 7.3°. It was suggested that the combination of these different frames may reduce the range of errors; some of these combinations in fact are implemented in a number of current navigation systems. Overall limb alignment and extension angle after standard surveys were found very repeatable over five independent observers [36], though these measurements were obtained in embalmed cadaveric specimens and in a single well reproducible knee position

The identification of the location for the centre of the ankle joint in knee surgical navigation has been investigated explicitly [50, 67]. The estimation technique based on the established midpoint of the most medial and most lateral aspects of the malleoli was shown to be accurate and reproducible in each anatomical plane. A number of methods introduced an inaccuracy in the mechanical axis of the shank smaller than 1° [56]. More complicated models for this joint [67, 78] are not necessary.

The estimation of the head of the femur, i.e. the hip joint centre, is a very important landmark since it is used in the definition of the femoral anatomical reference frame and, particularly, in the definition of the femoral and overall leg mechanical axes. An incorrect estimation of this point implies an incorrect definition of the femoral anatomical reference frame [21] which would result in abnormal estimation of the resection levels, final component malposition, and, ultimately, misalignment of lower limb mechanical axes, crucial for the long-term survival rate in TKA. The hip joint centre cannot be directly digitised but must be estimated by a motion trial of the femur with respect to the pelvis, i.e. with a functional approach [16, 30, 44]. With this technique, hip joint centre estimation errors are within 2–4 mm, but the real interest is in the effect on the femur mechanical axis. These position errors, on an average sized femur, may result in an axis deviation smaller than 1° [69]. The

mean maximum error over seven normal cadaveric hips was found to be 0.92° [60], even when using a technique without tracking the iliac crest, but with hip circle movements higher than 10°. This study also observed no statistical difference between iliac and no-iliac tracking, a traditional dilemma in navigation of TKA. In more recent studies [22, 29] using cortical pins to track hip joint motion, it was demonstrated that the best possible result for the hip centre estimation can be limited to 2 mm. A wide variety of surgical techniques have been proposed to estimate the centre of the hip and algorithms for computation [15, 47, 76]. However, a number of studies have shown, using mechanical analogues of the hip joint, that the error increases when reducing the range of motion [15, 29].

More recent systems offer the option of defining the flexion axis not from anatomical surveys or landmarking, recognised to be highly variable [37, 68, 70], but from the knee joint, i.e. tibiofemoral kinematics [1, 2, 69]. The assumption is that passive motion of the knee is suitable to establish an average axis of joint flexion, which can be used as the medial-lateral axis in defining the femoral anatomical reference frame [69, 78]. This option would also save other time-consuming and error-prone procedures but shall face the well-known issue of the varying instantaneous rotation axis throughout the flexion arc, both in normal and pathological knees. A first assessment of the reproducibility of a knee flexion axis kinematically derived from motion captured using a navigation system was performed on 12 cadaver knees and 4 arthroplasty surgeons and compared with that of posterior condylar and transepicondylar axes derived from digitised anatomical landmarks [31]. The variance of the former axis was found to be smaller than that of the latter axes when determined under neutral loading conditions, and also, under a knee distraction force, the 95 % confidence intervals for the standard deviation being respectively 2.14–2.71° and 1.96–2.47°; the variability of the kinematically derived axis increased under varus, valgus, and internal loading conditions for the knee. A most recent study with intraoperative measurements and postoperative computed tomography [52] claims, for a more correct femoral component placement, the superiority of the

calculated flexion axis with respect to the traditional posterior condylar axis, the Whiteside's
line, and the surgical transepicondylar axis, which
are based on landmark palpation. This is supported by another recent work [27] which has
shown the calculation of a functional flexion axis
consistent with the transepicondylar axis, particularly in the transverse plane, in arthritic knees and
from small ranges of knee motion. It has also been
pointed out that functional axes of knee flexion
can describe better motion at this joint than any
other geometry based [83].

The current navigation systems do not employ
robust procedures to verify possible errors in the
anatomical survey and landmarking, likely because
it can be difficult to recognise these and to correct
small inaccuracies, as most frequently occur.

2.2.3   Conventions and Protocols

In addition to the cautious procedures necessary for
tracking the technical frames and the critical
definitions for transporting these to the anatomical
frames, which have much more surgical value, a
number of conventions and protocols are utilised
within the software of the current navigation systems, in the form of mathematical algorithms. The
way to report joint motion is among the most debated
topics in human motion analysis [17] because reports
of knee kinematics are affected by the chosen convention, irrespective from the measured poses of the
femur and tibia. When knee kinematics is analysed
by surgeons and bioengineers, full awareness of the
joint convention is recommended. Kinematic results
from different navigation systems must be compared
very carefully because of the profound differences in
anatomical frame definitions and joint conventions.
International recommendations have been provided
by the International Society of Biomechanics [17,
35].

2.2.4   Spatial Registration Shape
Matching and Bone Morphing

In a number of image-free systems, bone models
must be registered in space for representing their

actual location and configuration throughout surgery. These models are either defined previously
by imaging the specific patient under surgery or
taken and modified from other sources, i.e. databases of bone models. In surgical navigation, registration is the process of matching, based on
anatomical   references,   any   radiograph,
fluoroscopy, or computed tomography scans, or
any possible relevant 3D model, to corresponding
actual anatomical structures of the patient under
surgery [4]; in other words, it is the operation
which gets to superimpose as best as possible
refined models to the current positions of corresponding bones. When these models are taken
from defined databases from populations of subjects, they can be allowed to deform according to
the patient specific morphology, i.e. bone morphing is applied. In both rigid registration and
bone morphing, when exact corresponding references are used, i.e. a limited number of defined
anatomical landmarks, the issues described in
Sect. 2.2.2 here apply as well. Alternatively,
when generic clouds of points are taken to match
on the scans/models and on relevant actual structures, larger errors are likely to occur. When the
bone models are registered in space, calculations
of joint kinematics, flexion, and mechanical axis
and even the thickness of bone resections are
facilitated because morphologic data are then
provided in addition to standard geometric data.
These techniques have also obviated the use of
preoperative or intraoperative imaging in most
cases [43]. Each of the procedures involved in
registration and morphing however is computa-
tionally demanding because the optimal final
location is estimated in a number of iterations
and inevitably involves inaccuracies.

The bone-morphing technique was introduced
[75] as a special global registration method: 3D
statistical deformable models were registered to
sparse data points digitised on the actual bones
by an optical 3D pointer. It was claimed an accurate, fast, and user-friendly method. Later, the
effect of a number of bone reconstruction parameters and of data sampling area on the accuracy of
a shape-based registration method for a computer
navigation system was assessed thoroughly
in vitro [55]. Using relevant surface bone models

from CT images, spatial registration to real bones was performed with errors smaller than 0.8 mm and 0.6° when 3-mm slice thickness, 1-mm reconstruction pitch, and 30 sampling points are used. A recent study [59] reported the reproducibility of bone morphing with final tracked 3D morphometric models obtained by elastic registration of statistical models to sparse point clouds digitised directly on the bone surface with a pointer. One expert and four trainee surgeons performed this protocol on a cadaveric knee ten times. Final femoral and tibial implant positioning parameters resulted in intra-surgeon standard deviations of less than 1.4° for rotation and 1.9 mm for translation for all surgeons in all directions except for tibial axial rotation. It was concluded that the information derived from registered 3D models is more accurate and reproducible than that derived from landmarking only.

2.2.5   Interfaces and Reporting

The procedures required by a navigation system should be presented to the operating surgeon with a clear and easy interface to minimise misunderstandings and to make the surgeon more aware of the effects of relevant actions. The large set of information collected and elaborated during a navigated TKA surgery can be returned to the surgeon for the benefit of the overall intervention in many different ways. This sort of development of navigation systems will continue for a long time, and perhaps its value has been underestimated.

A recent study was aimed explicitly at evaluating the effectiveness of software advancements of a navigation system in improving TKA component positioning and limb alignment [53]. Previous work from the same authors [1] had shown a statistically significant improvement in good knee alignments (11 %) from conventional to navigated techniques. Preoperative and postoperative x-ray measurements demonstrated further improvements when a new version of the software was used. Mean tourniquet time went from 74 min in conventional surgery to 90 min with the original

navigation software and back to 73 min with the advanced navigation software.

2.2.6   Performance of Osteotomy, Impaction, and Other Surgical Executions

Once the navigation system has planned the level and orientation of the osteotomies, then these must be performed with the sawblades, final bone preparation is executed, cement is then applied, and eventually the final components are implanted by hard impaction. In between, a number of trials and tests can be performed with the trial components. All these are additional surgical actions, all together termed 'the execution process' [39], mostly manually performed, which may affect considerably final component alignments, regardless of the accuracy with which the navigation-based plan had been designed. Even the manual adjustment of the saw guides, for example, can make difficult the targeting of the navigation goals. It has been shown recently that a significant improvement in guide positioning and corresponding accuracy of the final bone cuts, together with decreases in surgical time, can be achieved when adjustable cutting blocks are used [79].

The intraoperative deviations implied in the bone-cutting process of TKA were addressed explicitly as an important source of inaccuracy [6]. These were defined as the difference in spatial orientation between the cutting block before sawing and the corresponding achieved resection plane afterwards and measured by a CT-based navigation system. The mean difference over 50 computer-assisted TKAs was 1.4° in flexion/extension of the distal femoral cut, smaller than 1.0° elsewhere. To minimise these cutting errors, more robust surgical techniques and mechanical instruments would be sufficient, to enable a more stable fixation of the cutting blocks or even more appropriate preparation of instruments. Very similar results were found in another study [87], which also reported larger errors in bone cut resections through cutting slots (slotted cutting) than in those on the surface of a cutting guide (open cutting), attributed to the use of a thicker sawblade with higher stiffness in the latter method. Another interesting study [11] measured during surgical navigation the thicknesses of the real bone resections at the femur and tibia on both condyles and compared these with corresponding navigation plans: the mean difference was as small as 0.4, 0.2, and 0.1 mm respectively, but these become 1.7, 1.1, and 1.4 mm when the thickness of the sawblade is not considered in the calculation. 'Execution deviations', defined as the difference between planned targets and executed results, were reported in navigation-assisted minimally invasive TKAs [39]. In both femur and tibia resections in all anatomical planes, the mean resection deviations were all smaller than 0.8 mm and 0.7°. In a most recent study [54], the angular difference between the cutting surface and the corresponding preoperative plan in the sagittal and coronal planes, averaged over 20 knees, were respectively $1.6° \pm 2.2°$ in extension and $0.5° \pm 1.4°$ in valgus. Seventy percent of the knees were cut in an extended position with respect to the targeted alignment in the sagittal plane, and only 30 % of the knees had a malalignment of more than 1° in the coronal plane. These errors can be very different from knee to knee, as accounted for by the experience of the surgeon, mechanical accuracy and tolerance of the saw-blades and cutting jigs, movement of the fixation pins, correct tracking of the guide, sawblade thickness and oscillation, and quality of the bone. Using a computer-assisted technique, differently from the conventional ones, the surgeon is aware of any possible cutting error occurring at each point of the operation and can therefore correct these errors during surgery [6].

The alignment deviations caused by standard impaction of the tibial and femoral components have been shown to be considerable [19]. The alignment in three anatomical planes of the tibial and femoral bone resections first, and after final tibial and femoral component implantation with cement second, was measured during surgery by an instrumented probe of a navigation system. The alignment deviations between the bone resections and the subsequent implant placement were larger than 1° in the frontal plane of the femur and in the frontal and sagittal planes of the tibia respectively in 20, 11, and 33 % of the 91 knees analysed. The deviations were larger than 2° in 4, 3, and 9 % of the knees, respectively. Deviations as large as 3° were found at the tibia in the sagittal plane, i.e. posterior slope error. Also in the study which has analysed the overall 'execution deviations' [39], the bone resections were found to be less critical than the implant fixation, the mean coronal alignment, and degree of extension for the latter being respectively 0.7° (more in valgus) and 1.6° (decrease).

Execution deviations from planned alignment commonly occur also in navigated TKA, and this information should improve the awareness of the surgeons and the accuracy of the final results. The two main sources, i.e. bone resection and implant fixation, can also be combined, the latter being more difficult and less precise if the former is not well performed, i.e. errors in component-to-bone matching can more easily occur. The bone cement mantle is of course another source of deviation. Nevertheless, within a computer-navigated TKA, it is possible and recommended therefore to check carefully the final alignment of the prosthetic components before the cement hardens.

2.2.7 Concluding Remarks

The literature has demonstrated that a number of sources of error depend solely on the navigation system, position measurements, visibility, references, calculations, and conventions. Other errors depend on the surgeon's ability, such as landmarking and execution processes. The latter can be certainly limited by a more complete consciousness of the former errors and of relevant general procedures (anatomical survey, referencing, registration, etc.). Navigation systems will likely be enhanced by a more careful measure and analysis of all these errors, and perhaps by relevant compensation algorithms. A problem for a definite assessment of the accuracy of the final results after navigated surgery is that there are no techniques with the better accuracy and reproducibility to perform in real cases, any medical imaging-based procedure being affected by possibly even larger errors, with measurements frequently taken even with large manual intervention, as demonstrated in the literature.

2.3   System Validation Tests

To get overall and consistent information on the possible errors encountered in knee navigation surgery, in this section we present a series of published and unpublished results obtained with a single system (Stryker® Knee Navigation System software version 2.0, Stryker Leibinger GmbH & Co KG, Germany) and by a single staff of knee surgeons and biomedical engineers.

In a first paper [9], a Plexiglas grid with a surgical navigation tracker fixed rigidly to it, and with 33×33 small holes in known position with the same diameter as the pointer tip, was positioned horizontally at about 120 cm from the localiser. The position coordinates of each hole were collected by the pointer in the technical reference frame associated to the tracker. The full array of the collected points was optimally matched in space to the corresponding model of known relative positions by using the standard SVD calculation. In the grid digitisation test, the mean measured distance between the collected points and the known positions was 0.31 mm (range 0.78–0.14 mm), well within the nominal accuracy of the system, but mainly smaller than the resolution of this system.

A second test was performed to check the reproducibility of the anatomical reference frame definitions, presumed to be considerably affected by anatomical landmark digitisation. Ten anatomical surveys were performed in a single lower limb specimen by three surgeons, with different levels of experience in navigated TKA.

Almost all landmarks were highly reproducible on all planes. The most critical references, both inter- and intra-surgeon, were the proximodistal position of the medial malleolus and the mediolateral position of the ankle centre. As for

Table 2.1 Repeatability, from the most experienced (#1) to the least experienced (#3) surgeon

–	#1	#2	#3	Overall
Femur – sagittal plane	0.4°	0.6°	0.3°	0.3°
Femur – coronal plane	1.9°	1.1°	2.1°	1.1°
Femur – transverse plane	2.2°	1.1°	2.0°	1.2°
Tibia – sagittal plane	1.0°	0.5°	1.0°	1.0°
Tibia – coronal plane	3.5°	3.3°	5.8°	5.6°

the five orientation measurements of the relevant reference frames resulting from the survey repetitions analysed in this study, the confidence interval at 95 % for reproducibility is reported in Table 2.1. Except for the orientation in the coronal plane of the tibia, this interval is close to or smaller than 1°. The variation in orientation of the Whiteside's line with respect to the transepicondylar axis was 2.3°, 3.0°, and 3.2° in the order of decreasing experience and 1.6° on aggregate. These results demonstrated a very good repeatability in four out of the five alignments in TKA; in these four, very good performance was achieved also by the inexperienced young surgeon. The tibial varus/valgus remains a critical issue, and it is likely to be primarily affected, considering the present conventions utilised, by the estimation of the location of the ankle joint centre. From these observations it was deduced [33] that the accuracy of the system in itself in single-marker positioning is 0.3 mm and that intra- and inter-surgeon variations in landmark and axis calibrations are the largest part of error in defining anatomical reference frames. The latter variations were found in ad hoc experiments smaller than 2° in all five orientations of the osteotomy, except in the tibial frontal plane.

In another paper [8], in addition to the calibration grid, reproducibility of the definition of the patellar anatomical reference frame, expected to be affected by landmark digitisation, was assessed by performing digitisation of three relevant patellar landmarks ten times by two surgeons, both experienced with surgical navigation. The variability of the patellar frame in position along and orientation about the three anatomical planes was expressed as the confidence intervals at 95 %. The values at the confidence intervals in one of the two reproducibility tests were 5.7°, 7.1°, and 7.6°, respectively, in patellofemoral flexion, rotation, and tilt, and 0.7, 2.2, and 1.6 mm in the displacements along respectively the mediolateral, proximo-distal, and anteroposterior anatomical axes. With the other surgeon, these were respectively 7.5°, 6.4°, and 5.2° and 0.6, 1.7, and 1.0 mm.

The procedure for hip joint centre estimation should also be investigated carefully because of the necessary special functional technique, i.e. by means of trials of relative motion between the femur and the pelvis [16, 30, 44]. This additional acquisition is performed, in the various available systems, either with or without a pelvic tracker, i.e. in the pin-based or pin-less modality. The repeatability of this estimation process was performed on a sawbone model made of interileum-abdominal segment and a femur. To check for the instrument error only, the ball-and-socket, or spherical, articulation was obtained by a hip prosthesis, the stem being implanted in the femur, and the cup on the interileum-abdominal segment. Twenty estimations of the positions of the femur head centre in the femoral anatomical frame were obtained, ten in pin-less and ten in pin-based modality, both with the interileum-abdominal segment rigidly fixed to the workbench. The surface of the prosthetic femoral head was also digitised, whose optimum centre, estimated in the least-square sense, was considered as the reference goal for all the estimations (0.51-mm standard deviation). This goal point together with the epicondyles and the knee centre was used to define the femoral anatomical reference frame. Five circumduction trials with increasing amplitude and five with minimal amplitude were recorded. The estimations were found accurate along the anteroposterior and mediolateral directions of the femoral frame and less successful along the proximodistal in pin-based modality (up to 5-mm difference). Overall, the 3D difference was about 10 mm in the worst case along all femoral axes, irrespective of the two pin modalities. These estimations seem affected mostly by the number and distribution of the points on the sphere described by the circumduction (Fig. 2.2).

A final technical test utilised a mechanical hinge joint to assess the overall ability of the system to calculate the instantaneous helical axis, in this special case being a fixed axis of rotation. Two trackers were fixed into the fixed and moving arms, and position measurements were taken at three different angular velocities. The accuracy with which this axis was calculated was found −0.111° in slow, 0.115° in medium, and −0.004° fast motion, suitable for any calculation of kinematically derived axis of flexion.

In a most recent paper from these authors [32], it has been pointed out that despite the fact that nominal accuracy of this navigation system for tracker position and orientation is respectively about 0.5 mm and 0.5°, the relevant linear and angular measurements displayed to the surgeon in the operating theatre have a resolution of 1 mm and 0.5° respectively (see Fig. 2.3a, b).

For any characterisation of the overall navigation system and procedures within a specific single surgical context, the full series of validation tests is recommended.

2.4 Discussion

A new generation of surgical techniques and tools, known as surgical navigation systems, has been developed to help surgeons to obtain more accurate and reproducible TKA. Navigation systems can now also record important information intraoperatively such as final locations of the prosthesis components, ligament arrangements, joint kinematics and range of motion, laxity, and patellar tracking; this can be utilised at anytime after surgery for performance assessments. Surgical navigation can realise better preoperative surgical planning as well; however, the final results would rely largely on the soft tissue balance, which is a key issue for a good final function at the replaced knee [75] but hardly this is accounted for in plannings based fully on medical imaging.

Several good review articles summarise careful history, biomechanical principles, and perspective of these surgical navigation systems [4, 69]. In this present chapter, the various sources

Fig. 2.2 Snapshot from the
Stryker knee navigation
system, with the graphical
restitution at the display
during the hip joint centre
estimation: the clouds of
points described by the femur
tracker in the laboratory frame
are shown superimposed to
the best-fitting sphere; the
radius of this sphere is also
reported, together with the
standard deviation of the
estimation

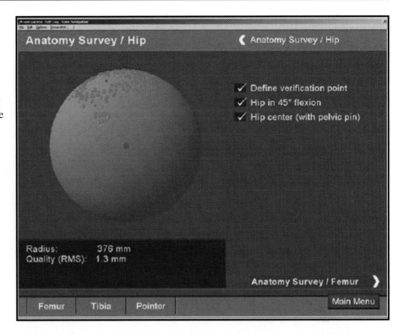

of error implied in the current surgical navigation
systems are enumerated and analysed. It is meant
that the perfect alignment of the prosthetic
components and the leg, with a minimum of relevant bone removal, is the primary goal of these
systems. The relevant expectation that an
improved alignment would result in better clinical outcomes and lower revision rates is still
debated and discussed in other chapters of this
book.

Many are the advantages of these systems, and
fewer are the disturbances: while providing valuable support to the surgery, the invasiveness and
extra-burden on the patient is very limited (particularly the image-free), as well as the disruption
for the surgeon; with both active and passive systems, the field of view is large, the compatibility
with (sterilisation, encumbrance, etc.) and the
constraints of the operating theatre have been
overcome, the learning curve is rapid. In addition, these systems now provide some support to
preoperative planning, including the selection of
the component size and positioning according to
patient-specific morphology and the alignment
procedures intraoperatively, according also to
soft tissue tensioning and knee joint natural kine-

matics. Finally, the capability of storing and
retrieving qualitative (images) and quantitative
(measurements) information is another appreciated feature.

Several issues are still problematic. The
repeatability of the identification of anatomical
landmarks by manual palpation and of axes by
visual inspection remains a concern. The estimation of the hip joint centre is still not fully convincing, particularly in those systems where the
pelvis is not tracked. A large debate exists on
what and how information should be reported to
the surgeon in the theatre; in addition to the necessarily friendly interface, both for requiring
actions and for reporting from these, it is definitely
crucial that the surgeon is more aware of the
actions to instruct the navigation system (anatomical calibrations, surface digitisation, joint
motion exercises, etc.) and in particular more
conscious about the most critical consequences
of relevant inappropriate performances. It has
been requested that additional measurements not
strictly associated to the standard procedures can
be allowed fully to the user, for taking complete
advantage of an expensive measurement system
which has direct access to the joint during its

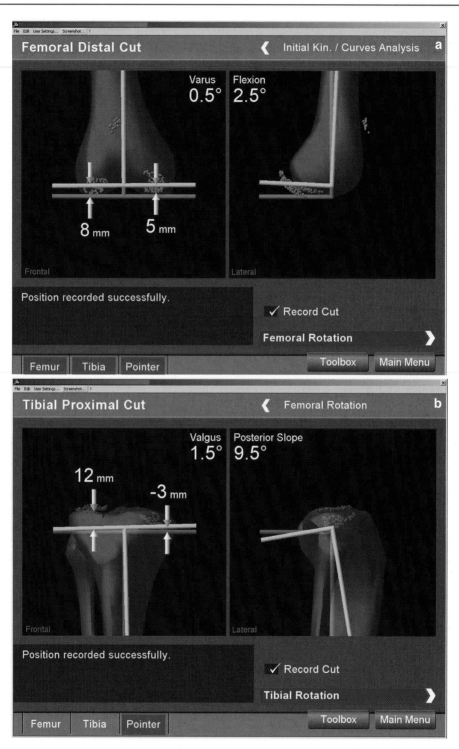

Fig. 2.3 a and **b** Snapshots from the Stryker knee navigation system, with diagrams of the at the distal femur (top, snapshot a) and the proximal tibia surgical plan (bottom, snapshot b), in the frontal (*left*) and sagittal (*right*) planes. Linear measurements are displayed with integer in millimetres; therefore, 1 mm is the minimum visible variance, i.e. resolution; angular measurements are displayed with one decimal figure, this being either 0 or 5, i.e. 0.5° is the resolution. The reference anatomical frame and the digitized points are also shown, on the distal femur (*green*) and on the proximal tibia (*blue*). The corresponding frames of the surgical instrumentation are also depicted (*yellow*).

replacement. A clear additional advantage would be the possibility to track the patella and the main ligamentous structures. Finally, the inclusion of knee joint models would definitely enhance further the potentials for the current navigation systems, importing into the standard geometrical or morphological criteria, ligament balancing [80], and , more in general, knee mechanical concepts and knowledge.

References

1. Anderson KC, Buehler KC, Markel DC (2005) Computer assisted navigation in total knee arthroplasty: comparison with conventional methods. J Arthroplasty 20(7 Suppl 3):132–138
2. Asano T, Akagi M, Nakamura T (2005) The functional flexion-extension axis of the knee corresponds to the surgical epicondylar axis: in vivo analysis using a biplanar image-matching technique. J Arthroplasty 20(8):1060–1067
3. Austin MS, Ghanem E, Joshi A et al (2008) The assessment of intraoperative prosthetic knee range of motion using two methods. J Arthroplasty 23(4):515–521
4. Bae DK, Song SJ (2011) Computer assisted navigation in knee arthroplasty. Clin Orthop Surg 3(4):259–267
5. Bar MC, Daubresse F, Hugon S (2011) The advantages of computer assistance in total knee arthroplasty. Acta Orthop Traumatol Turc 45(3):185–189
6. Bäthis H, Perlick L, Tingart M et al (2005) Intraoperative cutting errors in total knee arthroplasty. Arch Orthop Trauma Surg 125(1):16–20
7. Bauwens K, Matthes G, Wich M et al (2007) Navigated total knee replacement. A meta-analysis. J Bone Joint Surg Am 89:261–269
8. Belvedere C, Catani F, Ensini A et al (2007) Patellar tracking during total knee arthroplasty: an in vitro feasibility study. Knee Surg Sports Traumatol Arthrosc 15(8):985–993
9. Belvedere C, Ensini A, Leardini A et al (2007) Alignment of resection planes in total knee replacement obtained with the conventional technique, as assessed by a modern computer-based navigation system. Int J Med Robot 3(2):117–124
10. Belvedere C, Leardini A, Ensini A et al (2009) Three-dimensional patellar motion at the natural knee during passive flexion/extension. An in vitro study. J Orthop Res 27(11):1426–1431
11. Biant LC, Yeoh K, Walker PM et al (2008) The accuracy of bone resections made during computer navigated total knee replacement. Do we resect what the computer plans we resect? Knee 15(3):238–241
12. Biasca N, Schneider TO, Bungartz M (2009) Minimally invasive computer-navigated total knee arthroplasty. Orthop Clin North Am 40(4):537–563
13. Blakeney WG, Khan RJ, Wall SJ (2011) Computer-assisted techniques versus conventional guides for component alignment in total knee arthroplasty: a randomized controlled trial. J Bone Joint Surg Am 93(15):1377–1384
14. Brin YS, Livshetz I, Antoniou J et al (2010) Precise landmarking in computer assisted total knee arthroplasty is critical to final alignment. J Orthop Res 28(10):1355–1359
15. Camomilla V, Cereatti A, Vannozzi G et al (2006) An optimized protocol for hip joint centre determination using the functional method. J Biomech 39(6):1096–1106
16. Cappozzo A (1984) Gait analysis methodology. Hum Mov Sci 3:27–50
17. Cappozzo A, Della Croce U, Leardini A et al (2005) Human movement analysis using stereophotogrammetry. Part 1: theoretical background. Gait Posture 21(2):186–196
18. Casino D, Zaffagnini S, Martelli S et al (2009) Intraoperative evaluation of total knee replacement: kinematic assessment with a navigation system. Knee Surg Sports Traumatol Arthrosc 17(4):369–373
19. Catani F, Biasca N, Ensini A et al (2008) Alignment deviation between bone resection and final implant positioning in computer-navigated total knee arthroplasty. J Bone Joint Surg Am 90(4):765–771
20. Catani F, Digennaro V, Ensini A et al (2012) Navigation-assisted total knee arthroplasty in knees with osteoarthritis due to extra-articular deformity. Knee Surg Sports Traumatol Arthrosc 20(3):546–551
21. Cereatti A, Camomilla V, Vannozzi G et al (2007) Propagation of the hip joint centre location error to the estimate of femur vs pelvis orientation using a constrained or an unconstrained approach. J Biomech 40(6):1228–1234
22. Cereatti A, Donati M, Camomilla V et al (2009) Hip joint centre location: an ex vivo study. J Biomech 42(7):818–823
23. Chauhan SK, Scott RG, Breidahl W et al (2004) Computer-assisted knee arthroplasty versus a conventional jig-based technique A. randomised, prospective trial. J Bone Joint Surg Br 86(3):372–377
24. Cheng T, Pan XY, Mao X et al (2011) Little clinical advantage of computer-assisted navigation over conventional instrumentation in primary total knee arthroplasty at early follow-up. Knee 19(4):237–245
25. Cheng T, Zhang G, Zhang X (2011) Imageless navigation system does not improve component rotational alignment in total knee arthroplasty. J Surg Res 171(2):590–600
26. Chiari L, Della Croce U, Leardini A et al (2005) Human movement analysis using stereophotogrammetry. Part 2: instrumental errors. Gait Posture 21(2):197–211
27. Colle F, Bignozzi S, Lopomo N et al (2012) Knee functional flexion axis in osteoarthritic patients: comparison in vivo with transepicondylar axis using a navigation system. Knee Surg Sports Traumatol Arthrosc 20(3):552–558
28. Conti G, Cristofolini L, Juszczyk M et al (2008) Comparison of three standard anatomical reference

frames for the tibia-fibula complex. J Biomech 41(16): 3384–3389

29. De Momi E, Lopomo N, Cerveri P et al (2009) In-vitro experimental assessment of a new robust algorithm for hip joint centre estimation. J Biomech 42(8): 989–995

30. Della Croce U, Leardini A, Chiari L et al (2005) Human movement analysis using stereophotogrammetry. Part 4: assessment of anatomical landmark misplacement and its effects on joint kinematics. Gait Posture 21(2):226–237

31. Doro LC, Hughes RE, Miller JD et al (2008) The reproducibility of a kinematically-derived axis of the knee versus digitized anatomical landmarks using a knee navigation system. Open Biomed Eng J 2:52–56

32. Ensini A, Catani F, Biasca N et al (2012) Joint line is well restored when navigation surgery is performed for total knee arthroplasty. Knee Surg Sports Traumatol Arthrosc 20(3):495–502

33. Ensini A, Catani F, Leardini A et al (2007) Alignments and clinical results in conventional and navigated total knee arthroplasty. Clin Orthop Relat Res 457:156–162

34. Frantz DD, Wiles AD, Leis SE et al (2003) Accuracy assessment protocols for electromagnetic tracking systems. Phys Med Biol 48(14):2241–2251

35. Grood ES, Suntay WJ (1983) A joint coordinate system for the clinical description of three-dimensional motions: application to the knee. J Biomech Eng 105(2):136–144

36. Hauschild O, Konstantinidis L, Strohm PC et al (2009) Reliability of leg alignment using the OrthoPilot system depends on knee position: a cadaveric study. Knee Surg Sports Traumatol Arthrosc 17(10):1143–1151

37. Jenny JY, Boeri C (2004) Low reproducibility of the intra-operative measurement of the transepicondylar axis during total knee replacement. Acta Orthop Scand 75(1):74–77

38. Jenny JY, Boeri C, Picard F et al (2004) Reproducibility of intra-operative measurement of the mechanical axes of the lower limb during total knee replacement with a non-image-based navigation system. Comput Aided Surg 9(4):161–165

39. Kim TK, Chang CB, Kang YG et al (2010) Execution accuracy of bone resection and implant fixation in computer assisted minimally invasive total knee arthroplasty. Knee 17(1):23–28

40. Kim KI, Ramteke AA, Bae DK (2010) Navigation-assisted minimal invasive total knee arthroplasty in patients with extra-articular femoral deformity. J Arthroplasty 25(4):658.e17–22

41. Konyves A, Willis-Owen CA, Spriggins AJ (2010) The long-term benefit of computer-assisted surgical navigation in unicompartmental knee arthroplasty. J Orthop Surg Res 5:94

42. Koyonos L, Stulberg SD, Moen TC et al (2009) Sources of error in total knee arthroplasty. Orthopedics 32(5):317

43. Laskin RS, Beksaç B (2006) Computer-assisted navigation in TKA: where we are and where we are going. Clin Orthop Relat Res 452:127–131

44. Leardini A, Cappozzo A, Catani F et al (1999) Validation of a functional method for the estimation of hip joint centre location. J Biomech 32:99–103

45. Leardini A, Chiari L, Della Croce U et al (2005) Human movement analysis using stereophotogrammetry. Part 3. Soft tissue artifact assessment and compensation. Gait Posture 21(2):212–225

46. Lopomo N, Bignozzi S, Martelli S et al (2009) Reliability of a navigation system for intra-operative evaluation of antero-posterior knee joint laxity. Comput Biol Med 39(3):280–285

47. Lopomo N, Sun L, Zaffagnini S et al (2010) Evaluation of formal methods in hip joint center assessment: an in vitro analysis. Clin Biomech (Bristol, Avon) 25(3):206–212

48. Lustig S, Fleury C, Goy D et al (2011) The accuracy of acquisition of an imageless computer-assisted system and its implication for knee arthroplasty. Knee 18(1):15–20

49. Manzotti A, Cerveri P, De Momi E et al (2010) Relationship between cutting errors and learning curve in computer-assisted total knee replacement. Int Orthop 34(5):655–662

50. Marchant DC, Rimmington DP, Crawford RW et al (2005) An algorithm for locating the center of the ankle joint in knee navigation surgery. Comput Aided Surg 10(1):45–49

51. Mason JB, Fehring TK, Estok R et al (2007) Meta-analysis of alignment outcomes in computer-assisted total knee arthroplasty surgery. J Arthroplasty 22(8): 1097–1106

52. Matziolis G, Pfiel S, Wassilew G et al (2011) Kinematic analysis of the flexion axis for correct femoral component placement. Knee Surg Sports Traumatol Arthrosc 19(9):1504–1509

53. Molli RG, Anderson KC, Buehler KC et al (2011) Computer-assisted navigation software advancements improve the accuracy of total knee arthroplasty. J Arthroplasty 26(3):432–438

54. Nakahara H, Matsuda S, Moro-Oka TA et al (2011) Cutting error of the distal femur in total knee arthroplasty by use of a navigation system. J Arthroplasty 27(6):1119–1122

55. Nishihara S, Sugano N, Ikai M et al (2003) Accuracy evaluation of a shape-based registration method for a computer navigation system for total knee arthroplasty. J Knee Surg 16(2):98–105

56. Nofrini L, Slomczykowski M, Iacono F et al (2004) Evaluation of accuracy in ankle center location for tibial mechanical axis identification. J Invest Surg 17(1):23–29

57. Novak EJ, Silverstein MD, Bozic KJ (2007) The cost-effectiveness of computer-assisted navigation in total knee arthroplasty. J Bone Joint Surg Am 89(11): 2389–2397

58. Page SR, Deakin AH, Payne AP et al (2011) Reliability of frames of reference used for tibial component rotation in total knee arthroplasty. Comput Aided Surg 16(2):86–92

59. Perrin N, Stindel E, Roux C (2005) BoneMorphing versus freehand localization of anatomical landmarks: consequences for the reproducibility of implant positioning in total knee arthroplasty. Comput Aided Surg 10(5–6):301–309

60. Picard F, Leitner F, Gregori A et al (2007) A cadaveric study to assess the accuracy of computer-assisted surgery in locating the hip center during total knee arthroplasty. J Arthroplasty 22(4):590–595

61. Pitto RP, Graydon AJ, Bradley L et al (2006) Accuracy of a computer-assisted navigation system for total knee replacement. J Bone Joint Surg Br 88(5): 601–605

62. Rosenberger RE, Fink C, Quirbach S et al (2008) The immediate effect of navigation on implant accuracy in primary mini-invasive unicompartmental knee arthroplasty. Knee Surg Sports Traumatol Arthrosc 16(12):1133–1140

63. Sato T, Koga Y, Sobue T et al (2007) Quantitative 3-dimensional analysis of preoperative and postoperative joint lines in total knee arthroplasty: a new concept for evaluation of component alignment. J Arthroplasty 22:560–568

64. Schnurr C, Eysel P, König DP (2011) Do residents perform TKAs using computer navigation as accurately as consultants? Orthopedics 34(3):174. doi:10.3928/01477447-20110124-05

65. Shetty GM, Mullaji A, Lingaraju AP et al (2011) How accurate are orthopaedic surgeons in visually estimating lower limb alignment? Acta Orthop Belg 77(5): 638–643

66. Shinozaki T, Gotoh M, Mitsui Y et al (2011) Computer-assisted total knee arthroplasty: comparisons with the conventional technique. Kurume Med J 58(1):21–26

67. Siston RA, Daub AC, Giori NJ et al (2005) Evaluation of methods that locate the center of the ankle for computer-assisted total knee arthroplasty. Clin Orthop Relat Res 439:129–135

68. Siston RA, Giori NJ, Goodman SB et al (2006) Intraoperative passive kinematics of osteoarthritic knees before and after total knee arthroplasty. J Orthop Res 24(8):1607–1614

69. Siston RA, Giori NJ, Goodman SB et al (2007) Surgical navigation for total knee arthroplasty: a perspective. J Biomech 40(4):728–735

70. Siston RA, Patel JJ, Goodman SB et al (2005) The variability of femoral rotational alignment in total knee arthroplasty. J Bone Joint Surg Am 87: 2276–2280

71. Slover JD, Tosteson AN, Bozic KJ et al (2008) Impact of hospital volume on the economic value of computer navigation for total knee replacement. J Bone Joint Surg Am 90(7):1492–1500

72. Smith BR, Deakin AH, Baines J et al (2010) Computer navigated total knee arthroplasty: the learning curve. Comput Aided Surg 15(1–3):40–48

73. Spencer JM, Chauhan SK, Sloan K et al (2007) Computer navigation versus conventional total knee replacement: no difference in functional results at two years. J Bone Joint Surg Br 89(4):477–480

74. Stevens F, Conditt MA, Kulkarni N et al (2010) Minimizing electromagnetic interference from surgical instruments on electromagnetic surgical navigation. Clin Orthop Relat Res 468(8):2244–2250

75. Stindel E, Briard JL, Merloz P et al (2002) Bone morphing: 3D morphological data for total knee arthroplasty. Comput Aided Surg 7(3):156–168

76. Stindel E, Gil D, Briard JL et al (2005) Detection of the center of the hip joint in computer-assisted surgery: an evaluation study of the Surgetics algorithm. Comput Aided Surg 10(3):133–139

77. Stulberg SD (2003) How accurate is current TKR instrumentation? Clin Orthop Relat Res (416): 177–184

78. Stulberg SD, Loan P, Sarin V (2002) Computer-assisted navigation in total knee replacement: results of an initial experience in thirty-five patients. J Bone Joint Surg Am 84-A(Suppl 2):90–98

79. Suero EM, Plaskos C, Dixon PL et al (2011) Adjustable cutting blocks improve alignment and surgical time in computer-assisted total knee replacement. Knee Surg Sports Traumatol Arthrosc 2012 Sep;20(9):1736–41

80. Thoma W, Schreiber S, Hovy L (2000) Computer-assisted implant positioning in knee endoprosthetics. Kinematic analysis for optimization of surgical technique. Orthopade 29(7):614–626

81. Tigani D, Masetti G, Sabbioni G et al (2012) Computer-assisted surgery as indication of choice: total knee arthroplasty in case of retained hardware or extra-articular deformity. Int Orthop 36(7):1379–1385

82. Ulrich SD, Mont MA, Bonutti PM et al (2007) Scientific evidence supporting computer-assisted surgery and minimally invasive surgery for total knee arthroplasty. Expert Rev Med Devices 4(4):497–505

83. Van Campen A, De Groote F, Bosmans L et al (2011) Functional knee axis based on isokinetic dynamometry data: comparison of two methods, MRI validation, and effect on knee joint kinematics. J Biomech 44(15):2595–2600

84. Victor J, Van Doninck D, Labey L et al (2009) How precise can bony landmarks be determined on a CT scan of the knee? Knee 16(5):358–365

85. Weber P, Utzschneider S, Sadoghi P et al (2012) Navigation in minimally invasive unicompartmental knee arthroplasty has no advantage in comparison to a conventional minimally invasive implantation. Arch Orthop Trauma Surg 132(2):281–288

86. Yaffe MA, Koo SS, Stulberg SD (2008) Radiographic and navigation measurements of TKA limb alignment do not correlate. Clin Orthop Relat Res 466(11):2736–2744

87. Yau WP, Chiu KY (2008) Cutting errors in total knee replacement: assessment by computer assisted surgery. Knee Surg Sports Traumatol Arthrosc 16(7): 670–673

88. Yau WP, Leung A, Chiu KY et al (2005) Intraobserver errors in obtaining visually selected anatomic landmarks during registration process in nonimage-based navigation-assisted total knee arthroplasty: a cadaveric experiment. J Arthroplasty 20(5):591–601

89. Yau WP, Leung A, Liu KG et al (2007) Interobserver and intra-observer errors in obtaining visually selected anatomical landmarks during registration process in non-image-based navigation-assisted total knee arthroplasty. J Arthroplasty 22(8):1150–1161

Does Computer-Assisted Surgery Affect Clinical Outcome? A Review of the Literature

3

Petra J.C. Heesterbeek and Ate B. Wymenga

3.1 Introduction

A large number of pages have been written on the topic whether the use of computer-assisted surgery (CAS) improves accuracy and precision of component placement compared with conventional total knee replacement (TKR). Although not all of these papers are sufficiently powered by themselves, the results of the randomized clinical trials [1, 5, 6, 8, 13, 24, 26, 28, 30] and other studies were pooled into meta-analyses of Bauwens et al. and Mason et al. [2, 22]. These meta-analyses show that the use of CAS results in significant improvement in accuracy and precision of component orientation and mechanical axis after TKR [2, 22].

The question is whether a more precise component alignment with fewer outliers will result in better clinical outcome. As Laskin wrote eloquently: "Although it is philosophically difficult to argue against any system that increases accuracy, it is reasonable to question whether this improvement, which is often in the range of 1–1.5 degrees, will have a salutary effect on the

P.J.C. Heesterbeek, Ph.D. (✉)
Department of Research,
Sint Maartenskliniek,
Nijmegen, The Netherlands
e-mail: p.heesterbeek@maartenskliniek.nl

A.B. Wymenga, M.D., Ph.D.
Department of Orthopedics,
Sint Maartenskliniek,
Nijmegen, The Netherlands
e-mail: a.wymenga@maartenskliniek.nl

long-term implant survival" [19]. The goal of this chapter is to summarize the published evidence that helps answer this question.

3.2 Methodology

Because too few high-quality papers have been published on this topic and because the papers that have been published do not use the same outcome parameters, a meta-analysis could not be performed. The methodology used for this chapter is a description and summary of the findings in the literature. For this summary, PubMed was searched with the MeSH terms: "outcome assessment (health care)"; "surgery, computer-assisted"; "arthroplasty, replacement, knee"; and "survival analysis." Papers were selected based on their methodological quality in terms of a sound research question, good methodology without bias, and when appropriate, with sufficient statistical power.

3.3 Effect of Alignment on Clinical Outcome and Survival in Non-navigated TKR

Before we take a deeper look at the papers dealing with CAS and clinical outcome, we will first discuss some papers that attempt to relate alignment with function in primary, non-navigated TKR. Longstaff et al. used a concept of cumulative error scores in their study [21]. A summed amount of $\geq 6°$ of error in alignment of the components was considered bad; a total error of 5° or less, good. Analysis of their cohort of 159 TKR patients revealed a 2-day longer hospital stay for the patients having a bad cumulative error score compared to those having a good score. Furthermore, they reported a statistically significantly lower KSS score at 1-year follow-up for the "bad" group [21]. Results in the same direction have been reported by Fang et al. [11]. They performed a survival analysis on 6,070 knees (3,992 patients) and concluded that knees with the best survival had an anatomical axis between 2.4° and 7.2° of valgus, representing the mean of the study population with 1 SD. Knees outside this "neutral" range had statistically significantly worse survival after 20 years. Although no confidence intervals nor censored data were presented in their paper, the survival differences lie in the range of 2–4 % [11]. A more recent paper by Parratte et al. reported the opposite with a Kaplan-Meier survival analysis [25]. They divided their study population of 398 knees (280 patients) into two groups: neutrally aligned knees with a mechanical axis of 0°±3° and an outlier group. After adjusting for age and body mass index, there was not a significant independent association of alignment with revision. They therefore concluded that a postoperative mechanical axis of 0°±3° did not improve the 15-year implant survival rate [25]. The paper of Bonner et al. presented the same conclusion [4]. The authors found a very weak trend, with broad confidence intervals, toward improved survival with more accurate alignment of the mechanical axis, but this was not statistically significant. Their conclusion was that the benefits of alignment within 3° by the use of CAS may have been exaggerated and that a beneficial effect of CAS on long-term implant survival remains unproven [4].

3.4 Effect of Navigation on Clinical Outcome

An overview of relevant papers that have been published on the comparison of CAS versus conventional TKR and that have reported on clinical outcome is summarized in Table 3.1. Although there is a difference in the outcome scores that have been used, the general conclusion that can be drawn from the results is clear: there is no convincing evidence that the use of

CAS has a positive effect on clinical outcome. Whether this conclusion will stand for the next few years remains to be determined. Follow-up on patients that were enrolled in an RCT (as two groups already did [15, 29]) is an excellent method to obtain long-term follow-up of groups of patients without selection bias.

3.5 Effect of Navigation on Implant Survival

In addition to clinical outcome scores, it is a valid hypothesis that better alignment might affect implant survival. To conduct proper survival studies, a certain amount of time is necessary. CAS for TKR is still quite young, and this might be the main reason that there have been very few papers published yet on the effect of CAS on implant survival. A registry study of Gøthesen et al. has been published in 2011, and this study described the short-term outcome of 1,465 navigated TKRs in the period 2005–2008 [12]. Although there was no answer for causation, this Norwegian Arthroplasty Register study reported the interesting finding that, although the difference was small, improved implant longevity due to CAS might be unlikely, considering the inferior short-term results on a national basis. The failure mechanisms must be explored in greater detail in future, but it may be that a certain implant type causes this disappointing effect. A contrasting conclusion has been reported by the second study that mentioned implant survival in their report. The group of Hernández-Vaquero et al. did not perform a Kaplan-Meier survival analysis, but reported that after a follow-up of 8 years, there was no statistically significant difference in survival between CAS and conventional [15]. The survival rate for the TKR implanted using CAS was 94.74 %, and that of the conventional group was 81.08 % ($p=0.068$). Due to the rather small sample size for reporting survival rates, this nonsignificant difference might be the result of a type II error.

3.6 Discussion

This review shows that there is no convincing evidence to indicate an improvement in clinical outcome and survival following the use of CAS.

Table 3.1 Literature overview of comparative studies on CAS versus conventional techniques in TKR

Study	Longest follow-up (years)	Study type	Scores	Results
Ensini et al. [10]	2	RCT	Oxford	No differences
			Patella	No differences
			Satisfaction	No differences
Spencer et al. [29]	2	Follow-up of RCT	KSS	No differences
			WOMAC	No differences
			SF-36	No differences
			Oxford	No differences
			Patella	No differences
Ek et al. [9]	2	RCT	Oxford	No differences
			Patella	No differences
			Satisfaction	No differences
Choong et al. [7]a	1	RCT	IKS	No differences
			SF-12	No differences
Kamat et al. [18]	3	Retrospective cohort	Oxford	No differences
			KSS	No differences
Seon et al. [27]	2	RCT	HSS	No differences
			WOMAC	No differences
			ROM	No differences
Hernández-Vaquero et al. [15]	8	Follow-up of RCT	KSS	No differences
Ishida et al. [17]b	5	Retrospective matched cohort	KSS	Navigation better
			ROM	Navigation better
Lehnen et al. [20]c	1	Prospective cohort	KSS	Navigation better
			WOMAC	Navigation better
			Satisfaction	Navigation better

Oxford Oxford Knee Score, *Patella* Bartlett patella score, *KSS* Knee Society Score, *WOMAC* Western Ontario and McMaster Universities Arthritis Index, *SF-36* Short Form-36, *IKS* International Knee Score, *SF-12* Short Form-12, *HSS* Hospital for Special Surgery score
aChoong et al. reported differences between well-aligned knees and knees with a mechanical axis >3°, no differences between CAS and conventional TKR
bIshida et al. matched patients after 5 years of follow-up, only on implant type. It is unclear from their paper whether this might have caused selection bias
cLehnen et al. compared CAS with the use of a spring tensioner in one group with conventional surgery without the use of a spring tensioner in the other group. It is not clear which component caused the difference

Perhaps because TKR is a very successful operation with a high level of patient satisfaction and functional improvement, it may be difficult for CAS to show a significant improvement in the short term. It may be possible that improved alignment may decrease wear of the implant and improve the functional outcome in the long term, but so far, there is no trend in the published literature indicating this direction, and authors doubt whether there will be evidence [3].

It is clear and supported by the evidence that with CAS, the prosthesis components can be aligned more precisely during surgery [2, 22]. However, it is unknown whether these parameters, which can be determined more precisely, actually have sufficient influence to result in better clinical outcome. Although it might reasonably be assumed that a poorly aligned TKR might function less satisfactorily, other factors such as the soft-tissue envelope definitely need to be taken into account.

Several authors write in the discussion of their papers that perhaps the ability of CAS to provide all the information including soft-tissue management during surgery can result in an added value of navigation in TKR. It is commonly known that component malpositioning is not the only cause of long-term TKR failure. Instability, often representing a failure to correct a deformity or balance the flexion and extension spaces, can likewise lead to implant failure [19]. A navigation system can quantify the size of the extension and flexion spaces and the stability with the trial implants in position to help with appropriate modifications in order to get the soft tissues correctly balanced.

A concept that gets more and more attention is kinematic alignment of a TKR instead of alignment according to the mechanical axis. In contrast to mechanical alignment, the use of kinematic alignment with custom-fit cutting guides and a cruciate-retaining, symmetric medial and lateral femoral-tibial bearing surface aims to minimize the undesirable consequences of adduction and reverse axial rotation (external rotation) [16, 23]. The rationale behind kinematic alignment is that the three kinematic axes of the knee are being restored in order to achieve more normal contact kinematics without release of the collateral ligaments or lateral retinaculum [16]. Future randomized controlled trials are needed to help critically evaluate clinical function and survivorship between these different types of alignment of TKR.

What do we need to assess the effect of navigation on clinical outcome on the long-term follow-up? Because it is quite time consuming, it makes sense to follow-up on the patients from existing, and already published, high-quality RCTs. Selection bias by using CAS only on the difficult cases (as supported by some authors) is being ruled out in this strategy. The researchers must be able to track down all patients, because otherwise underpowered studies might be the result. It is already questionable whether studies that were powered on mechanical alignment as a primary outcome variable can provide enough evidence with clinical and functional outcome as secondary scores.

In the search for an answer, registries definitely have a place. In national registries, a high number of consecutive patients are included with all types of implants. When selection bias on the use of CAS can be ruled out, the data collected by registries provides valuable information. The Norwegian Arthroplasty Registry was the first to publish on the effect of CAS on survival; perhaps others will follow [12]. If surgeons in the future only have the tendency to use CAS in difficult cases, then cohort studies are no longer possible because of selection bias. RCTs can be the way to obtain an answer.

It becomes clear from Table 3.1 that there is a variety of clinical and functional outcome scores that are being used in trials. We have to ask ourselves whether we will be able to find an answer with the use of clinical scores [14]. Future trials should have high methodological standards (excluding bias, including randomization), longer and more standardized follow-up protocols to ensure high methodological and statistical power, and focus on meaningful and standardized outcomes in terms of functional recovery and quality of life. Also, economical parameters, length of hospital stay, and risk for readmission should be measured. Only then can a high-quality meta-analysis be performed in the hope of getting an answer to the question whether CAS leads to improved clinical outcome.

Conclusion

The literature does not provide evidence that the use of navigation in TKR leads to superior clinical outcome on the short- to midterm follow-up. High-quality long-term follow-up studies and implant registry analyses are required to answer whether the use of CAS through more accurate alignment will result in less wear and superior implant survival, but in the mean time, perhaps it is wise to use CAS for soft-tissue management.

References

1. Bathis H, Perlick L, Tingart M et al (2004) Alignment in total knee arthroplasty. A comparison of computer-assisted surgery with the conventional technique. J Bone Joint Surg Br 86:682–687
2. Bauwens K, Wich M, Ekkernkamp A et al (2007) Navigated total knee replacement. A meta-analysis. J Bone Joint Surg Am 89:261–269
3. Bellemans J (2009) Navigation and CAS: is D-day approaching? Knee Surg Sports Traumatol Arthrosc 17:1141–1142

4. Bonner TJ, Eardley WG, Patterson P et al (2011) The effect of post-operative mechanical axis alignment on the survival of primary total knee replacements after a follow-up of 15 years. J Bone Joint Surg Br 93:1217–1222
5. Chauhan SK, Scott RG, Breidahl W et al (2004) Computer-assisted knee arthroplasty versus a conventional jig-based technique. A randomised, prospective trial. J Bone Joint Surg Br 86:372–377
6. Chin PL, Yang KY, Yeo SJ et al (2005) Randomized control trial comparing radiographic total knee arthroplasty implant placement using computer navigation versus conventional technique. J Arthroplasty 20: 618–626
7. Choong PF, Dowsey MM, Stoney JD (2009) Does accurate anatomical alignment result in better function and quality of life? Comparing conventional and computer-assisted total knee arthroplasty. J Arthroplasty 24:560–569
8. Decking R, Markmann Y, Fuchs J et al (2005) Leg axis after computer-navigated total knee arthroplasty. J Arthroplasty 20:282–288
9. Ek ET, Dowsey MM, Tse LF et al (2008) Comparison of functional and radiological outcomes after computer-assisted versus conventional total knee arthroplasty: a matched-control retrospective study. J Orthop Surg (Hong Kong) 16:192–196
10. Ensini A, Catani F, Leardini A et al (2007) Alignments and clinical results in conventional and navigated total knee arthroplasty. Clin Orthop Relat Res 457: 156–162
11. Fang DM, Ritter MA, Davis KE (2009) Coronal alignment in total knee arthroplasty: just how important is it? J Arthroplasty 24:39–43
12. Gøthesen O, Espehaug B, Havelin L et al (2011) Short-term outcome of 1,465 computer-navigated primary total knee replacements 2005–2008. Acta Orthop 82:293–300
13. Hart R, Janecek M, Chaker A et al (2003) Total knee arthroplasty implanted with and without kinematic navigation. Int Orthop 27:366–369
14. Heesterbeek PJ, Wymenga AB (2010) PCL balancing, an example of the need to couple detailed biomechanical parameters with clinical functional outcome. Knee Surg Sports Traumatol Arthrosc 18:1301–1303
15. Hernández-Vaquero D, Suarez-Vazquez A, Iglesias-Fernandez S (2011) Can computer assistance improve the clinical and functional scores in total knee arthroplasty? Clin Orthop Relat Res 469: 3436–3442
16. Howell SM, Hodapp EE, Kuznik K et al (2009) In vivo adduction and reverse axial rotation (external) of the tibial component can be minimized. Orthopedics 32:319
17. Ishida K, Matsumoto T, Tsumura N et al (2011) Midterm outcomes of computer-assisted total knee arthroplasty. Knee Surg Sports Traumatol Arthrosc 19:1107–1112
18. Kamat YD, Aurakzai KM, Adhikari AR et al (2009) Does computer navigation in total knee arthroplasty improve patient outcome at midterm follow-up? Int Orthop 33:1567–1570
19. Laskin RS, Beksac B (2006) Computer-assisted navigation in TKA: where we are and where we are going. Clin Orthop Relat Res 452:127–131
20. Lehnen K, Giesinger K, Warschkow R et al (2011) Clinical outcome using a ligament referencing technique in CAS versus conventional technique. Knee Surg Sports Traumatol Arthrosc 19:887–892
21. Longstaff LM, Sloan K, Stamp N et al (2009) Good alignment after total knee arthroplasty leads to faster rehabilitation and better function. J Arthroplasty 24: 570–578
22. Mason JB, Fehring TK, Estok R et al (2007) Meta-analysis of alignment outcomes in computer-assisted total knee arthroplasty surgery. J Arthroplasty 22: 1097–1106
23. Nunley RM, Ellison BS, Zhu J et al (2012) Do patient-specific guides improve coronal alignment in total knee arthroplasty? Clin Orthop Relat Res 470: 895–902
24. Oberst M, Bertsch C, Wurstlin S et al (2003) CT analysis of leg alignment after conventional vs. navigated knee prosthesis implantation. Initial results of a controlled, prospective and randomized study. Unfallchirurg 106:941–948
25. Parratte S, Pagnano MW, Trousdale RT et al (2010) Effect of postoperative mechanical axis alignment on the fifteen-year survival of modern, cemented total knee replacements. J Bone Joint Surg Am 92:2143–2149
26. Saragaglia D, Picard F, Chaussard C et al (2001) Computer-assisted knee arthroplasty: comparison with a conventional procedure. Results of 50 cases in a prospective randomized study. Rev Chir Orthop Reparatrice Appar Mot 87:18–28
27. Seon JK, Park SJ, Lee KB et al (2009) Functional comparison of total knee arthroplasty performed with and without a navigation system. Int Orthop 33: 987–990
28. Sparmann M, Wolke B, Czupalla H et al (2003) Positioning of total knee arthroplasty with and without navigation support. A prospective, randomised study. J Bone Joint Surg Br 85:830–835
29. Spencer JM, Chauhan SK, Sloan K et al (2007) Computer navigation versus conventional total knee replacement: no difference in functional results at two years. J Bone Joint Surg Br 89:477–480
30. Victor J and Hoste D (2004) Image-based computer-assisted total knee arthroplasty leads to lower variability in coronal alignment. Clin Orthop Relat Res 428: 131–139

TKA: Measured Resection Technique

4

Andrea Ensini, Paolo Barbadoro, Alberto Leardini,
Claudio Belvedere, and Sandro Giannini

4.1 Introduction: Conventional Measured Resection Technique

Good clinical outcomes for total knee arthroplasty (TKA) can be obtained if the soft tissues are well balanced and the prosthetic components are properly oriented, combined with joint line restoration. The correct rotational alignment of the femoral component is critical because it determines patellar groove position and flexion gap stability. Improper alignment can also induce anterior knee pain, arthrofibrosis, and torsional stress on the tibial component that could lead to wear or loosening [1–3, 7, 8].

Measured resection technique is based on the surgical identification of bony landmarks to obtain the best position of the femoral component,

leaving the soft tissue balancing until after trial component implantation. Here are the main surgical landmarks:

- *Posterior condylar axis*: the line connecting the posterior condyles, which was used as a reference for primary TKAs before 1986 (the same posterior osteotomy from both femoral condyles) [1].

- *Surgical transepicondylar axis*: The line connecting the lateral epicondylar prominence and the sulcus of the medial epicondyle, where the deep fibers of the medial collateral ligament are attached [3]. It is perpendicular to the mechanical axis of the femur and perpendicular to the mechanical axis of the tibia when the knee is flexed to 90°. It was defined as a reference for the rotation of the femoral component in TKA when other landmarks cannot be used [3], particularly in prosthetic revisions and in primary TKA with dysplasia of the distal femur [3]. Sometimes, it is difficult to identify accurately [1].

- *Clinical transepicondylar axis*: The line connecting the lateral epicondylar prominence and the most prominent point of the medial epicondyle, where the superficial fibers of the medial collateral ligament are attached. It is difficult to identify the prominence of the medial epicondyle. This is externally rotated to the posterior condylar axis, about 3.5° (±2°) for varus or neutral knees; this is more externally rotated 4.4° (±1.8°) for valgus knees [7].

- *Posterior condylar angle*: The angle between the posterior condylar axis and the surgical

A. Ensini, M.D. (✉) • P. Barbadoro, M.D.
Department of Orthopaedic Surgery, Istituto Ortopedico
Rizzoli, University of Bologna,
via di Barbiano 1/10, Bologna 40136, Italy
e-mail: andrea.ensini@ior.it; paolobarba@hotmail.it

A. Leardini, Ph.D. • C. Belvedere, Ph.D.
Movement Analysis Laboratory,
Istituto Ortopedico Rizzoli,
via di Barbiano 1/10, Bologna 40136, Italy
e-mail: alberto.leardini@ior.it; claudio.belvedere@ior.it

S. Giannini, M.D.
Department of Orthopaedic Surgery, Istituto Ortopedico
Rizzoli, University of Bologna,
via di Barbiano 1/10, Bologna 40136, Italy

Movement Analysis Laboratory,
Istituto Ortopedico Rizzoli,
via di Barbiano 1/10, Bologna 40136, Italy
e-mail: sandro.giannini@ior.it

F. Catani, S. Zaffagnini (eds.), *Knee Surgery using Computer Assisted Surgery and Robotics*,
DOI 10.1007/978-3-642-31430-8_4, © ESSKA 2013

transepicondylar axis [3]. There is an internal rotation of the posterior condylar axis with respect to the surgical transepicondylar axis. Berger et al. [3] demonstrated a mean of this angle of 3.5° (±1.2°) of internal rotation for males and a mean of 0.3° (±1.2°) for females.

- *Anteroposterior axis (Arima axis or Whiteside's line)*: A line through the deepest part of the patellar groove anteriorly and the center of the intercondylar notch posteriorly. This axis is easily identified intraoperatively with the knee flexed. This is the best reference for the rotation of femoral components in a valgus TKA to avoid patellar instability. After 1986, this was used as a reference for rotational alignment of the femoral component for primary TKAs. The femoral surfaces were resected in a line perpendicular to the anteroposterior axis to establish rotational alignment of the femoral component. This line results approximately 4° (3–5°) externally rotated with respect to the posterior condylar axis [1]. The resection of the posterior condyles results in slightly more resection of the medial femoral condyle than that of the lateral condyle in normal knees; the resection of the medial condyle is much more than that of the lateral condyle in the valgus knees [1, 8].

TKA based on measured resection technique is recommended to place the femoral component parallel to the transepicondylar axis, perpendicular to the anteroposterior axis, or approximately 3–4° externally rotated to the posterior condylar axis.

In the knee with a normal condylar shape, the resection of the femoral condyles with a slight external rotation in respect to the posterior condylar axis would result in correct rotational alignment of the implant relative to the other landmarks. However, valgus knee resections relative to the surgical transepicondylar axis or perpendicular to the anteroposterior axis result in minimal resection of the lateral femoral condyle, which may be viewed as an extreme external rotation of the femoral resection surfaces, but, in this case, is correct. Indeed, in a severe valgus knee, a resection parallel to the posterior condylar axis could lead to malposition of the femoral component in

an excessive internal rotation and in consequent medialization of the patellar groove in the extended position [1, 8].

Some authors [7] considered the anteroposterior axis difficult to define in the arthritic knee, due to trochlear wear and intercondylar osteophytes, in case of severe trochlear dysplasia and in some varus knees. They considered the surgical transepicondylar axis as a good landmark for rotational alignment of the femoral component when the proximal tibia cut is performed at right angles to its mechanical axis.

A double checking of the rotation by using the anteroposterior axis and the transepicondylar axis should ensure a correct rotation of the femoral component in most total knee replacements [7].

4.2 Navigated Measured Resection Technique

4.2.1 Preoperative Surgical Planning

Accurate surgical planning is fundamental in navigated TKA. This planning is performed through an accurate clinical examination of the deformity and with a correct preoperative x-ray examination.

A clinical examination of the deformity can give the best solutions for the individual patient; for this reason, the deformity must be considered not only in the coronal plane but also in the sagittal and transverse planes. The evaluation of the deformity in the coronal plane is the most important factor to consider in the preoperative evaluation because the amount of this deformity will affect the amount of surgical correction. Moreover, manual correction of the deformity has to be considered: in case of a correctable deformity, only with right femoral and tibial bone cuts, it could be possible to obtain a well-aligned limb. on the other hand, when the deformity is fixed, some degree of soft tissue release could be considered. When a mediolateral laxity as well as those related to the bone defect is present, a more constrained prosthetic implant could be considered. The deformity on the sagittal plane must be considered too during preoperative planning.

In severe flexion contracture, not related to bone anterior impingement, a more distal than posterior femoral cut could be performed associated with a reduction of the tibial posterior slope or an extension of the femoral component. All these procedures can correct this kind of deformity, avoiding a gap unbalancing related to an eventually excessive resection of the proximal tibia. In case of genu recurvatum, a reduction of the extension gap could correct this deformity, but a more constrained prosthesis design could be considered [6]. The deformity on the transverse plane is difficult to recognize and is often related to previous femoral or tibial fractures. In this case, a preoperative CT of the lower limb could be useful to plan their correction.

The x-ray evaluation is performed by means of a weight-bearing lower-limb radiograph in anteroposterior (AP) projection, particularly of the knee in AP and latero-lateral (LL) projections, and a merchant view of the knee. Compared to the conventional technique, with the navigation technique, it is not necessary to measure the femoral valgus angle because the distal femoral cut is directly planned on the femoral mechanical axis, but it is useful to measure the deformity of the knee on a lower-limb AP radiograph. Moreover, if a natural inclination of the slope for the tibial cut is used, the inclination of the tibial plateau in the LL view has been measured to replicate it intraoperatively with navigation.

4.2.2 Surgical Navigation: Stryker Knee Navigation System

Navigation was introduced in TKA surgery in order to obtain better accuracy in component alignment. This better accuracy is obtained through specific steps that have to be executed with a lot of accuracy. During the learning curve, it is necessary to perform all the steps with caution so that the results of this procedure are acceptable and the surgeon does not become discouraged. The original scope of surgical navigation, as described in the previous chapters, is:

- To plan intraoperatively the positioning of the components
- To verify, during all the steps of surgery, the accuracy of all the osteotomies performed
- To assess the preoperative and postoperative knee kinematics

All surgical navigation systems are able to perform these phases during TKA, and it is possible to apply these systems both with "measured resection technique" and with "gap-balancing technique." Below, the measured resection technique is described using the Stryker knee navigation system, version 4.0 through the following steps:

1. Initial setting
2. Anatomical survey
3. Intra-operative planning
4. Jigs navigation
5. Verification of resections
6. Soft tissue balancing
7. Final kinematics

4.2.2.1 Initial Setting

Before starting surgery, it is necessary to insert the patient data. These data include patient demographic data, the etiology and the entity of knee deformity, the kind of prosthesis used, and the name of the surgeon. Recording these data is important for future statistical analysis; it should be always possible to find them in the final report of every single patient.

When a surgeon approaches the surgical navigation, he has to set up his personal surgical profile. For this reason, the surgeon can define if his surgical technique provides femur first or tibia first or an anterior or posterior femoral reference; moreover, it is possible to set up the inclination of the tibial posterior slope and the thickness of the femoral or tibial resections. At the end, the surgeon can choose what kinematic curves to record of the knee with deformity, during trials or at the end of the surgical procedure.

Before starting with the surgical approach, the supports for tibial and femoral trackers have to be fixed to the distal femur and to the proximal tibia. With an Ortholock anchoring device, it is possible to obtain very good bone fixation without interference of the surgical approach (Fig. 4.1).

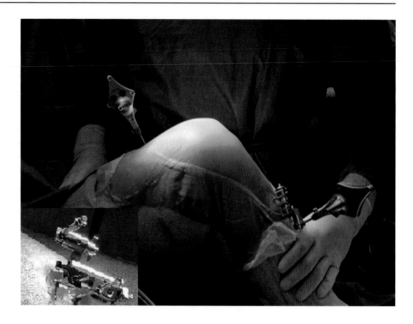

Fig. 4.1 A left knee with the tibial and femoral trackers (Ortholock anchoring device). In the bottom left, particularly illustrated is the pin fixation of the device

Usually, in the femur, the two bi-cortical 3-mm diameter pins are inserted from the lateral side of the femur, while in the tibia, the pins are inserted below the tibial tubercle. The Ortholock system allows one to direct the trackers in order to obtain better visualization by the camera and moreover to always recognize the position of the bone segment or of the navigation jigs during knee motion, or the knee is always in a particular position related to the surgical procedure. After trackers and pointer activation, it is possible to bring the camera in line with the knee joint so that all instruments are centered in the working volume signified by the gray circles in the "Setup System" dialog (Fig. 4.2).

4.2.2.2 Anatomical Survey

This is one of the basic steps of navigation, especially in the imageless-based systems; in fact, all the surgical femoral and tibial references have been defined by digitizing some anatomical landmarks. The accuracy of these references is strictly related to the accuracy of our landmarks digitization. Moreover, it is very important to know how the reference axis and plane have been defined by the software. Below, the femoral and tibial references are shown for the Stryker knee navigation system, version 4.0

Femur Anatomical Survey
By digitizing femoral landmarks, the following axes and references are defined:
- Mechanical femur axis
- Femoral rotation axis
- Reference for resection level in the distal and posterior femur
- Reference for anterior notching
- Reference for automatic sizing, implant positioning, and for mediolateral overhang

The mechanical femur axis is defined by the line from the hip center and the knee center. The hip center is calculated through a slow and smooth circumduction of the hip, avoiding pelvic motion, while the femur center is directly digitized with the tip's pointer at the center of the trochlear sulcus anterior just above the intercondylar notch (Fig. 4.3). The mechanical femur axis is defined as the reference for varus/valgus and flexion/extension alignments.

The femoral rotation is defined as the average rotation axis calculated by the digitized transepicondylar axis (medial and lateral epicondyle) and femoral AP axis. The medial and lateral epicondyles are directly digitized with the tip's pointer respectively at the sulcus of the medial epicondyle and onto the most prominent point of the lateral epicondyle. The femoral AP axis is calculated by

Fig. 4.2 The tibial tracker, the femoral tracker, and the pointer are visible in the camera; we can see all the three elements inside to the gray circle in the "Setup System" dialog

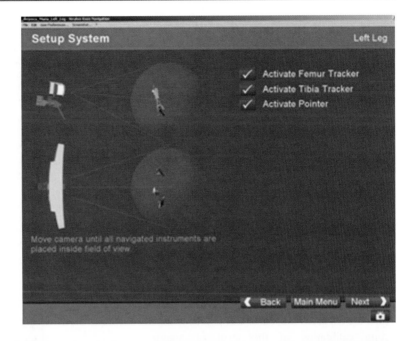

Fig. 4.3 Digitalization of the femur center. The pointer is at the center of the trochlear sulcus anterior just above the intercondylar notch

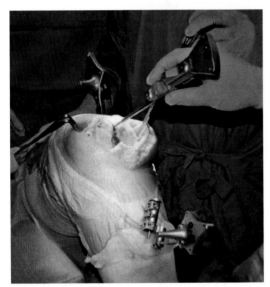

aligning the pointer's axis with the most posterior point of the trochlea and the most anterior point of the intercondylar notch, also referred to as Whiteside's line [1, 8] (Fig. 4.4).

The reference for the distal femur resection level is the most prominent distal point of the

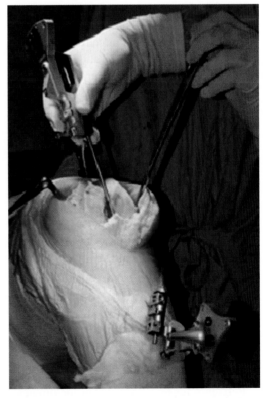

Fig. 4.4 Digitalization of the femoral anteroposterior axis

digitized condyle. The system calculates the length of the perpendicular line from the reference point to the distal resection plane both in the medial and lateral condyle. It is important that the most distal aspect of the condyle has been included in the point cloud digitized and that the pointer has not left the surface of the bone during digitization, in order to avoid wrong resection thickness. The same procedure is performed to calculate the reference for the posterior resection level; in this case, the length from the most posterior point of the medial and lateral condyle to the posterior resection plane is considered.

The reference for anterior notching is defined during point acquisition of the anterior aspect of the distal femur. The point cloud of this digitization includes the portion of the anterior aspect below the expected saw blade exit points, to avoid wrong calibration of the level of anterior notching.

The reference for automatic sizing and femoral implant positioning, as in conventional technique, are the anterior cortical bone and the posterior femoral condyles. Anterior or posterior references can be used for femoral implant positioning. Based on the selected implant family and the digitized axes and bone morphology, the software calculates the optimal size and position of the femoral implant. The goal of the calculations is to achieve the best anterior match while keeping the implant size as small as possible. Moreover, with the required digitization of the medial and lateral overhang in the femoral regions, the software will provide, in numerical value, the average medial/lateral overhang or uncovered bone cut.

Tibial Anatomical Survey

By digitizing tibial landmarks, the following axes and references are defined:
- Mechanical tibia axis
- Tibial rotation axis
- Reference for resection level in the proximal tibia

The mechanical tibia axis is defined by the line from the tibia center and the calculated ankle center. The tibia center is directly digitized with

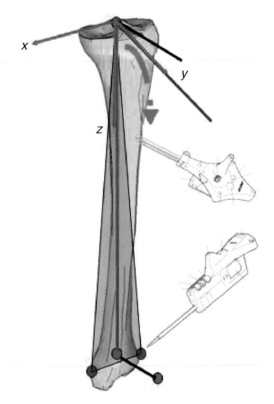

Fig. 4.5 Illustration of the tibial reference frame. The mechanical axis is the *blue line* from the tibia center and the calculated ankle center

the tip's pointer onto the middle of the interspinous sulcus anteriorly near the anterior midfootprint of the ACL attachment, while the ankle center is calculated by dividing the digitized transmalleolar axis according to the ratio of 56 % lateral to 44 % medial. The transmalleolar axis is the line between the most prominent point of the medial and lateral malleolus directly digitized with the tip's pointer. The mechanical tibia axis so defined is the reference for varus/valgus and flexion/extension alignments (Fig. 4.5).

The tibial rotation axis is calculated by aligning the pointer's axis with the midpoint of the posterior cruciate ligament (PCL) and the medial third of the tibial tuberosity. This axis is the reference for rotational alignment of the tibial component.

The reference for the proximal tibial resection level is the most recessed point of the digitized compartment. The system calculates the length of the perpendicular line from the reference point to

Fig. 4.6 Illustration of the intraoperative planning with the knee in extension. It is possible to see the femoral size and the medial and the lateral extension gaps

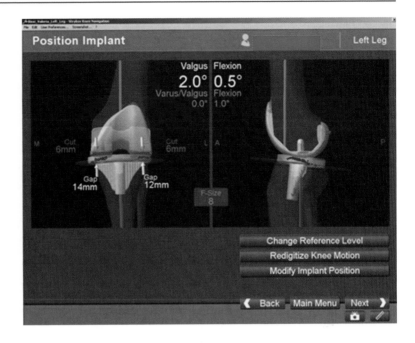

the tibial resection plane both in the medial and lateral compartment. It is important that the lowest aspect of the compartment has been included in the point cloud digitized and that the pointer does not digitize below the lowest anatomical point, in order to avoid wrong resection thickness.

4.2.2.3 Intraoperative Planning

At the end of patient registration, the software will calculate the size and position for the best fitting implant and place it on the virtual femur. Varus/valgus and rotational alignments, as well as the reconstruction of the posterior and distal condyles, are achieved in accordance with the principles of measured resection technique. Optimal femoral implant size and position are calculated in the following manner: first, the software virtually positions the smallest implant size on the digitized femur. For positioning, varus/valgus and rotational alignments are set to 0°respectively to the calculated mechanical axis and to the average rotation axis calculated by the digitized transepicondylar axis (medial and lateral epicondyle) and femoral AP axis. The distal and posterior condyles are reconstructed in accordance with the principles of measured resection technique. After positioning the smallest implant

size, the software iterates this process for all available implant sizes. In addition, different flexion angles as well as AP shift are applied. Once the intraoperative planning is displayed on the screen, the surgeon can decide whether to accept or modify it, changing femoral size or position. As described in Figs. 4.6 and 4.7, it is possible to change the orientation of the femoral component, to shift it in craniocaudal or anteroposterior direction, and to change the femoral size. Usually, the varus/valgus and rotational alignments are not changed, even if it were possible. Whenever a change in the position or in the size of the femoral component is performed, it is possible to verify the result of this change with respect to the gap balancing, if this caused an anterior notching or if there is a mediolateral overhang of the component with respect to the bone.

During this phase, keep in mind the preoperative deformity is crucial because the surgeon can adjust the intraoperative planning to correct the deformity; for example, with a severe flexion deformity, a greater distal femoral cut with reduction of femoral flexion can be planned with respect to a standard posterior cut. At the end of this phase, the "Planned Femoral Implant" dialog appears on the screen, summarizing size,

Fig. 4.7 Illustration of the intraoperative planning with the knee in flexion. It is possible to modify the femoral size, the flexion of the component, and the AP position. Moreover, the surgeon can check as the new implant position can influence the flexion gap, or if there is some anterior notching

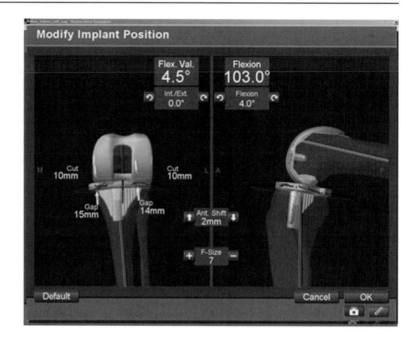

Fig. 4.8 Snapshot of the planned femoral implant of the Triathlon cruciate-retaining TKA. The surgeon can see the size and the alignment of the femoral component

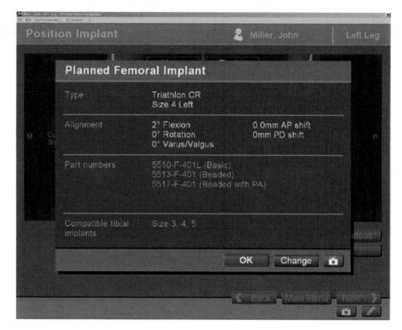

alignment, and position of the calculated femoral implant (Fig. 4.8).

4.2.2.4 Jig Navigation

When the intraoperative planning has been ended, the surgeon starts with the cutting jig navigation following his preferred technique. In this case,

the femur-first technique will be shown. During the evolution of navigation hardware, more and more handy cutting jigs have been built in order to reduce the time of surgery. In the early days of the introduction of surgical navigation, the conventional cutting blocks, i.e. that with intramedullary rod for the femur and/or extramedullary

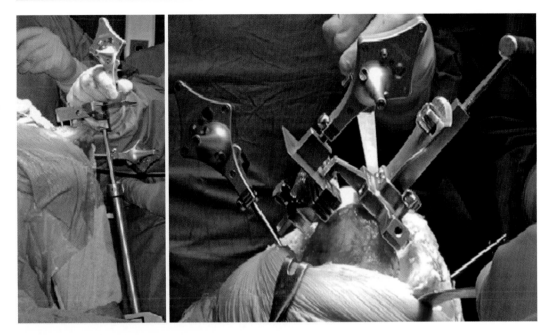

Fig. 4.9 Surgical navigation with conventional cutting jigs

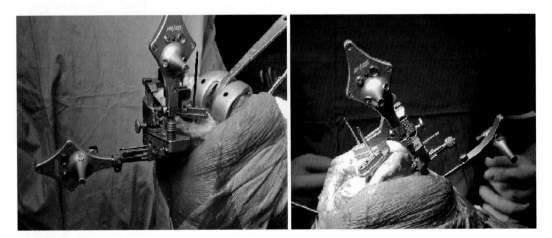

Fig. 4.10 Surgical navigation with dedicated cutting jigs

rod for the tibia, were navigated by inserting a proper plane probe suitably instrumented with a tracker into the cutting slot. This mode of surgical navigation required a lot of time related both to navigation and to the positioning of conventional femoral and tibial guides (Fig. 4.9). After dedicated jigs were developed, the positioning of these guides was performed without any conventional instrumentation (Fig. 4.10). The jig orientation is adjusted with micrometer screws; one is

able to check the alignment in the coronal and sagittal plane and the amount of the resections. After a lot of surgical navigation procedures, acquiring some experience with navigated jigs, the "free-hand technique" can be used, obtaining a very fast and accurate positioning of the cutting guides. This technique provides the manual orientation of the jig controlled directly on the monitor by the first operator, while an assistant fixes the jig with drilling pins (Fig. 4.11). With the

Fig. 4.11 Surgical navigation with free-hand technique for the distal femur resection

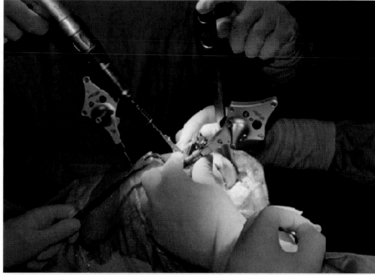

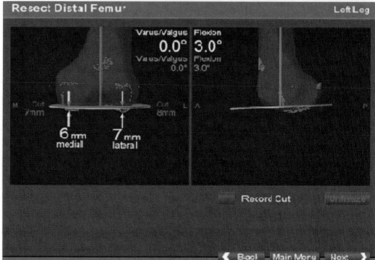

same technique, "dedicated mini jigs" could also be used for navigated mini invasive surgical technique (Fig. 4.12).

Usually, the distal femoral resection is performed at 0° with respect to the femoral mechanical axis, with 0–5° of flexion, in order to avoid anterior notching of the femoral cortex, and with 8 mm of resection depth from the most distal femoral condyle, to restore the thickness of the distal part of the femoral component; in this case, a Scorpio NRG implant (8 mm of thickness) has been used. In some particular cases, the amount of the distal femoral resection can be modified: when a patella baja is present, it is recommended to reduce the amount of this resection and to increase the proximal tibial resection, while in a flexed knee, it is recommended to increase this resection with respect to the femoral posterior cut and to reduce the femoral flexion.

The femoral rotation and the AP positioning of the 4-in-1 cutting block are performed by the "navigated drill templates for AP alignment" (Fig. 4.13). The navigated drill templates can replace the conventional AP sizer. By this dedicated jig, it is possible to check the position of the femoral component as previously planned matching the position of the yellow line (jig orientation) to the green (planning orientation) lines. Before

Fig. 4.12 Dedicated femoral mini jig for navigated mini invasive technique

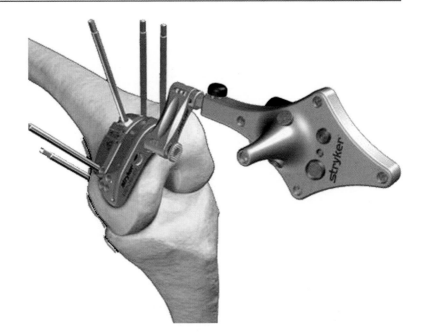

fixing the jig, the system confirms the presence of anterior notching. In this case, it is possible to translate anteriorly the guide, checking the posterior resection that could be too large.

The proximal tibial resection (Fig. 4.14) is performed at 0° with respect to the tibial mechanical axis, with 0–10° of posterior slope trying to restore the natural slope of the tibial plateau as measured on the LL knee radiograph, and with about 10 mm of resection depth from the most normal tibial condyle.

The tibial rotation can be navigated following the orientation calculated during the anatomical tibial survey, but we prefer to align the tibia by using the trial components and leave the tibial component to self-align with respect to the femoral trial.

4.2.2.5 Verification of Resections

The real advantage of navigation is the possibility to check every single step during surgery and so have the possibility to change the orientation of all osteotomies. Usually, with conventional instrumentation, only a visual inspection, and therefore the experience of the surgeon, allows verification of the accuracy of every single bone cut, whereas with navigation, this checking is provided through the numerical data of the

software. Sometimes, as demonstrated by Bäthis et al. [2], it can be differences from the guide orientation and the correlate bone cut, and these differences are very difficult to see with only a visual inspection.

The verification of osteotomies orientation during navigation is performed with a dedicated "resection plane probe," which can be used both for the distal femoral and proximal tibial bone cuts (Fig. 4.15). The orientation and the amount of the posterior femoral bone cut must be recorded by using the "posterior plane probe." In this way, it will be possible to check if the planned osteotomies correspond to the real bone cuts and possibly make some changes. Once all these bone cuts are recorded, gap monitoring will be possible with apposite distractor or more easily with trial component (Fig. 4.16).

4.2.2.6 Soft Tissue Balancing

The soft tissue balancing, as with conventional technique, is usually performed with a trial component after bone resection, also with navigated technique. In more detail, the soft tissue balancing is performed two times.

Before performing the bone cuts when landmark calibration during anatomical survey phase and preoperative knee kinematics are recorded,

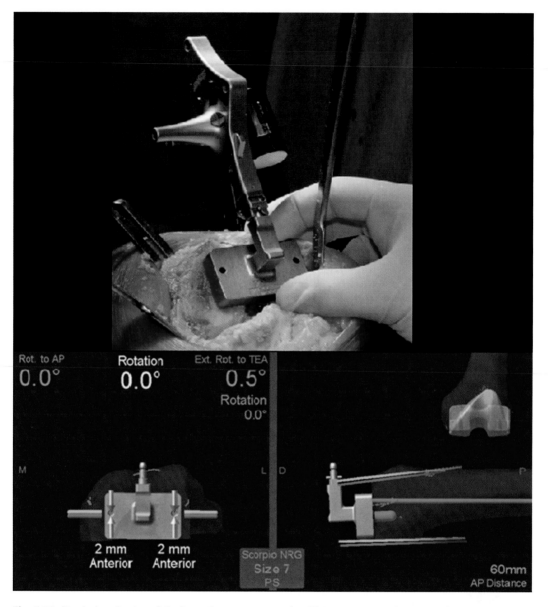

Fig. 4.13 Surgical navigation of the femoral component rotation. The surgeon can orientate the femoral component with respect to the AP axis, the transepicondylar axis, or the mean of the two values

the knee deformity is checked, evaluating if it is fixed or correctable. In the first case, the deformity is not related only to the bone defect but also to medial or lateral soft tissue contracture, and therefore, some amount of soft tissue release is performed before the intraoperative planning. Before performing this release, it is necessary to remove all osteophytes mostly in the posterior condyles and in the tibial plateau because these could give contractures that do not exist. With navigation, it is possible to check and record this deformity at all degrees of flexion and verify if this deformity is correctable and eventually to perform a calibrated medial or lateral soft tissue release, avoiding excessive laxity of the collateral ligaments (Fig. 4.17). When the complete correction of the deformity is obtained, the intraoperative planning is performed.

Fig. 4.14 Surgical
navigation with
free-hand technique for
the proximal tibial
resection

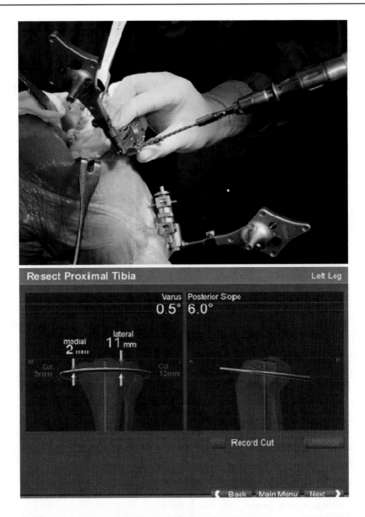

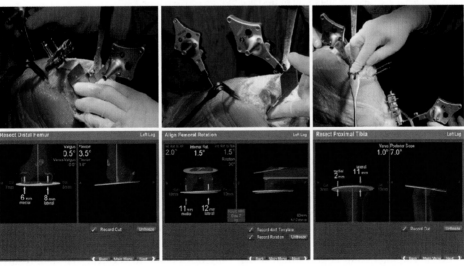

Fig. 4.15 Verification of the osteotomies orientation; respectively of the distal femur resection, posterior femoral resection and proximal tibial resection

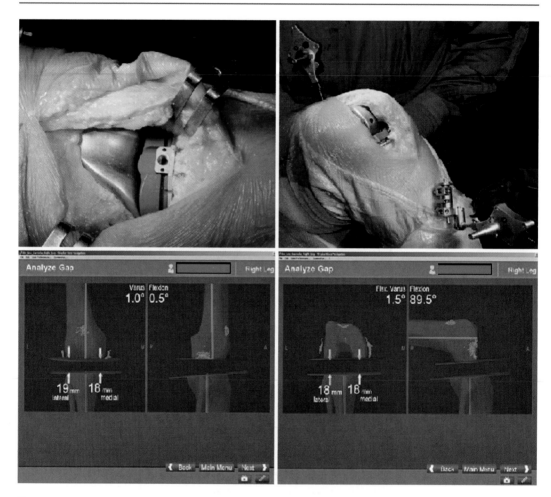

Fig. 4.16 Navigation assessment with trial components. The surgeon can analyze in extension and in flexion the medial and the lateral gaps and the alignment of the knee

In the second time, soft tissue release is performed with trial components. When the release has been performed in the right way, as shown above, and planning has been followed, this second phase is not necessary. Sometimes, some degree of deformity remains after trial component positioning, and therefore, following navigation, this second phase of soft tissue release is performed. The release of the medial collateral ligament is performed on its anterior part if the varus deformity is prevalent in flexion and on its posterior part if the varus deformity is prevalent in extension. In the fixed valgus deformity, a release of the iliotibial band is performed if the deformity is prevalent in extension, whereas a release of the lateral posterior capsule, lateral

collateral ligament, or popliteus tendon if the deformity is prevalent in flexion [5].

After the soft tissue release, the stability and the flexion and extension gap are checked again, and if some degree of instability is present, a thicker insert can be implanted.

4.2.2.7 Final Kinematics

When all the definitive components have been cemented, the final knee kinematics is recorded (Fig. 4.18). It is possible to record the final alignment in extension, the knee kinematics during flexion, and the collateral ligament tension during flexion and to compare the final results with the preoperative. It is possible to perform some further soft tissue release because sometimes the

Fig. 4.17 Diagram of the deformity in a varus knee during the range of motion. This deformity is completely correctable in extension, but not in flexion. Probably a soft tissue release could be performed only to correct the flexion medial contracture

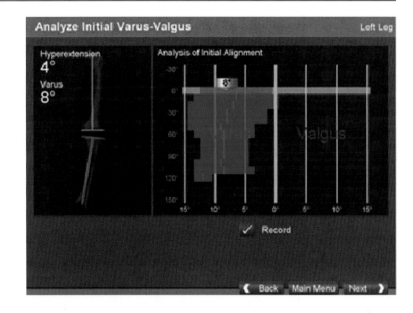

Fig. 4.18 Analysis of final alignment. The knee is close to 0°, with a good stability during all the range of movement

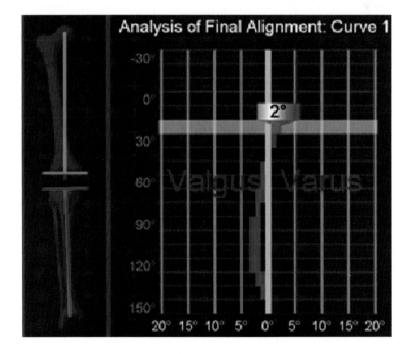

alignment of the definitive components could be different with respect to the trial components [4]. At the end, all the data related to the preoperative deformity, to the planning, to the bone cuts orientation, and to the final kinematics are recorded in the final report. The report of these data is useful both for clinical research and for documentation in medical-legal issues.

References

1. Arima J, Whiteside LA, McCarthy DS et al (1995) Femoral rotational alignment, based on the anteroposterior axis, in total knee arthroplasty in a valgus knee. J Bone Joint Surg Am 77(9):1331–1334
2. Bäthis H, Perlick L, Tingart M et al (2005) Intraoperative cutting errors in total knee arthroplasty. Arch Orthop Trauma Surg 125(1):16–20

3. Berger RA, Rubash HE, Seel MJ et al (1993) Determining the rotational alignment of the femoral component in total knee arthroplasty using the epicondylar axis. Clin Orthop Relat Res 286:40–47

4. Catani F, Biasca N, Ensini A et al (2008) Alignment deviation between bone resection and final implant positioning in computer-navigated total knee arthroplasty. J Bone Joint Surg Am 90(4):765–771

5. Hungerford DS, Krackow KA, Kenna RV (1984) Management of fixed deformity at total knee arthroplasty. In: Hungerford DS, Lennox DW (eds) Total knee arthroplasty a comprehensive approach. Williams & Wilkins, Baltimore

6. Meding JB, Keating EM, Ritter MA, Faris PM, Berend ME (2003) Genu recurvatum in total knee replacement. Clin Orthop Relat Res 416:64–67

7. Poilvache PL, Insall JN, Scuderi GR et al (1996) Rotational landmarks and sizing of the distal femur in total knee arthroplasty. Clin Orthop Relat Res 331:35–46

8. Whiteside LA, Arima J (1995) The anteroposterior axis for femoral rotational alignment in valgus total knee arthroplasty. Clin Orthop Relat Res 321:168–172

Computer Assisted Surgery (CAS): Ligament Balance

5

Claudio Carlo Castelli, Valerio Gotti,
and Mario Iapicca

5.1 Introduction

The goal of the total knee arthroplasty (TKR) procedure is to restore a stable, painless, and functional joint as long as possible.

These outcomes are achieved as follows:

- A good alignment of the axis of the limb and a perfect position of the prosthetic components (Fig. 5.1)
- Balanced and symmetric flexion and extension gaps: ligament balance [7, 18] (Fig. 5.2)

By now, all the CAS systems in TKA are image-free and are based on absolutely equal parameters in all software. The reproducibility and accuracy of the parameters, mentioned above, depend on any software and on the surgeon's experience and ability, and he is the only one responsible for the procedure.

At the beginning, it is the surgeon who has to enter the following data:

- Geometrical:
  - Hip centre of rotation
  - Knee and ankle centre (femoral and tibial anatomical axis)
  - Femoral and tibial rotation axis
- Morphological:
  (based on the virtual digitizing of the femoral and tibial articular surfaces and their bone landmarks)
  On the femoral side:
  - Anterior cortex
  - Posterior cortex
  - Epicondylar axis
  - Whiteside line
  - Distal condyles (Fig. 5.3a)
  On the tibial side:
  - Tibial plateau surface
  - Highest and deepest areas
  - Tibial rotational axis (TTA medial third – PCL tibial insertion) (Fig. 5.3b)
- Kinematic
  This data is still controversial and debated, but it is an essential and extremely important step to standardize a valuable functional outcome.

5.2 Intraoperative ligament balance quantitative evaluation

The intraoperative ligament tension has been evaluated in different ways during all these years.

C.C. Castelli (✉) • V. Gotti • M. Iapicca
Department of Orthopaedic Surgery and Trauma,
Ospedali Riuniti di Bergamo, Largo Barozzi 1,
Bergamo 24128, Italy
e-mail: ccastelli@ospedaliriuniti.bergamo.it;
vgotti@ospedaliriuniti.bergamo.it;
miapicca@ospedaliriuniti.bergamo.it

F. Catani, S. Zaffagnini (eds.), *Knee Surgery using Computer Assisted Surgery and Robotics*,
DOI 10.1007/978-3-642-31430-8_5, © ESSKA 2013

Fig. 5.1 Limb alignment by CAS

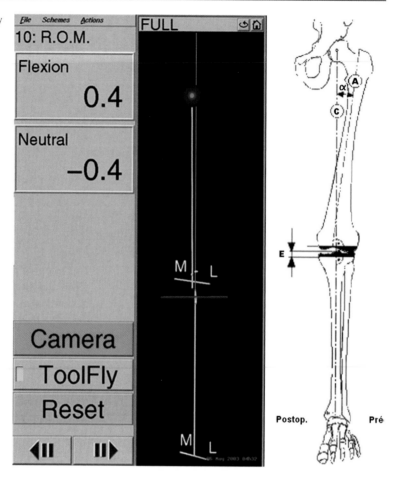

5.2.1 Gap Based

The goal was to reach balanced and symmetrical flexion and extension gaps through a controlled resection by spacer blocks.

Advantages: Easy procedure, uncomplicated instrumentation, traditional surgical technique (easier for the surgeon) (Fig. 5.4a).

Disadvantages: The spacer blocks just give a static evaluation of the extension and 90° flexion gaps, but the stability or laxity and the ligament tension are still based on the surgeon's experience.

By this technique, the tension is not correlated to the gap, and because of that, it cannot be related to the perfect reproducibility of CAS [10, 11].

5.2.2 Force Based

In order to get symmetric gaps, this technique needs tensors that give a well-known tension; this is easily integrated in CAS (Fig. 5.4b).

Disadvantages: The applied force is constant independent of the sex, age, disease, or morphology of the patient. Ligament tension obviously

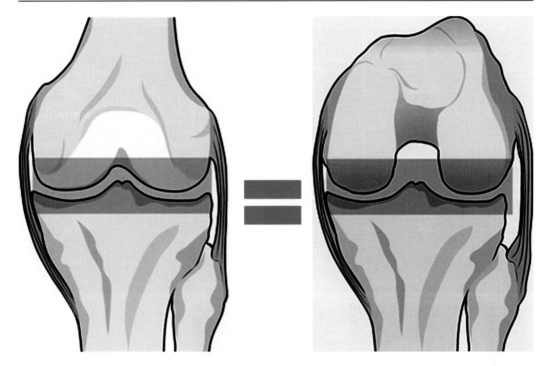

Fig. 5.2 Rectangular flexion and extension gaps

depends on these different factors. The same force applied to different patients may lead to over- or under-resection.

5.2.3 CAS-Assisted Advanced Ligament Balance

Starting from that, it has been necessary to evaluate the ligament tension through different tools, which had to be integrated in navigation systems in order to obtain accurate and reproducible data.

The Fishkin papers can be considered as the starting point: He worked on the relationship between applied force (Newton) and the ligament elongation in mm in knees affected by degenerative arthritis [9, 12, 15] (Fig. 5.5).

This is just a starting point: The viscoelastic properties of the ligaments must also be considered; the graphic below shows the correlation curve between strain (MPa) and stress (%). There are three different areas:

- *Toe area*: Shows an exponential correlation related to the force in order to obtain just the physiological flattening of the ligament bundles with no tension yet.
- *Elastic area*: The relation between σ and ϵ is linear, and the ligament bundles are all parallel in increasing and decreasing tension and in lengthening.
- *Failure area*: Starting from the yielding point, where the bundles start to fail progressively and very little force is needed to obtain an extensive lengthening (total ligament failure: $\sigma = 75$ – MPa; $\epsilon = 15$ %) (Fig. 5.6).

In order to obtain the correct ligament balance, the surgeon has to work on the first two areas.

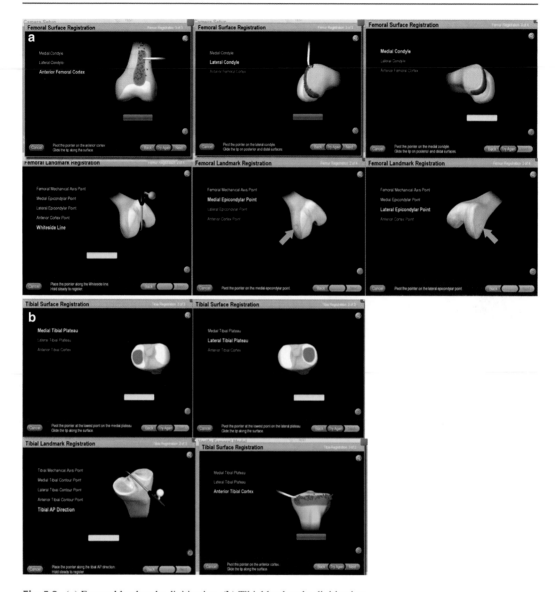

Fig. 5.3 (**a**) Femoral landmarks digitization. (**b**) Tibial landmarks digitization

Starting from these assumptions, a prototype tensor "hydraulic knee analyzer – HKA®" was tested on ten cadaver knees [3, 4] (Fig. 5.7).

The first issue that came out was to choose the correct tool in order to measure all the different tensions (bar) and different gaps (mm) at the same time in the medial and lateral compartments during 90° of flexion and complete extension: A closed hydraulic system with a manometer was used.

A balanced flexion and extension gap has a precise relationship with the pressure applied on the medial and lateral compartments in all the tests performed: The pressure in flexion was measured in four bars (65.6 N) and six bars (98.4 N) in extension.

Once these results were obtained, the authors started using this procedure on patients.

The tibia-first technique was used. The above-mentioned system uses the tibial resection as

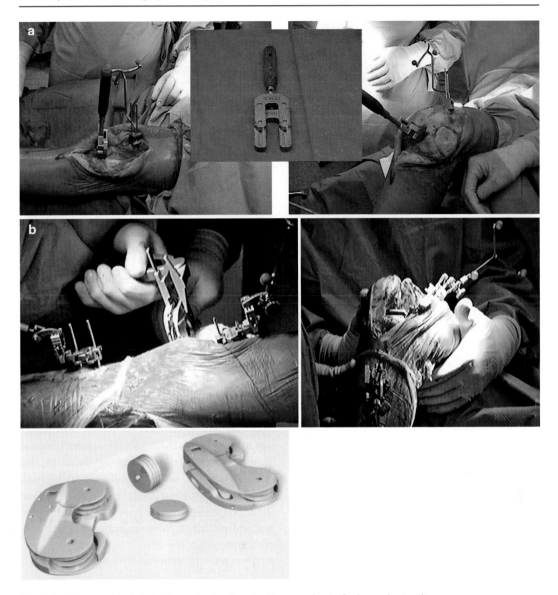

Fig. 5.4 (**a**) Spacer block in flexion and extension. (**b**) Tensor spring in flexion and extension

reference to obtain virtual intraoperative planning (Fig. 5.8).

In full extension, we position the HKA® pumping the pressure up to six bars; then, we check the alignment to see if the deformity has been corrected; if not, we perform a step-by-step release of soft tissues led by CAS.

Once the desired alignment is obtained, we store the preliminary extension gap on the computer.

Now the HKA® is positioned at 90° flexion and is pumped up to four bars. The computer is checked to achieve the correct gap by proper sizing and positioning of the femoral component on sagittal and frontal planes. As a reference, we use the correct gap monitored by the anatomical landmark (normally Whiteside line).

The rotation of the femoral component is obtained by using a functional parameter.

Fig. 5.5 Fishkin's curve load elongation [9]

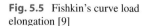
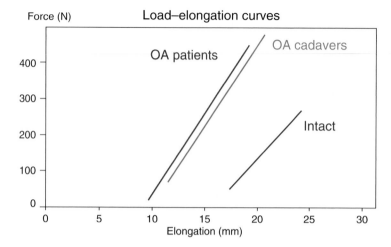

Fig. 5.6 Stress strain curve of the ligaments

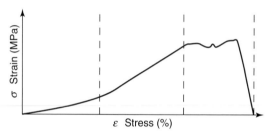

From the computer, we get a view of a rectangular flexion gap with the tibial resection used as reference and also by checking the anatomical landmark (normally Whiteside line). In controversial and difficult cases, the surgeon chooses the best compromise [5].

To decide the correct femoral size, besides the morphological landmarks, we use the virtual flexion gap given by HKA. Once the correct size is obtained on the A/P plane, we consider the minimum thickness referring to the specific geometry of the prosthesis. At the same time, the system correlates the extension to the flexion gap in order to decide the distal femoral resection, avoiding an unacceptable variation of the joint line.

A few of the latest generation systems provide us with virtual planning on the screen, by showing us the amount of joint line movement on all planes of the space (Fig. 5.9).

We do emphasize that, at this moment, the only resection performed is the tibial one, and all the other planned resections are just virtual. We have the chance to modify the size of the femoral component and its position on the three planes of the space in order to achieve balanced and symmetrical gaps, before resecting the distal femoral bone.

Then, the surgical procedure follows the usual conventional steps, even if we continue to check full flexion-extension movement for the correct alignment and articular tension, thanks to the navigator and HKA.

By analysing the results and checking the x-ray alignment, KSS, SF-36 and WOMAC, we can conclude that, considering a homogeneous patient morphotype, operated by the same surgeon, with the same prosthesis, navigation enables one to obtain better results very close to the ideal results when compared to the traditional surgical procedure whose results are much less homogeneous.

This kind of analysis is limited because it does not consider the advanced ligament balance concept, so new postoperative evaluation tests are needed to better evaluate the joint stability.

Different options can be considered; in 2006, we proposed a method to improve the evaluation of joint laxity in TKA by creating a fluoroscopic stress test method [6].

An x-ray transparent table, high enough to use a fluoroscopic device at different angles, has been designed. The patient sits on the table with his limb on a board hinged to the table at the level of the knee joint. The board flexes the knee at 0°, 45° and 90°. The knees are strapped in jaws adaptable to each knee. The joint rotation is dominated by an elastic band, passing through the jaws. A

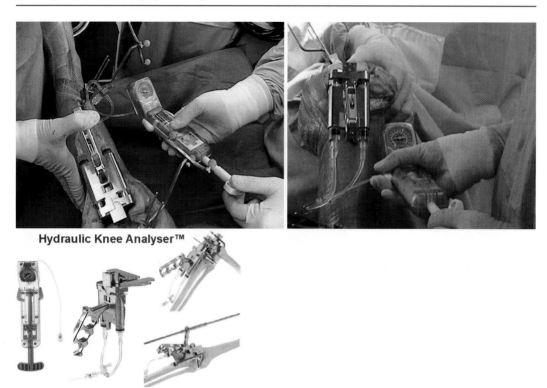

Fig. 5.7   Hydraulic knee analyzer – HKA® in flexion and extension

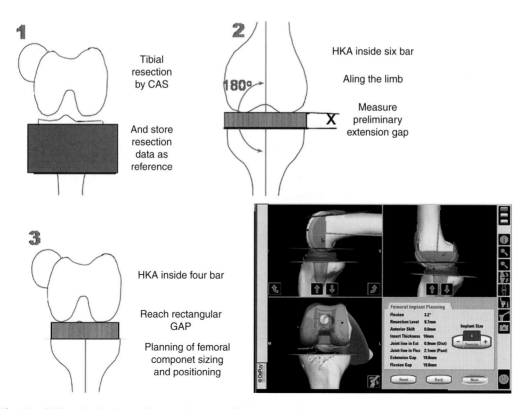

1

Tibial resection by CAS

And store resection data as reference

2

180°

X

HKA inside six bar

Aling the limb

Measure preliminary extension gap

3

HKA inside four bar

Reach rectangular GAP

Planning of femoral componet sizing and positioning

Femoral Implant Planning

Flexion   3.2°
Resection Level   9.7mm
Anterior Shift   0.0mm
Insert Thickness   10mm
Joint line in Ext 0.9mm (Dist)
Joint line in Flex 2.1mm (Post)
Extension Gap   19.8mm
Flexion Gap   19.8mm

Implant Size

Fig. 5.8   CAS-assisted advanced ligament balance: tibia-first technique and intraoperative virtual planning

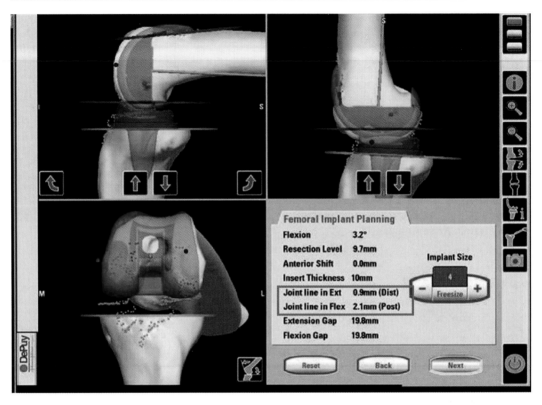

Fig. 5.9 Measure of movement of the joint line in the intraoperative virtual planning

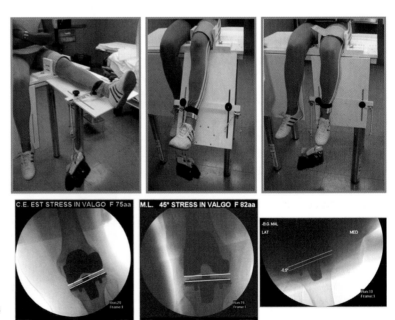

Fig. 5.10 Fluoroscopic stress test method [6]

fluoroscopic image is checked at three different angles of flexion without any stress applied and then with 5 kg (50 N) applied at the level of the ankle in varus and valgus stress (Fig. 5.10).

To validate this method, a study has been carried out on three patients with the same primary TKA (Innex®). For each joint position, two images have been shot; for each angle, the authors did some shots with an adjustment grid so that every image is reworked by specific software to correct the optical deformation.

As suggested by an independent and external examiner (Istituto Ricerche Farmacologiche M. Negri – Milano), 50 images have been selected and randomized, organizing them in 16 series, in different serial orders. Four raters examined independently four series each using a drawing vector software (ImageJ) outlining the tangent to the most prominent points of the condylar curve and of the tibial plateau. The software automatically calculated the angle of the two lines. A comparison between the results of each rater has been carried out.

A mathematical model of the prosthesis extracted from the CT scan has been used to compare the real angle with the angle calculated on the prosthesis shadow.

The results show that the CAS and "Advanced Ligament Balance" group obtained:

• A better reproducibility (statistically significant).
• Patients treated by navigation surgery showed better clinical results correlated to better stability (low laxity) at 45° flexion at varus/valgus stress.

This method is reliable, simple, cheap, user friendly, and well tolerated by the patients.

It is useful to detect instability in knee flexion which may otherwise be overlooked in the clinical tests.

Thanks to the most recent software, it is possible to make kinematic evaluations at the beginning and at the end of the surgical procedure through the varus/valgus stress test which was formerly made with the surgeon's hands at the end of TKA. The values obtained are measured and memorized by the computer that gives us the possibility to check the pre- and post-surgery difference curves of stability and mobility (Fig. 5.11a, b).

This data enables us to evaluate the patient's preop and post-op kinematics. It is a data bank where we can check all the values regarding the correct ligament tension for every single patient in order to recreate the same tension with patients of the same morphotype, gender, age, etc.

The surgeon's experience still plays an essential role in identifying the patient's specific features, to adapt the "standard" surgical technique to the anatomy and kinematics of the patient. The new research trends are directed to patient-based surgery, a method in which the correct surgical positioning is obtained by the patient's specific parameters. In order to correlate the effect of the patient's anatomical and kinematic variables and the intraoperative decision workflow performed by skilled surgeons, with the follow-up of TKA patients, a multicentre study, performed in Italy coordinated by the SIGASCOT society, including six surgeons was started in October 2009. Each surgeon performed 20 computer-assisted TKA with BLUIGS system (Orthokey LLC, Lewes, Delaware). [2] The following data is recorded (Fig. 5.12):

• Anatomic variables (limb alignment, angles between transepicondylar line, Whiteside line and posterior condyle line)
• Kinematic variables (functional flexion axis, varus-valgus laxity range at 0° and 30° of flexion, flexion and extension gap)
• Intraoperative data (ligament release, implant positioning and size)
• Clinical data acquired preoperatively and after 6-month follow-up (KOOS score, KSS score, SF-36 score, HSS patellar score, knee functional score)

Anatomical data is correlated with preoperative kinematics to see if bone morphology influences knee kinematics. Anatomical and kinematic variables are correlated with

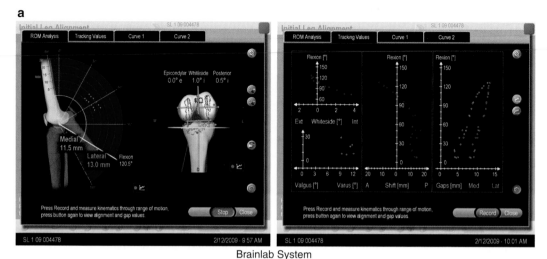

Fig. 5.11 Kinematic curve: (**a**) Brainlab® system (**b**) Orthokey® system

intraoperative data to see if constitutional bone morphology and kinematics influence surgical strategy. Preoperative kinematic data is correlated to preoperative clinical scores to see whether clinical scores are affected by patients' kinematics. Repeatability of functional flexion axis and interobserver variability of transepicondylar axis were also calculated; we computed transepicondylar axis variability because we used this axis as the main anatomical reference, and since it was a surgeon dependent landmark, we wanted to evaluate whether there was a significant difference in intraoperative acquisitions among the study participants.

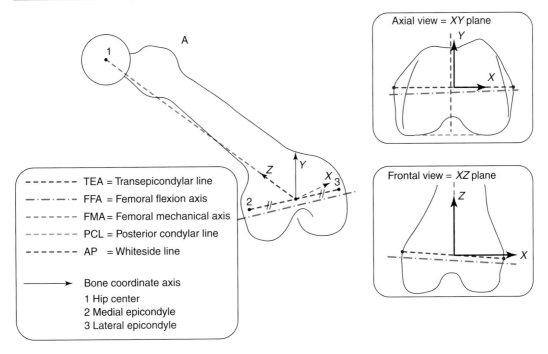

Axial view = *XY* plane

Frontal view = *XZ* plane

TEA = Transepicondylar line
FFA = Femoral flexion axis
FMA = Femoral mechanical axis
PCL = Posterior condylar line
AP   = Whiteside line

Bone coordinate axis
1 Hip center
2 Medial epicondyle
3 Lateral epicondyle

Fig. 5.12   Reference axes legend

At present, the primary indicator for a successful TKA remains the achievement of correct limb alignment. This parameter however is not able to describe alone the complex interaction between limb alignment, ligament balance, joint kinematics and clinical results.

Computer-assisted surgery has the potential to quantify more precisely pre- and post-operative joint parameters. This quantification permits us to better describe how patients' constitutional features can influence the surgical result. Our preliminary results, obtained at time zero during surgery, suggest that limb alignment and constitutional bone morphology are not correlated with clinical scoring. Joint laxity in extension has been found to be correlated with clinical scoring. From a kinematic point of view, the femoral flexion axis showed good repeatability, tested on the acquisitions of six different surgeons. This kinematic axis is a reliable reference for femoral component positioning in TKA (Fig. 5.13).

The low variability of transepicondylar axis confirmed that the acquisitions made from different operators were homogeneous and that the navigation system can improve the surgeon repeatability in TKA implantation, compared to traditional instrumentation.

A kinematic derived test such as laxity is more correlated with clinical scoring with respect to limb alignment. In addition, the flexion axis of the knee, acquired intraoperatively by means of navigation, showed excellent results. The continuation of this study with additional data acquisitions and with clinical results at follow-up may permit us to definitively identify or confirm which kinematic and anatomical parameters are correlated with a good surgical result at follow-up and, therefore, define a more patient-specific surgical workflow.

Other authors [1, 8, 13, 14, 16, 17] are still looking for different solutions from the above mentioned ones, even if there are still unanswered questions about the bulky tensors and their harm to the anatomical tissues of the knee, a possibility could be the miniaturization of the tools adopted right now connected to the CAS System.

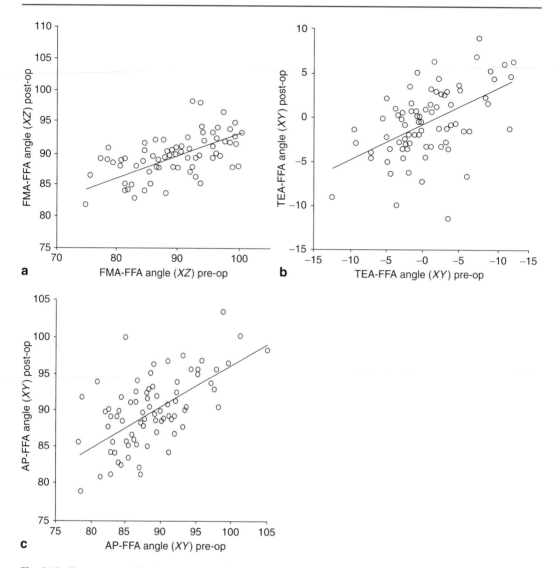

Fig. 5.13 Pearson correlation between pre- and postoperative angles of *FFA* with *FMA* (**a**), *TEA* (**b**) and *AP* (**c**) line orientation

References

1. Bignozzi S, Briard JL, Marcacci M (2004) Clinical validation of a novel spring loaded tensioning device and computer assisted navigation. In: 4th Annual of CAOS – international proceeding, Chicago
2. Bignozzi S, Castelli CC, Gotti V et al (2010) Multicentric functional evaluation of TKA by mean of navigation technology. In: 10th Annual of CAOS – international proceeding, Paris
3. Castelli C, Barbieri F, Gotti V (2003) L'instabilità articolare nelle protesi totali di ginocchio: ruolo della navigazione nell'ottenimento del bilancio legamentoso. GIOT 29(Suppl):S450–S452
4. Castelli C, Barbieri F, Gotti V (2003) Ct free TKA application and soft tissue balancing: the new concept. In: 6th EFORT congress, Helsinki
5. Castelli C., Gotti V, Barbieri F (2003) Choice of femoral component rotational alignment in tkr-ct less navigation system's role. In: 3rd Annual of CAOS – international proceeding, Marbella
6. Castelli C, Barbieri F, Gotti V (2006) A validated method to asses fluoroscopically the varus-valgus stability in flexion TKA. In: 6th Annual of CAOS – international proceeding, Montreal
7. Clayton M, Thompson TR, Mack RP (1986) Correction of alignment deformities during total knee arthroplasties. Clin Orthop Relat Res 202:117–124

8. Crottet D, Maeder T, Fritschy D (2004) A force sensing device for ligament balancing in total knee arthroplasty. In: 4th Annual of CAOS – international proceeding, Chicago

9. Fishkin Z, Miller D, Ritter C (2002) Changes in human knee ligament stiffness secondary to osteoarthritis. J Orthop Res 20:204–207

10. Jenny JY, Lefevbre Y, Vernizeau M (2002) Validation d'un protocol experimental d'étude optoélectronique de la cinématique active continue de l'articulation du genou in vitro. Revue de chir Orthop 88:790–796

11. Jenny JY, Lefevbre Y, Vernizeau M (2002) Etude de la cinématique active continue de l'articulation fémoro-patellaire d'un genou normal ou porteur d'une prothése in vitro. Revue de chir Orthop 88:797–802

12. Kennedy JC, Hawkins RJ, Willis RB (1976) Tension studies of human knee ligament. J Bone Joint Surg Am 58(3):350–355

13. Krackow KA (2003) Fine tuning your next total knee: computer assisted surgery. Orthopedics 26(9):971–972

14. Marmignon C, Lemniei A, Cinquin P (2004) A computer assisted controlled distraction device to guide ligament balancing during TKA. In: 4th Annual of CAOS – international proceeding, Chicago

15. Sinha RJ, Sheik B, Halbrecht J (1999) Collateral ligament strain after total knee arthroplasty. American Academy of Orthopaedic Surgeons – annual meeting, Anaheim

16. Sparmann M, Wolke B, Czupalla H (2003) Positioning of total knee arthroplasty with and without navigation support. A prospective, randomized study. J Bone Joint Surg Br 85(6):830–835

17. Viskontas DG, Srinskas TV, Chess DG (2004) Computer assisted gap equalization in TKA. In: 4th Annual of CAOS – international proceeding, Chicago

18. Winemaker MJ (2002) Perfect balance in total knee arthroplasty: the elusive compromise. J Arthroplasty 17(1):2–10

Robotics in TKA

6

J. Bellemans

6.1 Introduction

Robotic technology was introduced in orthopaedics in the late 1980s, and the first robotic-assisted hip replacement was performed on a human patient in 1992.

Subsequently, the first robotic system for clinical use was commercialized in 1994 under approval of the European Union [1].

Although most of the initial research and development was performed by schools and centres in Germany, the enthusiasm has since spread out not only over the whole European continent but also over North America and the rest of the world. Today, for example, robots are not only used in hip arthroplasty but also in knee arthroplasty and cruciate ligament surgery, with different commercial systems available.

Generally speaking, robots can be categorized in three groups: (1) passive, (2) active, or (3) semi-active [5].

Passive robots hold the guide or jig in the correct place, but the actual cutting or drilling is performed by the surgeon or the operator.

Active (autonomous) robots not only hold the cutting tool, they also autonomously make the appropriate cuts. The involvement of the surgeon is limited to the planning phase, whereas the practical execution is performed by the robot under vigilance of the surgeon, who usually has an alarm button to switch off the system when needed.

Semi-active or so-called haptic robots combine both principles, whereby the robot guides the cutting tool within a predefined trajectory (e.g. a plane on the proximal tibia), within which the surgeon can work under the constraints provided by the robot.

6.2 Autonomous Robots

The first systems that became commercially available for knee surgery were active robots.

Unfortunately, they were not a huge success despite the initial enthusiasm by the early believers in this technology. These active robots required a high degree of safety and reliability and needed to give the surgeon adequate feedback about the ongoing process, such as the cutting path with respect to the preoperative planning, cutting forces, and bone motion, in order to allow him to appropriately detect if something was going wrong and intervene if necessary.

Several systems that fulfilled these requirements were commercially available for knee arthroplasty, i.e. the ROBODOC system® (Integrated Surgical Systems, Davis, CA), the CASPAR system® (U.R.S. Ortho Rastatt, Germany), and the BRIGIT system® (Zimmer, Warsaw, USA) (Fig. 6.1).

J. Bellemans, M.D., Ph.D.
Department of Orthopaedic Surgery, University Hospital
Pellenberg, Katholieke Universiteit Leuven,
Weligerveld 1, Pellenberg 3012, Belgium
e-mail: johan.bellemans@uz.kuleuven.ac.be

F. Catani, S. Zaffagnini (eds.), *Knee Surgery using Computer Assisted Surgery and Robotics*,
DOI 10.1007/978-3-642-31430-8_6, © ESSKA 2013

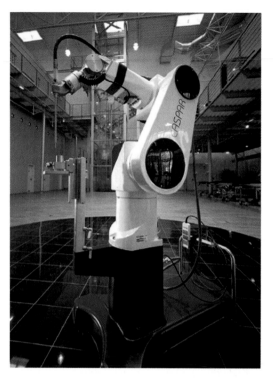

Fig. 6.1 CASPAR autonomous robot system® (U.R.S. Ortho Rastatt, Germany)

Each of these systems had a comparable application protocol, which consisted of four steps: (1) placement of the fiducial marker pins, (2) spiral CT scanning of the patient's leg [2], (3) preoperative planning and virtual implantation [3], and (4) the actual surgical implantation [4, 7].

Just as in classical computer-navigated TKA, fiducial markers were applied to the femoral and tibial bones for spatial orientation and geometric calculations.

With the pins in place, a spiral CT scan was obtained. The femoral head, the knee joint, ankle joint, and the pins were scanned, usually while the patient was still under spinal or epidural anaesthesia.

Next, the virtual implantation was performed on the screen by selecting a specific implant and size and positioning it onto the corresponding bone while changing or playing with the component translation and/or rotation until a satisfactory position was achieved.

Once the optimal position for the components was obtained, the milling area could be specified and adapted in order to avoid milling into the soft tissue regions, thereby reducing soft tissue trauma. (Fig. 6.2)

Finally, all data were saved and transferred to the robot control unit.

Subsequently, the surgical implantation could be performed through a standard incision and medial parapatellar arthrotomy. The leg is flexed and rigidly connected to the robot, by two transverse Steinman pins inserted, respectively, through the proximal tibia and the distal femur. These two pins were connected to a frame which was linked to the robot, while several retracting devices were mounted onto this frame for optimal exposure and soft tissue retraction.

In order to detect and control undesired motion of the leg during the robotic surgery, reflective markers were attached to this frame as well, which were continuously monitored by an infrared camera system and which would immediately stop the robot in case any type of undesired motion was detected.

After verification of the fiducial markers, the robotic action was started by the surgeon. The robot used a milling cutter to perform the bone resection, together with constant water irrigation for cooling purposes and for cleaning the milling debris. The surgeon maintained control over the milling process by a manually held button, which shut off the robotic action as soon as the button was depressed. At any stage during the procedure, the surgeon could switch to a conventional implantation technique when desired.

We have published our experience with such an autonomic robot system in 2007 in Clinical Orthopaedics and Related Research [2].

Twenty-one cases of robot-assisted TKA using the CASPAR system had been performed at our institution between 2000 and 2002 with an intense learning curve not only for the surgeon but even more for the nursing staff and the radiologists involved. Unlike any other new operating technique, this type of robotic surgery indeed posed many challenges during the learning process. Not only the important increase in operating time but also the sense of helplessness towards computer technology and software dysfunction (caused by the operator or not) was a

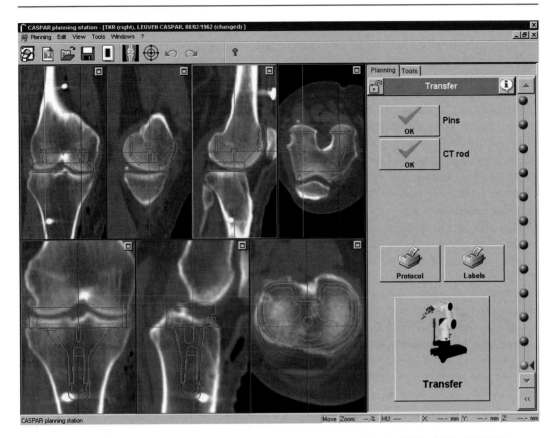

Fig. 6.2 Preoperative planning of the resection trajectory and component position for TKA with the CASPAR system

constant area of concern and frustration during the learning phase, which required an adequate dose of perseverance for the team to succeed.

Despite this hard learning curve, however, excellent results were obtained in all cases that were finished successfully, with overall frontal alignment on full leg standing x-rays within the 1° error of neutral alignment. In three of the cases, the robotic process was aborted because of technical difficulties with the recognition of the reflective markers' position, leading to a continuous error signalling on the screen. Each of these cases was successfully finished by converting to a conventional technique.

Comparable experiences to ours have in the meantime been reported by other groups. Siebert et al. published their results on 70 cases using the CASPAR system, with a mean difference between planned and obtained tibiofemoral alignment of 0, 8°. Some outliers were noted, with a maximum of 4° compared to the planned alignment [6, 12].

An average operating time of 135 (80–220) min was necessary to perform the surgery.

Borner et al. recently reported their results with the ROBODOC system and the Duracon total knee prosthesis in their first 100 cases. In only 5 % of the cases, the procedure needed to be abandoned and switched to a conventional technique due to technical problems. Alignment was within the 3° margin for all cases, and operating time took between 90 and 100 min after the initial learning curve [3].

Despite the excellent accuracy obtained with these autonomous systems, they did not become generally adopted.

Their complexity and excessive financial cost (500K euro) was considered unjustifiable by most surgeons and hospitals.

It is for these reasons that most research groups and companies involved in orthopaedic robotics have started focussing more on semi-active (haptic) robotic systems.

6.3 Semi-Active (Haptic) Robots

Haptic (semi-active) robots may have a better future than fully autonomous robots.

Haptic robots guide the cutting tool within a predefined trajectory (e.g. a plane on the proximal tibia), within which the surgeon can work under the constraints provided by the robot. As such they combine the intraoperative versatility and adaptability of navigation systems together with the advantages of almost perfect machining and bone preparation. Such semi-active robots could theoretically be much cheaper and more user-friendly than the current active robot systems and therefore much more successful in daily application. It is therefore logical that today a number of groups are working with semi-active robots in knee arthroplasty and are exploring their potential role.

The Robotic Arm Interactive Orthopaedic (RIO) System® (MAKO, Fort Lauderdale, USA) is a system which has been used for performing unicompartmental knee arthroplasty. [8, 9]

During bone resection, the system steers and controls the surgeon's action based upon his preoperative planning, both through an auditory as well as haptic feedback mechanism. As such the surgeon is prevented from resecting outside his preoperative plan.

The Acrobot system® (Acrobot, London, UK) is a similar device that was developed in conjunction with engineers and surgeons at Imperial College.

Both systems have been in clinical use for a number of years now, and their initial results have recently been published.

Cobb et al. reported their experience with the Acrobot system in a prospective randomized study compared with conventional UKA. The operation lasted on average 16 min longer in the Acrobot group, but the alignment was much better with 100 % of cases within the 2° deviation from the planned alignment, whereas this was only the case in 40 % of the conventional group. A trend was also noted towards improvement in performance with increasing accuracy based on the Western Ontario and McMaster Universities Osteoarthritis index and the American Knee Society Scores at 6 weeks and 3 months [4].

Recently, Roche et al. demonstrated excellent radiographic accuracy with the RIO system and the potential to use the technology in a mini-invasive setting [11].

An important downside of these systems still remains their cumbersome and voluminous bulky nature (they are positioned next to the operating table), as well as their exorbitant cost.

In an attempt to overcome these disadvantages, a number of smaller mini-robotic systems

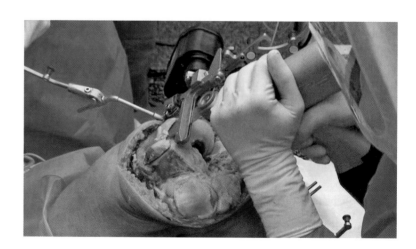

Fig. 6.3 Semi-autonomous Praxiteles® system (Praxim, Grenoble, France) for TKA. The mini-robot is attached to the bone and guides the resection guide

have been developed that can be mounted onto the bone [5, 10, 13] (Fig. 6.3).

These mini robots provide an additional advantage over the existing haptic systems with ease of use and financial cost and are currently being investigated in clinical trials both in Europe as well as North America.

Time will tell which systems will become adopted by the surgical community and will likely depend on technical feasibility, operational comfort, clinical outcome, and last but not least, financial cost.

References

1. Bargar W (2004) Robotic hip surgery and current development with the Robodoc system. In: Steihl JB, Konermann WH, Haaker RG (eds) Navigation and robotics in total joint and spine surgery, vol 15. Springer, Berlin/Heidelberg/New York/Tokyo, pp 119–121
2. Bellemans J, Vandenneucker H, Vanlauwe J (2007) Robot assisted total knee arthroplasty. Clin Orthop Relat Res 464:111–116
3. Borner M, Wiesel U, Ditzen W (2004) Clinical experiences with Robodoc and the Duracon total knee. In: Steihl JB, Konermann WH, Haaker RG (eds) Navigation and robotics in total joint and spine surgery, vol 51. Springer, Berlin/Heidelberg/New York/Tokyo, pp 362–366
4. Cobb J, Henckel J, Gomes P et al (2006) Hands-on robotic unicompartmental knee replacement: a prospective, randomized controlled study of the Acrobot system. J Bone Joint Surg Br 88:188–197
5. Lang J, Mannava S, Floyd A et al (2011) Robotic systems in orthopaedic surgery. J Bone Joint Surg Br 93:1296–1299
6. Mai S, Iorke C, Siebert W (2004) Clinical results with the robot assisted Caspar system and the search-evolution prosthesis. In: Steihl JB, Konermann WH, Haaker RG (eds) Navigation and robotics in total joint and spine surgery, vol 50. Springer, Berlin/Heidelberg/New York/Tokyo, pp 355–361
7. Park S, Lee C (2007) Comparison of robotic assisted and conventional manual implantation of a primary total knee arthroplasty. J Arthroplasty 22:1054–1059
8. Pearle A, Kendoff D, Stueber V et al (2009) Perioperative management of unicompartmental knee arthroplasty using the MAKO robotic arm system. Am J Orthop 38:16–19
9. Pearle A, O'Loughlin P, Kendoff D (2010) Robot assisted unicompartmental knee arthroplasty. J Arthroplasty 25:230–237
10. Plaskos C, Cinquin P, Lavallee S et al (2005) Praxiteles: a miniature bone-mounted robot for minimal access total knee arthroplasty. Int J Med Robot 1:67–79
11. Roche M, Augustin D, Conditt M (2010) Accuracy of robotically assisted UKA. J Bone Joint Surg Br 92S:127
12. Siebert W, Mai S, Kober R et al (2002) Technique and first clinical results of robot-assisted total knee replacement. Knee 9:173–180
13. Wolf A, Jaramaz B, Lisien B et al (2005) MBARS: mini bone-attached robotic system for joint arthroplasty. Int J Med Robot 1:101–121

Soft Tissue Management in PCL-Retaining TKA

7

Nicolas Haffner and Peter Ritschl

7.1 Introduction

As soon as conservative measures such as physical therapy as well as medication (e.g., NSAIDs or DMOADs) fail to alleviate pain in the osteoarthritic knee, surgery comes into play. If symptoms show an acute onset and clinical and radiological findings display only mild osteoarthritic changes, arthroscopy might be the first choice of treatment. If clinical and radiological changes are limited to one compartment (medial or lateral) only, the orthopedic surgeon should aim for a correction osteotomy or a unicondylar knee replacement. In all other cases such as severe bi- or tricompartmental osteoarthritis, total knee replacement is the only choice of treatment. It is a well-described and evidence-based procedure that is able to reduce pain and restore quality of life. To date, there is no gold standard for the implantation of a TKA.

Navigation and its use in TKA has evolved in the late 1990s of the last century but its broader application has been limited. Due to recent industrial developments such as the implementation of patient-matched cutting blocks, navigation is now experiencing a renaissance. In regard to navigation, we have to differentiate between image-based and image-free navigation systems. Whereas patient-matched cutting blocks (PMCB) have to be considered as image-based navigation, most of the orthopedic world would consider image-free techniques as the classical or the conventional navigation. Image-based navigational systems rely on CT or NMR data, which is acquired preoperatively, to guide the surgeon during the operative procedure. In contrast, using image-free navigational systems, the data is collected intraoperatively, and the bony landmarks that are detected are transmitted to a computer. So far the literature has not shown any clinical advantage of using navigational systems in TKA, besides the reduction of outliers in the frontal alignment (varus/valgus of 3°). In regard to the sagittal plane, there are conflicting results in the literature as to whether the use of navigational systems is able to reduce outliers. The reconstruction of the tibial slope shows no statistical differences compared to the conventional TKA [24].

Degenerative changes in the knee occur on the basis of primary or secondary osteoarthritis. The deformities seen in arthritic knees and in the overall alignment of the leg can be due to bony angulation or ligament imbalance.

Bony deformity can be located at the joint level itself, at the metaphysis or the diaphysis of the bone. Deformities at the articular surface and at the metaphyseal level can be managed during the implantation of the artificial joint. Diaphyseal angulations greater than 20° require a separate operative procedure such as a correction osteotomy [27].

N. Haffner, M.D. • P. Ritschl, M.D., Ph.D. (✉)
Orthopedic Clinic Gersthof,
Wielemansgasse 28, Vienna A-1180, Austria
e-mail: nicolas.haffner@wienkav.at;
peter.ritschl@wienkav.at

Soft tissue management during total knee arthroplasty (TKA) includes soft tissue release, component alignment [28], femoral component rotation [11], as well as flexion and extension gap balancing.

As there are no set standards regarding when to perform soft tissue releases in TKA, the following issues will be addressed in this chapter:

1. When are soft tissue releases traditionally performed during TKA?
2. The force-controlled soft tissue balancing technique
   A modification of the gap balancing technique as a novel approach to integrate soft tissue releases during the implantation of a TKA using a NAV/CAS system
3. Surgical techniques of soft tissue release in varus and valgus deformities
4. Sagittal plane balancing in PCL-retaining TKA

7.2   When Are Soft Tissue Releases Performed During TKA?

Generally there are two main strategies for TKA implantation: The measured resection technique and the gap technique (bone-referenced versus ligament-balanced technique).

The measured resection technique was introduced by Hungerford et al. [13]. This technique is also called the femur-first technique and starts with the bony cuts of the femur. The principle of this technique is to resect the amount of bone which is later replaced by the thickness of the prosthesis. Bony landmarks are used to guide resections equal to the distal and posterior thickness of the femoral component. Ligament releases are performed at the end of the procedure if needed in flexion and extension.

The gap technique was introduced by Insall et al. [16]. It is also known as the tibia-first technique where the tibia cut is performed first. It is essential to perform ligament releases before the femoral bone cuts. In extension, ligament releases are executed if necessary to obtain a rectangular extension gap, whereas in flexion no releases are done. In flexion, a potential asymmetry in the gap is corrected with femoral rotation, and equal collateral ligament tension in extension and flexion is guiding the level and the position of the bone cuts.

In conclusion, the timing of the soft tissue releases during the surgical procedure is different according to the chosen implantation methods.

Using the measured resection technique, the operative algorithm follows two general steps:

Step one:

Bone cuts are executed according to the anatomical landmarks.

For the distal femoral cut, the cutting jig is aligned to the anatomical axis mostly using an intramedullary alignment rod. To align the tibia cut, an extramedullary alignment device is usually applied. For both the femoral as well as for the tibial alignment, a vice versa intra- or extramedullary adjustment rod is available. For rotational alignment, the transepicondylar axis, the anteroposterior line or Whiteside's line, and the posterior condyles are used as a reference.

Step two:

Implantation of the trial components (or spacer blocks, laminar spreaders, and other tensioning devices) and balancing of the knee [23]. Therefore, the measured resection technique leaves the soft tissue releases to the end of the surgical procedure independently using navigation or conventional instrumentation.

Using the gap technique, the operative algorithm is somewhat reversed:

Step one:

After the tibia cut is done, tight ligamentous structures are released in extension to align the leg. For this surgical step, laminar spreaders or tensioners are used. In flexion, these or similar devices are inserted in the flexion gap to tension the ligaments. As a consequence of this balanced gap technique and in contrast to a measured resection technique, the rotation of the femoral component can vary freely within the restrictions of the soft tissue structures. No further releases are performed in flexion [14, 15].

Step two:

After tensioning the ligaments, the anterior and the posterior cuts are performed parallel to the tibia cut.

In contrast to the measured resection technique, the gap technique puts ligament balancing at the beginning of the surgical procedure.

There is no clear evidence about which of these methods yields better results in terms of stability and minimizing polyethylene wear. The measured resection technique is used more widely than the gap technique. For both techniques, excellent results have been reported.

Dennis compared the "lift-off" of both methods. The results showed that lift-off greater than 1 mm occurred in 60 and 45 % of the PCL-retaining and PCL-substituting TKA using measured resection versus none in the gap-balanced group. The authors of this article conclude that rotation of the femoral component using a gap balancing technique resulted in better coronal stability, which will improve functional performance and reduce polyethylene wear [9].

In a comparative study using a navigation system, Sabbioni reported that the results of imaging and the number of outliers were not statistically different ($P=0.56$) for the mechanical axis and prosthetic positioning between the two groups. The gap technique showed a statistically significant alteration of the postoperative joint line value when compared to the measured resection technique ($P=0.036$). The mean elevation of the joint line was 4.09 mm for the gap group and 3.50 mm in the measured resection group [25].

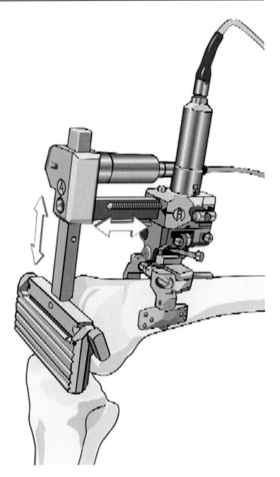

Fig. 7.1 The mini-robot brings the 5-in-1 cutting block or the saw guide in the calculated position. After the position is accepted, the surgeon carries out the bone cuts

7.3 The Integration of Gap Balancing Using a NAV/CAS System and Force-Controlled Soft Tissue Balancing Technique

The force-controlled soft tissue balancing technique is a modification of the gap technique and uses the Galileo Navigation System (Galileo S&N®).

The navigation system allows the surgeon to integrate soft tissue balancing, component positioning, and sizing of the femoral prosthesis into the implantation procedure. The Galileo® Navigation System uses a computer-assisted femoral cutting device – a so-called mini-robot, so that the femoral cuts can be carried out (Fig. 7.1). It is a passive system, which means that the cuts are done by the surgeon and not the robot. Every implantation step is visualized on the screen and can be accepted or changed by the surgeon before the surgical step is taken.

Furthermore, the surgeon has the ability to plan the femoral prosthesis in terms of rotation, AP position, and size. Before doing the bone cuts, all three factors can be calculated and visualized on the screen, and each one of them can be changed if desired to potentially gain a superior balanced knee.

Figures 7.3, 7.4, and 7.5 demonstrate the individual steps of the force-controlled soft tissue balancing technique. The surgical procedure is illustrated using a "double spring" ligament tensioner which allows a force-controlled tensioning of the medial and lateral compartment of the knee (Fig. 7.2).

The first step is to balance the knee in extension (Fig. 7.3). In case of a fixed varus or valgus deformity, a ligament release is done.

The second step is to define the gap in flexion and to plan the femoral prosthesis (Fig. 7.4a, b).

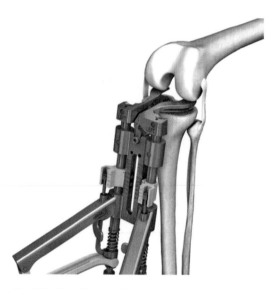

Fig. 7.2 "Double spring" compartment-specific, quantitative, force-controlled ligament tensioner

The planning of the femoral component consisting of determining the femoral rotation, the size, and the AP position is step three (Fig. 7.4b). Rotational alignment is indicated separately with figures visible for the gap balancing or the measured resection technique. The surgeon should be aware of the fact that the everted patella has an influence on the gap symmetry [22].

Step four deals with the synchronization of the gaps in terms of their width (Fig. 7.5a left, b right).

The force-controlled soft tissue balancing technique is therefore a modification of the gap technique, where the whole process of ligament and gap balancing is integrated in the implantation procedure.

In our opinion, this technique offers advantages over the classic gap balancing technique.

First of all, every surgical step is calculated and then visualized by the computer. The figures seen on the screen can be judged for their plausibility before any cut is carried out.

The force-controlled gap balancing allows individualization of the measured forces applied in flexion and extension. Generally at our institution, 160 N are applied in extension and 140 N in flexion (80/80 in extension and 70/70 in flexion for each compartment). In obese patients, this can be adapted to 180 and 160 N each [31]. In a recent paper from Heesterbeek et al., it was found that a tension of 100 N in flexion might be too tight in some individuals for spreading out the

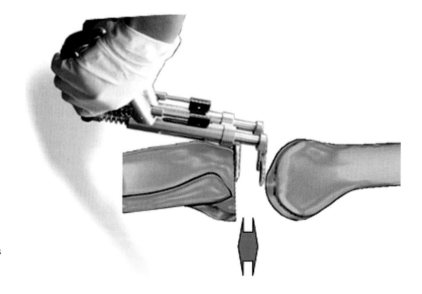

Fig. 7.3 Balancing the knee in extension. The ligament tensioner is spread out 80 N on the medial and lateral compartment of the knee. In case that the navigation system reveals an imbalance of the knee joint, a soft tissue release is carried out to obtain a correct mechanical axis

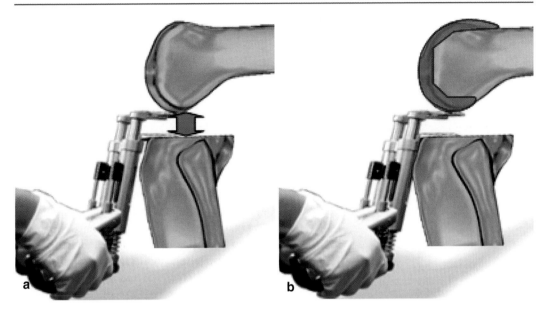

Fig. 7.4 Defining the width of the flexion gap by tensioning the medial and lateral compartment with 70 N each (**a**). Thereafter, the femoral component is defined in terms of size, AP position, and rotation (**b**)

flexion gap. All together there seems to be a great interpatient variability. Due to several factors such as age, activity level, gender, weight, soft tissue stiffness, and genetic factors influencing the individual stability of the knee, further research needs to be done in order to find the individual stability point in flexion and extension. In contrary to the classic gap technique, this individual approach of balancing the knee is done much more carefully using the force-controlled soft tissue balancing technique. In addition, the technique shows higher reproducibility [10].

Another advantage of using the NAV/CAS system is that the AP position of the femoral component can be shifted ½-mm steps in both directions, and the flexion gap can be precisely adjusted to accommodate the prosthesis. Hence, overstuffing of the femoropatellar joint or notching of the anterior femoral cortex will be avoided, and there are no limitations as to the use of an anterior or posterior referenced system.

Flexion alignment of the femoral component can also influence the width of the gap. The authors of a recent article found that the amount of the resected bone of the posterior medial con-

dyle decreased approximately 1 mm for every 2° of additional flexion in all TKA systems [28].

During the registration process, the flexion position of the femoral prosthesis is indicated on the screen and can be set to the desired value, which avoids hyperflexion or hyperextension of the femoral component.

For rotational alignment, both the figures of the anatomical landmarks as well as the values calculated by the gap technique are visualized on the screen. The decision whether the surgeon wants to follow the measured resection or the gap technique should be made according to the plausibility of the indicated figures on the screen.

The surgeon has to take into consideration that using the measured resection technique, bony landmarks can be difficult to palpate and therefore the registration of these points is relatively uncertain [18]. On the other hand, rotational alignment can vary greatly using the gap technique. In a recent paper, femoral component rotation was measured intraoperatively with a tensor applied in flexion. The tension applied was 150 N and a great variability ranging from −4° (internal rotation) to 13° (external rotation) was found [11].

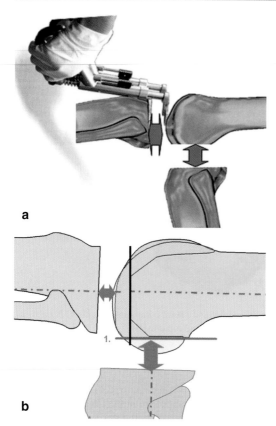

a

b

Fig. 7.5 (**a**) After performing the posterior femoral cut, the definitive width of the flexion gap under the tension of 140 N (70 N on the medial and lateral side) is achieved. To synchronize the width of the gaps, the extension gap is spread out to 160 N (80 N on the medial and lateral side). The computer calculates the distal femoral cut, which is then performed according to the calculation. The black resection line in (**b**) demonstrates the calculated resection level for the distal femoral cut

After the definitive space of the flexion gap is determined, the width of the extension gap is synchronized under the force conditions of 80/80 N on each compartment. The computer calculates the resection level, and the cut is performed (Fig. 7.5a, b).

7.4   Surgical Techniques of Soft Tissue Release

Although numerous techniques to establish balanced soft tissue tension have been proposed, there is no consensus regarding the optimal method or sequence of releases [4, 30].

There are basically four surgical techniques to release tight structures in the coronal plane:
1. A subperiosteal detachment of stabilizing ligamentous structures from the underlying bone, which is generally called the "soft tissue release." A proponent of this method is L. Whiteside. The releases are generally done according to a fixed sequence.
2. The "pie crust technique" is a multiple puncturing technique to release soft tissues used mainly in valgus deformities.
3. "Tightest structure first" release.
4. Ligament advancement procedures.

Leo Whiteside follows the measured resection technique. This means that he starts with the bone cuts. The alignment of the components of the implant is done separately on the femur and tibia based on anatomic landmarks in extension and flexion, regardless of ligament contracture or stretching.

When alignment, sizing, and positioning of the implants are correct and all osteophytes are removed, the ligaments can be assessed.

Ligaments contribute differently to joint stability in flexion and extension. Therefore, ligament releases are performed in order of their stabilizing function in flexion, extension, or both [30].

According to his algorithm, in a fixed varus deformity, if the knee is tight medially in flexion, the anterior portion of the medial collateral ligament is released. When the knee is tight medially in extension only, the posterior portion of the medial collateral ligament and possibly the posterior medial capsule are released. The posterior cruciate ligament is preserved when the entire medial collateral ligaments are released. Further structures that can be released medially are the semimembranosus tendon and other tendons of the superficial pes anserinus (sartorius, gracilis, semitendinosus).

In valgus knees which are tight in flexion and extension, the lateral collateral ligament and popliteus tendon are released. Those knees that remain tight only in extension have a release of the iliotibial band. Posterior capsular release is done only, if necessary, for persistent lateral ligament tightness. If all static lateral stabilizing structures require release, the biceps femoris muscle, the gastrocnemius muscle, and the deep fascia can support the knee until capsular healing occurs. Because external rotational and posterior constraints are not provided by these secondary lateral stabilizing structures, a more congruent tibial polyethylene component may be necessary to provide stability [29, 30].

In contrast using the gap technique releases are done only in extension to align the knee. No releases are performed in flexion.

In a cadaver study, Krackow looked at the effect of sequential varus releases. Each release sequence was tested in full extension, in 45° and in 90° of flexion to compare any differences obtained in the joint gaps. After releases of the posteromedial capsule oblique ligament complex, the superficial medial collateral ligament (MCL), the pes anserinus, and semimembranosus tendons, valgus rotation increased to 6.9° in full extension and 13.4° in 90° of flexion. The largest increase (3.2°) in valgus rotation occurred after the superficial MCL was released. Initial release of the superficial MCL led to a more gradual correction with release of subsequent structures. Changes seen in 90° of flexion were significantly greater than those in full extension. This might explain a certain amount of flexion instability of TKA, since a significantly larger correction is obtained in flexion [20].

The pie crust technique as a release technique for the valgus knee was introduced by Insall et al. [17]. This release is performed with a laminar spreader distracting the femorotibial joint space. First, a transverse incision is made through the arcuate complex at the level of the tibial bone cut. Next, multiple stab incisions are made through the lateral structures like the iliotibial band [1, 6]. Attention should be paid to the peroneal nerve which might be in danger due to its location [7].

As a modification of this technique, Bellemans recently described the lengthening of the medial collateral ligament with a multiple needle puncturing technique in a moderate varus deformity using a 19-gauge needle. Until now this technique was not applicable for balancing the medial side due to the risk for iatrogenic transection of the medial collateral ligament. In order to avoid that and for better control of the release, the trial implants or laminar spreader is left in the joint

space to progressively stretch out the medial soft tissue sleeve. After doing so, multiple needle punctures into the tensioned fibers, while applying a continuous valgus stress, are performed. According to Bellemans technique, punctures are conducted every 3–5 mm in either direction (proximal/distal and anterior/posterior) [2].

The "tightest structure first" release balances the knee, by dissecting the tightest structure first. There is no strict sequence in performing this release. There is only one publication about this technique.

The authors of this article were using a balanced gap technique. The effect of each ligament release was investigated using a navigation system, while the knee was distracted with a tensor in extension and flexion. The authors concluded that in PCL-retaining TKA, a stepwise "tightest structure first" protocol for ligament releases in extension with the balanced gap technique results in an effective, gradual, alignment correction in extension, while femoral rotating effects in flexion were limited [12].

The ligament advancement procedures have been described by Krackow [19]. This method should be reserved for special indications on the medial and lateral side. Some reports show good results [3, 4].

7.5   Sagittal Plane Balancing in TKA

Total knee arthroplasty instrumentation systems differ greatly in sagittal plane balancing, either using an anterior or posterior referenced system. In an anterior referenced system, changes in femoral size will affect the flexion gap tightness. Therefore, femoral size selection is important to assure sagittal plane balance. In posterior referenced systems, femoral size changes do not affect the flexion gap but influence the width of the femoropatellar articulation space [21]. Most of the instrumentation systems today allow for shifting the cutting block in either direction to provide an optimized gap balancing. Using the Galileo® Navigation System, this computer-assisted shifting is possible in ½-mm steps.

Clinically a properly balanced PCL is of great importance in PCL-retaining TKA. A too lax PCL has the risk of AP – instability which can result in pain, effusion, impaired function of the extensor mechanism, and last but not least in enhanced PE wear. A too tight PCL decreases the range of motion especially the flexion ability, increases the pressure on the dorsal aspect of the PE insert which enhances PE wear, and can therefore affect implant fixation due to posterior loading [10, 26].

Two intraoperative tests of PCL tension, the *pullout lift-off* (POLO) for fixed bearings and *slide-back* for mobile bearings have been reported [26].

Pullout test: If a curved or dished stemless tray can be pulled out in 90° flexion of the knee, PCL tension and flexion stability are too lax, and the tibial polyethylene thickness should be replaced by a higher one.

Lift-off test: After the pullout test, the extensor mechanism is reduced to its anatomical position. An everted extensor mechanism may produce a false-positive lift-off test. The knee is flexed between 90° and 100°. If the trial component lifts off the anterior tibial surface, the PCL is too tight. Lift-off occurs because the tight PCL pulls the femoral component posteriorly against the posterior upslope of the PE tray. When the lift-off test is positive, a selective femoral release is necessary leaving the trials in place. The effect on lift-off can be observed as the release progresses.

Slide-back test: A trial insert is placed between the femoral and tibial components without the stabilizing post that confines its mobility in rotating platform designs. The knee is flexed 90°, and one notes the anterior-posterior position of the insert on the tray. If the PCL is too tight, the insert will slide posteriorly on the tray. If it is too loose, the insert will slide forward over the front of the tray. In a well-balanced PCL, the insert should be located 1 to 3 mm posterior to the front of the tibial tray.

Christen et al. examined the relationship between the size of the flexion gap and the anterior translation of the tibia in flexion. For implantation of a posterior cruciate ligament (PCL)-retaining TKA, they used a double spring compartment-specific, quantitative, force-controlled ligament tensioner (BalanSys). The tension force used was lying between 100 and 200 N. They showed that each increase of 1 mm in the flexion gap in the tensed knee resulted in a mean anterior tibial translation of 1.25 mm. An additional thickness of polyethylene insert of 2 mm results thereafter in an approximate increase in tibial anterior translation of 2.5 mm [5].

An important question is where the ideal femoral and tibial contact point should be. In a recent paper, the medial contact point in the natural knee in 90° of flexion was determined to be at 68 % (±6.6 %) of the AP diameter of the tibia measured below the tibia-plateau simulating a bone resection in TKR [8]. According to this paper flexion gap balancing has narrow margins. The question of whether the surgeon should aim for a little too tight or a little too loose flexion gap is difficult to answer. If it is too tight the contact point is shifted dorsally creating higher pressure levels on the polyethylene and the dorsal aspect of the tibial tray. Clinically this leads to decreased ROM and pain. On the other hand, a knee that has a loose flexion gap results in a more anterior contact point on the tibia. Thereafter, the lever arm of the patella will be decreased, and some AP instability may occur, thus creating potentially higher shearing forces which could lead to an enhanced PE wear. Heesterbeek et al. prefer a slightly looser flexion gap in order to balance the knee [10].

Conclusion

Soft tissue management in posterior cruciate-retaining TKA is a complex issue. It includes soft tissue release, component alignment in the frontal and sagittal plane, femoral component rotation, correct bony resection, and synchronization of the flexion and extension gap in terms of their width. The timing of soft tissue releases is strongly dependent on the way in which the TKA is performed. Using the measured resection technique, soft tissue releases are performed at the end, whereas using the gap technique they are done at the beginning of the surgical procedure. With the application of NAV/CAS systems, soft tissue releases and other important factors for gap balancing are integrated into the implantation procedure. The visualization of different balancing factors at the same time on the screen helps the surgeon to balance the gaps in an optimal way.

Soft tissue quality depends on a variety of individual factors such as age, gender, weight, activity level, and genetic factors, and therefore, its management must also be equally individualized. Recent papers show that there is a great interpatient variability considering soft tissue stiffness. One way to address these individual parameters is the intraoperative registration of different factors by computer models. Navigation has introduced the integration of registered data into surgery. We truly believe that through this integration we are able to balance the knee more individually than conventional surgery would do. Further research needs to be done to prove that. Meanwhile, the industry is asked to design more intelligent instrumentation systems to address these patient-specific factors to obtain a truly individual TKA in the future.

References

1. Aglietti P, Lup D, Cuomo P et al (2007) Total knee arthroplasty using a pie-crusting technique for valgus deformity. Clin Orthop Relat Res 464:73–77
2. Bellemans J, Vandenneucker H, Van Lauwe J et al (2010) A new surgical technique for medial collateral ligament balancing: multiple needle puncturing. J Arthroplasty 25(7):1151–1156
3. Brilhault J, Lautman S, Favard L et al (2002) Lateral femoral sliding osteotomy lateral release in total knee arthroplasty for a fixed valgus deformity. J Bone Joint Surg Br 84(8):1131–1137
4. Buechel FF (1990) A sequential three-step lateral release for correcting fixed valgus knee deformities during total knee arthroplasty. Clin Orthop Relat Res 260:170–175
5. Christen B, Heesterbeek PJ, Wymenga AB et al (2007) Posterior cruciate ligament balancing in total knee replacement: the quantitative relationship between tightness of the flexion gap and tibial translation. J Bone Joint Surg Br 89(8):1046–1050
6. Clarke HD, Fuchs R, Scuderi GR et al (2005) Clinical results in valgus total knee arthroplasty with the "pie crust" technique of lateral soft tissue releases. J Arthroplasty 20(8):1010–1014
7. Clarke HD, Schwartz JB, Math KR et al (2004) Anatomic risk of peroneal nerve injury with the "pie crust" technique for valgus release in total knee arthroplasty. J Arthroplasty 19:40
8. De Jong RJ, Heesterbeek PJ, Wymenga AB (2010) A new measurement technique for the tibiofemoral contact point in normal knees and knees with TKR. Knee Surg Sports Traumatol Arthrosc 18(3):388–393
9. Dennis DA, Komistek RD, Kim RH et al (2010) Gap balancing versus measured resection technique for total knee arthroplasty. Clin Orthop Relat Res 468(1):102–107
10. Heesterbeek PJ (2011) Mind the gaps: clinical and technical aspects of PCL-retaining total knee replacement with the balanced gap technique. Acta Orthop Suppl 82(344):1–26
11. Heesterbeek PJ, Jacobs W, Wymenga AB (2009) Effects of the balanced gap technique on femoral component rotation in TKA. Clin Orthop Relat Res 467(4):1015–1022
12. Heesterbeek PJ, Wymenga AB (2010) Correction of axial and rotational alignment after medial and lateral releases during balanced gap TKA. A clinical study of 54 patients. Acta Orthop 81(3):347–353
13. Hungerford DS, Kenna RV, Krackow KA (1982) The porous-coated anatomic total knee. Orthop Clin North Am 13(1):103–122
14. Insall JN, Binazzi R, Soudry M, Mestriner LA (1985) Total knee arthroplasty. Clin Orthop Relat Res 192:13–22
15. Insall J, Ranawat CS, Scott WN, Walker P (1976) Total condylar knee replacement: preliminary report. Clin Orthop Relat Res 2001;388:3–6
16. Insall JN et al (1993) The gap technique (S. 742). In: Insall JN (ed) Surgery of the knee, 2nd edn. Churchill Livingstone, New York
17. Insall JN et al (1993) Ligament releases (S. 779–789). In: Insall JN (ed) Surgery of the knee, 2nd edn. Churchill Livingstone, New York
18. Jenny JY, Boeri C (2004) Low reproducibility of the intra-operative measurement of the transepicondylar axis during total knee replacement. Acta Orthop Scand 75(1):74–77
19. Krackow KA (1990) Deformity. In: Krackow KA (ed) The technique of total knee arthroplasty. CV Mosby, Baltimore, pp 249–372
20. Krackow KA, Mihalko WM (1999) The effect of medial release on flexion and extension gaps in cadaveric knees: implications for soft-tissue balancing in total knee arthroplasty. Am J Knee Surg 12(4):222–228
21. Manson TT, Khanuja HS, Jacobs MA et al (2009) Sagittal plane balancing in the total knee arthroplasty. J Surg Orthop Adv 18(2):83–92
22. Mayman D, Plaskos C, Kendoff D et al (2009) Ligament tension in the ACL-deficient knee: assessment of medial and lateral gaps. Clin Orthop Relat Res 467(6):1621–1628
23. MihalkoWM SKJ, Krackow KA et al (2009) Soft-tissue balancing during total knee arthroplasty in the varus knee. J Am Acad Orthop Surg 17(12):766–774
24. Pak LC, Kuang YY, Seng JY et al (2005) Randomized controlled trial comparing radiographic total knee arthroplasty implant placement using computer naviga-

tion versus conventional technique. J Arthroplasty 20(5): 618–626

25. Sabbioni G, Rani N, Del Piccolo N et al (2011) Gap balancing versus measured resection technique using a mobile-bearing prosthesis in computer-assisted surgery. Musculoskelet Surg 95(1):25–30

26. Scott RD, Chmell MJ (2008) Balancing the posterior cruciate ligament during cruciate-retaining fixed and mobile-bearing total knee arthroplasty: description of the pull-out lift-off and slide-back tests. J Arthroplasty 23(4):605–608

27. Tria AJ Jr (2004) Management of fixed deformities in total knee arthroplasty. J Long Term Eff Med Implants 14(1):33–50

28. Tsukeoka T, Lee TH (2011) Sagittal flexion of the femoral component affects flexion gap and sizing in total knee arthroplasty. J Arthroplasty 27(6): 1094–1099

29. Whiteside LA (1999) Selective ligament release in total knee arthroplasty of the knee in valgus. Clin Orthop Relat Res (367):130–140

30. Whiteside LA (2002) Soft tissue balancing: the knee. J Arthroplasty 17(Suppl):23–27

31. Wyss T, Schuster AJ, Christen B et al (2008) Tension controlled ligament balanced total knee arthroplasty: 5-year results of a soft tissue orientated surgical technique. Arch Orthop Trauma Surg 128(2): 129–135

Soft Tissue Management in Computer-Assisted Cruciate-Retaining Total Knee Replacement

8

Petra J.C. Heesterbeek and Ate B. Wymenga

8.1 Introduction

Many authors state that computer-assisted surgery has, besides precise implant positioning during total knee replacement (TKR), the potential to evaluate soft tissue management. It has been thought that a TKR procedure with a ligament-guided approach might benefit more from the use of navigation than bone-referenced techniques [12]. The balanced gap technique, or the classic alignment method, was introduced by Insall and Freeman in the 1970s [9] and originated with those surgeons aiming for functional replacement by resecting the PCL (posterior cruciate ligament) [16]. This technique also builds from a tibia cut perpendicular to the mechanical axis of the tibia. In extension, this approach is partly comparable to the measured resection technique; the thickness of the implant determines the amount of resected bone. However, the specific philosophy of the gap technique is that the ligaments are tensioned after the initial soft tissue correction. Thereafter, gap resection is performed [17]. During flexion, this technique differs the most from the measured resection, or bone-referenced technique: the soft tissues are tensioned with laminar spreaders or tensors and determine the rotation of the femoral component. Theoretically, this technique results in stable and balanced (i.e. rectangular) extension and flexion gaps.

At present, surgical instruments often include a tensor or spreader to distract the extension and flexion gaps. Insall introduced a prototype of the modern spreader in his publication in 1976 and described it in more detail in 1985 [8, 9]. At that time, Freeman also described a spreader [15]. The balanced gap technique used for all patients described in this chapter was the balanSys™ system (Mathys Ltd, Bettlach, Switzerland). The instrumentation for this system uses either conventional (manual) alignment references or computer navigation. Improving implant alignment was not the primary purpose for using navigation; rather, we used it as a measurement device to investigate the relative movements, positions, and alignment of femur and tibia, and the effects of soft tissue management.

With this specific balanced gap technique with only releases in extension and fully accepting the variable femur rotation in flexion, a number of issues came up:

1. What are the effects of collateral ligament releases on varus and valgus laxity after TKR?
2. What are the axial and rotational alignment changes after stepwise medial or lateral collateral ligament releases in balanced gap TKR?

P.J.C. Heesterbeek, Ph.D. (✉)
Department of Research,
Sint Maartenskliniek,
Nijmegen, The Netherlands
e-mail: p.heesterbeek@maartenskliniek.nl

A.B. Wymenga, M.D., Ph.D.
Department of Orthopedics, Sint Maartenskliniek,
Nijmegen, The Netherlands
e-mail: a.wymenga@maartenskliniek.nl

F. Catani, S. Zaffagnini (eds.), *Knee Surgery using Computer Assisted Surgery and Robotics*,
DOI 10.1007/978-3-642-31430-8_8, © ESSKA 2013

3. Is the postoperative patella position affected by the variation in femoral component rotation in balanced gap TKR?
4. What is the relation between the applied distraction force in flexion and change of the tibia and femur position relative to each other when the PCL is intact?

8.2   Methods

We analysed the data presented in this chapter from a prospective case series of 50 patients who received a cruciate-retaining total knee implanted with computer-assisted surgery. The navigation system was used for the intraoperative measurements. A special "research" mode was installed on the computer by the company and enabled us to record data for research purposes at certain stages during the TKR procedure. The results and study patients were reported earlier in more detail in various papers by Heesterbeek et al. [2, 4, 5, 7].

There are several possible approaches, but the surgical technique used in the studies of this series started with determination of the femur and tibia axis and determination of the joint surfaces of femur and tibia. After that, a proximal tibia cut 6–8 mm below the unworn compartment perpendicular to the mechanical axis, with a dorsal slope of 7°, was performed. After osteophyte removal, a bi-compartmental tensor was inserted into the knee in extension. Frontal alignment of the leg is controlled by ligament tension and checked on the computer screen.

Releases of the collateral ligaments were performed at this stage when necessary to achieve correctly frontal leg alignment. The tightest structures were released first, and releases were performed only in extension until the leg alignment was neutral (mechanical axis). No additional releases were performed in flexion thereafter. All releases performed were registered and catalogued into lateral releases or medial releases including either the posteromedial capsule (PMC) or the superficial medial collateral ligament

(SMCL) in order to study the effect on alignment and femoral rotation.

Subsequently, the tensor was inserted into the joint at 90° flexion to balance the PCL; 100 N was used in all patients. The femur rotated freely guided by the ligaments; if the medial side was looser, then the femur exorotated. In the other extreme, if the lateral side was looser, then the femur showed endorotation. Hence, the tension in the soft tissue structures determined the posterior femoral cut, and therefore, rotation of the femoral component could vary. Thereafter, the ventral and dorsal femoral cuts were performed parallel to the tibial resection. The aim was to cut approximately 9 mm of the posterior medial femur condyle, which is the implant thickness, and this was checked on the computer screen (Fig. 8.1).

In case the computer screen predicted a bone cut of the medial posterior condyle larger than the implant thickness, a recut of the tibia was considered. This could be simulated on the computer screen. The joint line of the femur in flexion on the medial side is restored with this technique. The amount of bone resection of the lateral side is variable with this technique.

For examining the effects of gap distraction on movement of the femur and tibia, the flexion gap was distracted with a double-spring tensor with 100 and 200 N after the tibia had been cut. Movements of the femur and tibia during gap distraction were recorded by the navigation system. The dynamics of the flexion gap were described by the change in gap height, anterior translation, medial-lateral displacement, and femoral rotation when the flexion gap was distracted. We hypothesized that flexion gap dynamics might be different for knees with a steep or a flat PCL, and therefore, we additionally digitized the insertion points of the PCL during the anatomic landmark definition stage of the surgical protocol. PCL elevation was calculated as the angle between the digitized PCL (line between insertion points on femur and tibia) and the transverse plane of the tibia.

Next, the distal femoral cut was performed parallel to the tibia cut with 150-N distraction. The amount of bone resection could vary a few

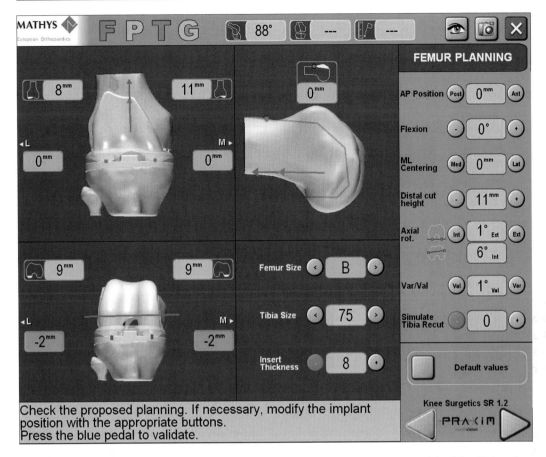

Fig. 8.1 Screenshot where the distal cut is larger (11 mm) than the implant thickness, a recut of the tibia with less slope could solve this problem

millimetres and so could the joint line in extension on the femur. The tibia rotation was set at 1/3 of the tuberosity, and patellar tracking was checked. No resurfacing of the patella was done in this series.

After implantation, the varus and valgus laxity in extension and flexion was measured with the navigation system using a spring-loaded device with application of 15-Nm force moment. Postoperative varus–valgus laxity was determined at 6 months after surgery by stress radiographs. For varus–valgus laxity in extension, the Telos device (Fa Telos, Medizinisch-Technische GmbH, Griesheim, Germany) was used; for varus-valgus laxity in flexion, we used the Flexilax, a custom-made stress device. The same amount of stress (15 Nm) was applied as during

the intraoperative measurements. The 3D motion captured by the navigation system from all measurements during surgery was extracted from the system. With a custom-written MATLAB program, all desired parameters were calculated from the recorded navigation data.

For all patients, patellar (skyline) radiographs were performed preoperatively and at the 2-year follow-up. Patellar tilt and displacement were measured using the Lateral Patellar Tilt and the Patellar Displacement measurement techniques, with 10° and 4 mm as cutoff points for tilt and displacement, respectively [3]. A logistic regression analysis was performed on femoral component rotation and preoperative patella position to identify predictors for postoperative patellar tilt and displacement.

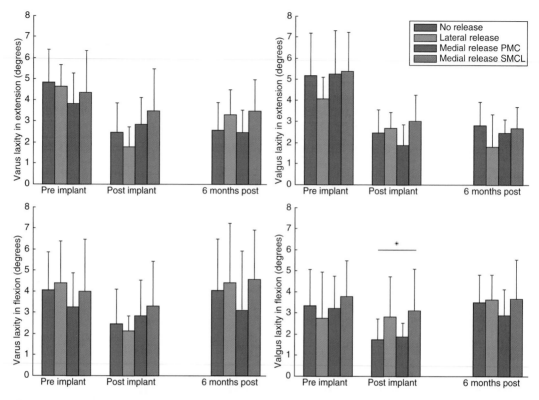

Fig. 8.2 Mean varus and valgus laxity in extension and flexion by release group (This figure has been adapted from earlier work of the authors [5])

8.3 Results

8.3.1 What Are the Effects of Ligament Releases on Varus and Valgus Laxity After TKR?

At surgery, before and after implantation of the prosthesis, there was no difference in varus or valgus laxity in extension and flexion between knees that did not need a ligament release, knees with a lateral release, knees with medial SMCL releases, and knees with medial PMC releases (Fig. 8.2). At 6 months after surgery, varus or valgus laxity in extension and flexion was not significantly different between the release categories. In other words, perioperative releases of the collateral ligaments did not result in increased varus or valgus laxity.

8.3.2 What Are the Axial and Rotational Alignment Changes After Stepwise Medial or Lateral Releases in Balanced Gap TKR?

In more than half of the patients, one or more releases were necessary. There was no significant difference in the alignment-correcting effect of a release depending upon the sequence in which this structure was released (Fig. 8.3a–d). Of all the releases that were performed, the effects were the greatest for the extension gap. When the posteromedial condyle was released, this led to a minor effect on leg axis in extension and on femoral rotation in flexion. Release of the superficial medial collateral ligament corrected the leg axis in extension a few degrees and had a small effect on femoral rotation in flexion. On the lateral side, release of the iliotibial tract led to a small

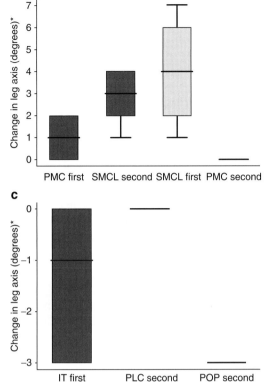

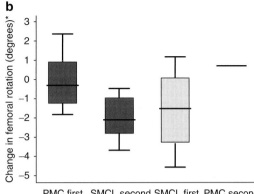

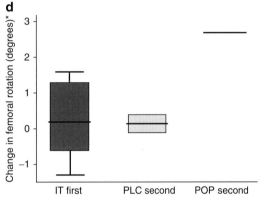

Fig. 8.3 (**a**) Box plot of change in leg axis after PMC release (*n*=15) and subsequent SMCL release (*n*=9) and after SMCL release (*n*=4) and subsequent PMC release (*n*=1). (**b**) Box plot of change in femur rotation after PMC release (*n*=15) and subsequent SMCL release (*n*=9) and after SMCL release (*n*=4) and subsequent PMC release (*n*=1). (**c**)Box plot of change in leg axis after IT release (*n*=7) and subsequent PLC release (*n*=2) or POP release (*n*=1).(**d**) Box plot of change in leg femur rotation after IT release (*n*=7) and subsequent PLC release (*n*=2) or POP release (*n*=1) (This figure has been adapted from earlier work of the authors [7]) *negative values indicate exorotation

correction of leg alignment in extension. The "tightest structure first" approach worked with the balance gap technique: all patients achieved neutral leg alignment, and the effects on femoral rotation remained limited.

8.3.3 Is the Patella Position Affected by the Variation in Femoral Component Rotation in Balanced Gap TKR?

Although femoral component rotation varied from 3° endorotation to 12° exorotation (Fig. 8.4),

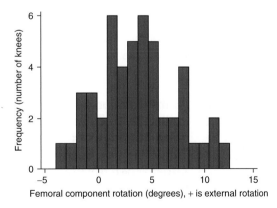

Fig. 8.4 Histogram presenting the variation in femoral component rotation. Femoral component rotation is calculated using the posterior condyles as reference

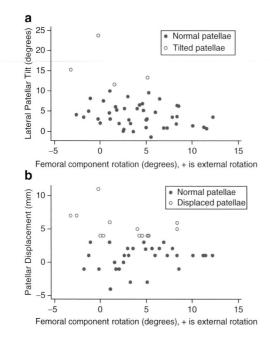

Fig. 8.5 (**a**) Lateral Patellar Tilt versus femoral component rotation (*n* = 46). Femoral component rotation is referenced to the posterior condyles (This figure has been
adapted from earlier work of the authors [6]). (**b**) Patellar
Displacement versus femoral component rotation (*n* = 46).
Femoral component rotation is referenced to the posterior
condyles (This figure has been adapted from earlier work
by the authors [6])

we could not statistically relate it to postoperative
tilt or displacement. The only statistically
significant predictor found was preoperative
patellar displacement; a preoperatively displaced
patella led in 50 % of the cases to a postoperatively displaced patella (Fig. 8.5).

8.3.4 What Is the Relation Between the Applied Distraction Force in Flexion and Change of the Tibia and Femur Position Relative to Each Other When the PCL Is Intact?

During flexion gap distraction, the greatest displacement was seen in the anterior-posterior
direction. The least amount of movement was
seen in the medial-lateral direction, and rotation of the femur remained limited. Mean ratio

between gap height increase and tibial translation was 1–1.9. PCL elevation angle significantly
affected the ratio between gap height increase
and anterior tibial translation; in knees with a
steep PCL, AP translation increased more for
each mm of increase in gap height (gap/AP
ratio was 1:2.3 [SD 0.63]) compared to knees
with a flat PCL (gap/AP ratio was 1:1.7 [SD
0.50]) (Fig. 8.6).

There was no significant difference in mean
ratio of gap height increase and anterior tibial
translation between knees with a collateral ligament release and knees without, although knees
with a release had a greater increase in PCL elevation as the distracting force increased from 100 to
200 N. When the flexion gap is distracted with a
bi-compartmental tensor, every extra mm that the
flexion gap is distracted can be expected to move
the tibia anteriorly by at least 1.7 mm (flat PCL)
or even more if the PCL is oriented steeply relative to the transverse plane of the tibia (Fig. 8.7).

8.4 Discussion

8.4.1 Collateral Ligament Releases and Varus–Valgus Laxity

In contrast to what was expected, collateral ligament releases made during surgery did not lead
to increased varus-valgus laxity. It had been
hypothesized that releases of the MCL, an
important medial stabilizer, would lead to
increased valgus laxity if stress was applied, but
this effect was not confirmed. Two possible
mechanisms to elucidate this discrepancy can be
suggested. Firstly, it is possible that distraction
and recruitment of the (remaining) peripheral
soft tissue envelope results in sufficient stability.
A second possible mechanism may be that after
a medial release, the central structure, the PCL,
prevents laxity along with a lateral compartment
that is completely filled and has been tensioned
with an implant.

Because of the in vivo nature of the study
setup, we could not detect whether released ligaments reattach to the bone. It is possible that after
a release in extension, ligament insertions shift

a

b

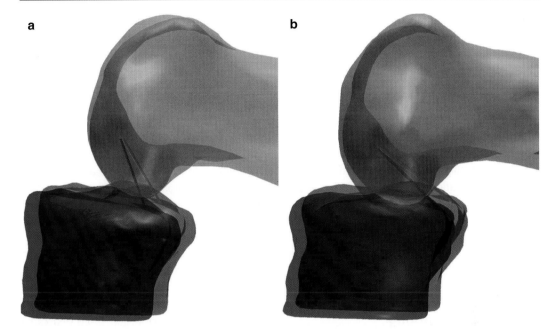

Fig. 8.6 3D illustration of two knees in sagittal view (no fibula). The situation with 100 N of tension is shown in *red* and that with 200 N is shown in *blue*. The amounts of gap height increase and anterior tibial translation are vis-ible and different for the knee with a steep PCL (**a**) and the knee with a flat PCL (**b**). Note the increase in PCL eleva-tion after 200 N has been applied (*blue* PCL) (This figure has been adapted from earlier work by the authors [4])

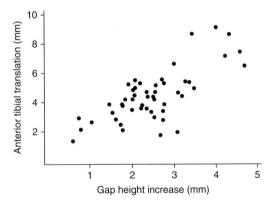

Fig. 8.7 Scatter plot of change in gap height versus change in anterior tibial translation

due to the distracting force during flexion. It may, however, not be important since the knees were stable immediately after surgery. It should be noted that extensive lateral releases including complete detachments of the lateral collateral ligament and popliteal tendon were not analysed in this study; in such cases, the results could be different. Although it remains, to a certain extent, a black box mechanism, the balanced gap

approach can be safely used, and those collateral ligament releases needed to align the leg in exten-sion will not lead to an increase in varus–valgus laxity.

8.4.2 Axial and Rotation Alignment Changes After Stepwise Medial or Lateral Releases

Interestingly, the collateral ligament releases per-formed in extension for alignment correction did not lead to great effects on femoral rotation in flexion which contradicts the findings in the lit-erature [10, 11, 13, 14]. Apparently, in flexion, gap distraction causes recruitment of all the sur-rounding soft tissue structures, and the effect of one released collateral ligament on femoral rota-tion remains small. Also, the PCL as the central structure holds the flexion gap together. Whereas in a cadaver study a single release would lead to much more laxity, it is plausible that in a clinical situation other structures comprising the soft tissue envelope in combination with the tendons, muscles, and skin ensures stability.

The method of releasing the tightest structure first, described, is actually a patient-specific approach in which the surgeon only releases the tightest structure at that moment and receives immediate feedback through the screen of the navigation system. In this case series, this stepwise technique has been applied and shown to work in combination with the balanced gap technique; we are confident that the effects found are not limited to the balanced gap technique but can also be applied during a measured resection technique. Probably the PCL, the secondary medial stabilizer, being intact during surgery is the important prerequisite.

8.4.3 Patellar Tracking

Using radiographic measurements, femoral component rotation as a predictor for patellar malposition after balanced gap TKR was investigated. This was not found to be the case; femoral component rotation was not a predictor for either patellar tilt or patellar displacement. Only preoperative patella position was identified as a risk factor for postoperative patellar displacement, although the confidence interval was broad.

The most intriguing finding was that femoral component rotation has much less effect on patella position than has commonly been suggested in the literature. Could this be the effect of the balanced gap technique or do other mechanisms play a role? With a measured resection technique, in theory, one would expect more knees with a certain amount of flexion laxity. Knees that are laterally loose in flexion would show a lift off of the lateral condyle in flexion and thereby endorotate the femur component in relation to the tibia. Theoretically, this could cause more patella subluxation, although in daily practice this mechanism has not actually been observed as a clinical phenomenon.

Probably a better explanation, as Berger reported [1], is that both femoral and tibial component rotations play a role. Only the combination of an endorotated tibial component with an endorotated femoral component can be detrimental for patellar tracking. In most cases, an endorotated femoral component alone, as we have found, is not enough to produce problems. Furthermore, the three degrees of maximum endorotation as found in the present work is probably not enough to produce patella problems as has been suggested in various experimental studies conducted on this topic. Therefore, we feel that the surgical technique is safe with respect to patellar tracking, certainly for PCL-retaining implants and if careful attention is given with regard to the tibial component rotation.

8.4.4 PCL Balancing

Our intraoperative measurements have shown that balancing the flexion gap is an extremely delicate technique; a few millimetres more or less gap distraction can make a difference and that directly influences gap balancing. This is much more critical than we had anticipated before this study. In addition to gap distraction, variation in PCL elevation angle also has been shown to play a role in PCL balancing. With the bi-compartmental tensor, a highly variable ratio up to 1–2.3 was found. Hence, a 2-mm change in bone cut or PE-insert thickness can change the tibiofemoral contact point 4 mm and make a difference between a perfectly balanced PCL and one that has been too tightly balanced. It is clear that balancing is difficult due to the great inter-patient variation in gap height increase and anterior tibial translation. For a PCL-retaining TKR, the question remains as to how one should balance the PCL. Although thus far, we have not yet found an optimal force with which to distract the gap; by using the navigation system, we have gained more insight into the dynamic character of the flexion gap.

8.4.5 Future Perspectives

Although a number of questions were answered in the above studies, many new questions came up. The optimal force for distracting the knee during TKR is not clearly defined and should be investigated further. Our impression is that the used forces of 150 N in extension and 100 N in flexion could be lower, but the appropriateness should be confirmed in clinical studies. Midflexion laxity of the normal natural knee should be defined better and midflexion laxity should be analysed further in TKR procedures. Computer-assisted surgery techniques can be used to register this laxity and help with a correct implant position in order to create the required laxity. New techniques such as the measurement of intraoperative stress–strain curves of the soft tissue around the knee could help to determine an individualized ideal distraction force. As for PCL balancing, computer-assisted surgery can help to distract the knee and create such gaps that the correct tibiofemoral contact point for the individual patient can be created, and new software should be developed for this. Patellar tracking during TKR can be measured more accurately with computer-assisted systems with trackers on the patella, and also the alignment of the femur component with the trochlear groove can be included in these systems in order to control all relevant geometrical implant positions in detail and restore the joint surfaces. Ideally, the surgeon should be guided by a navigated technique towards a replaced knee with correct femur, tibia and patella implant positions; a patient-individualized ligament tension for joint distraction; a clear-defined laxity in extension, midflexion and flexion, a correct tibiofemoral contact point of the medial femur condyle with a balanced PCL; and a correct patellar tracking.

Conclusion

A navigation system is perfectly suited as an intraoperative measurement tool for studying soft tissue effects during a TKR. It is accurate, not extra time-consuming, and gives a lot of 3D data that provide additional insight into the knee. With this project, we showed that varus–valgus laxity is not increased by ligament releases and laxity in extension. Collateral ligament releases needed to align the leg in extension can be performed with a gradual effect using the "tightest structure first" approach, and the effect on axial alignment and femoral rotation is limited. The balanced gap technique leads to a relatively broad range of femoral component rotation. This variable femoral component rotation does not predict postoperative patellar malposition, whereas a preoperatively existing patellar malposition was identified as a risk factor. PCL balancing by flexion gap distraction has definitive consequences for the relative tibiofemoral position, and it is dependent on the PCL elevation angle. The balanced gap TKR implantation technique is a safe and effective approach to create a stable TKR in flexion and extension and correct patella position after surgery.

References

1. Berger RA, Crossett LS, Jacobs JJ et al (1998) Malrotation causing patellofemoral complications after total knee arthroplasty. Clin Orthop Relat Res 356: 144–153
2. Heesterbeek P (2011) Mind the gaps! Clinical and technical aspects of PCL-retaining total knee replacement with the balanced gap technique: an academic essay in Medical Science. Acta Orthop Suppl 82:1–26
3. Heesterbeek PJC, Beumers MPC, Jacobs WCH et al (2007) A comparison of reproducibility of measurement techniques for patella position on axial radiographs after total knee arthroplasty. Knee 14:411–416
4. Heesterbeek P, Keijsers N, Jacobs W et al (2010) Posterior cruciate ligament recruitment affects anteroposterior translation during flexion gap distraction in total knee replacement. An intraoperative study involving 50 patients. Acta Orthop 81:471–477
5. Heesterbeek PJ, Keijsers NL, Wymenga AB (2010) Ligament releases do not lead to increased postoperative varus-valgus laxity in flexion and extension: a prospective clinical study in 49 TKR patients. Knee Surg Sports Traumatol Arthrosc 18:187–193
6. Heesterbeek PJ, Keijsers NL, Wymenga AB (2011) Femoral component rotation after balanced gap total knee replacement is not a predictor for postoperative patella position. Knee Surg Sports Traumatol Arthrosc 19:1131–1136
7. Heesterbeek PJ, Wymenga AB (2010) Correction of axial and rotational alignment after medial and lateral releases during balanced gap TKA. A clinical study of 54 patients. Acta Orthop 81:347–353
8. Insall JN, Binazzi R, Soudry M et al (1985) Total knee arthroplasty. Clin Orthop Relat Res 192:13–22

9. Insall J, Ranawat CS, Scott WN et al (1976) Total condylar knee replacement: preliminary report. Clin Orthop Relat Res 120:149–154

10. Krackow KA, Mihalko WM (1999) The effect of medial release on flexion and extension gaps in cadaveric knees: implications for soft-tissue balancing in total knee arthroplasty. Am J Knee Surg 12:222–228

11. Krackow KA, Mihalko WM (1999) Flexion-extension joint gap changes after lateral structure release for valgus deformity correction in total knee arthroplasty: a cadaveric study. J Arthroplasty 14:994–1004

12. Lehnen K, Giesinger K, Warschkow R et al (2011) Clinical outcome using a ligament referencing technique in CAS versus conventional technique. Knee Surg Sports Traumatol Arthrosc 19:887–892

13. Matsueda M, Gengerke TR, Murphy M et al (1999) Soft tissue release in total knee arthroplasty. Cadaver study using knees without deformities. Clin Orthop Relat Res 366:264–273

14. Mihalko WM, Whiteside LA, Krackow KA (2003) Comparison of ligament-balancing techniques during total knee arthroplasty. J Bone Joint Surg Am 85-A(Suppl 4):132–135

15. Moreland JR, Thomas RJ, Freeman MA (1979) ICLH replacement of the knee: 1977 and 1978. Clin Orthop Relat Res 145:47–59

16. Robinson RP (2005) The early innovators of today's resurfacing condylar knees. J Arthroplasty 20:2–26

17. Vail TP, Lang LE (2006) Surgical techniques and instrumentation in total knee arthroplasty. In: Insall JN, Scott WN, editors. Surgery of the knee. vol 4. Churchill Livingstone Elsevier, Philidelphia, pp 1455–1521

UKA: Standard

9

Fabio Catani, Vitantonio Digennaro,
Gianluca Grandi, and Andrea Marcovigi

9.1 Introduction

Unicompartmental knee arthroplasty (UKA) has encountered a growing interest of the orthopedic community since its introduction in the first years of 1970s (UKA). The long-term outcome of UKA depends on patient selection, age, gender, and level of activity [18, 22, 25]. Despite satisfying clinical and radiological outcomes of UKAs procedures [26, 47, 48], many cases with need for further intervention were also reported [38]. Polyethylene implant failure [2, 29, 39], deterioration of the lateral compartment within a few years following the UKA, pain in the contralateral or patellofemoral compartment [5], and aseptic loosening [31] could affect implant survival.

Further surgical treatment options such as total knee arthroplasty, high tibial osteotomy, arthroscopy with debridement or chondroplasty or microfracturing, and interpositional arthroplasty [41] could be performed for medial compartment arthritis; for this reason, the ideal indication for UKA is still a debated topic [3]. Inadequate implantation is overall recognized as

the main factor for early failure [6, 11]. Thus, it is generally agreed that accuracy of implant positioning and reconstruction of the mechanical lower limb are major requirements for achieving good long-term results in UKA. Unlike total knee arthroplasty (TKA), where there is a general agreement on the positioning of the components, there are different opinions regarding the ideal component positioning of the UKA prosthesis and lower limb mechanical axis [9, 23, 25, 37].

However, regardless of the UKA instrumentation system, it is generally agreed that instrumentation should allow the surgeon to place the prosthesis in the position they decide. Most UKA systems offer limited and potentially inaccurate instrumentation and substantially rely on surgeon's judgment regarding prosthesis placement, and inaccurate implantation rates of about 30 % have been reported for such instrumentation [23, 49]. Moreover, introduction of minimally invasive surgery (MIS) has necessitated to adapt the instruments with the limited space available. It has been suggested that minimally invasive UKA is not as accurate as open UKA in terms of component alignment or postoperative limb alignment, although minimally invasive surgery (MIS) has improved clinical results by reducing operative trauma and increasing the speed of recovery.

Image-free computer navigation systems have been developed to improve reproducible accurate implant positioning and precise reconstruction of the mechanical leg axis, regardless of preoperative deformity, and it was widely applied in total knee replacement [14, 16, 46]. The surgeon could

F. Catani (✉) • V. Digennaro • G. Grandi • A. Marcovigi
Department of Orthopedics and Traumatology,
Modena University Hospital, University of Modena and
Reggio Emilia, Via del Pozzo 71, Modena 41125, Italy
e-mail: fabio.catani@unimore.it;
digennaro_1977@libero.it; piedecavo@hotmail.com;
dott.marcovigi@gmail.com

F. Catani, S. Zaffagnini (eds.), *Knee Surgery using Computer Assisted Surgery and Robotics*,
DOI 10.1007/978-3-642-31430-8_9, © ESSKA 2013

verify real-time measurements for the femoral and tibial cuts with functional axes and kinematics analysis during surgery. Because less invasive exposure needs a graphic visualization support [21, 36] of the surgical site, the use of these systems has been increasingly recommended during the last years also in UKA [20, 23]. Some authors hypothesized that the navigation system would produce better and more reproducing results with respect to prosthetic position and mechanical lower limb alignment in UKA than the conventional instrumented technique [24].

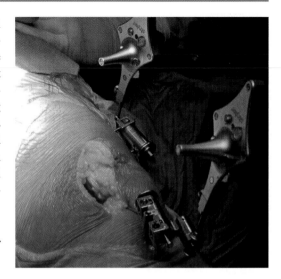

Fig. 9.1 Positioning of the femoral and tibial trackers

9.2 Indications

Several studies claim that an accurate patient selection is essential to reduce perioperative complications and to achieve optimal long-term results. Although the evolution in materials and techniques determines a nonstop revision of the ideal parameters, the indications that could be found in the literature are quite uniform, especially for some key factors [15, 36]. Increasing numbers of UKAs are being performed throughout the world, with some centers claiming that approximately 30 % of their patients are candidates for this procedure.

Indications

- Unicompartmental osteoarthritis of the knee non-involving the other compartments. Especially in older patients, a contralateral or patellofemoral low-grade degeneration (<I–II grade in Ahlbäck classification) could be tolerated if asymptomatic.
- Avascular necrosis of the femoral condyle.
- Range of movement > 100°, with a flexion contracture <10°. Some authors state that the indication could be extended to higher deformities as long as their cause could be removed during the intervention (e.g., osteophytosis).
- Mechanical axis deviation included between 15° valgus and 10° varus. The deformity must be *correctable*.
- *Cartier's angle* < 5°. *Cartier's angle* is the angle subtended between tibial joint line and tibial mechanical axis measured on an A/P radiography [10].
- Absence of anterior laxity.

- *Integrity of ACL.* A major theoretical concern in ACL-deficient knee undergoing UKR is the increased anterior translation of the tibia which may lead to premature polyethylene wear.
- *Age > 60* patients with low activity level.
- *Age > 50* patients in order to delay total knee replacement.
- *Weight.* Not yet defined.

Contraindications

- Obesity with a severe varus deformity
- Osteoporosis
- Inflammatory or autoimmune diseases (RA), even if only the knee is to be operated
- Severe combined laxity
- Not crystalline disease

9.3 Surgical Technique

The navigation system generally used was a CT-free, wireless computer navigation system with trackers fixed to the femur and tibia; the system did not require the use of an IM rod.

At the beginning of surgery, navigation trackers were rigidly fixed through two pins on the medial side of the distal femur and proximal tibia, just below the anterior tuberosity (Fig. 9.1). The location of the hip joint center was identified as the average center of a large and three-planar femur-

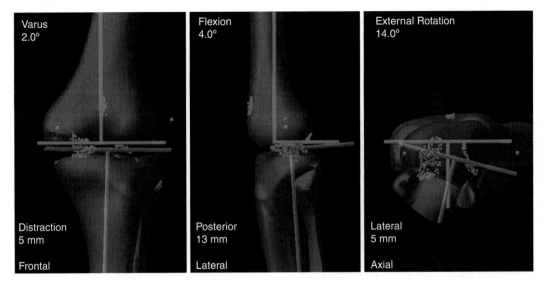

Fig. 9.2 Visualization of knee deformity on the navigation system screen before surgery

to-pelvis rotation. The standard anatomical survey with the navigation system, which entailed calibration of anatomical landmarks and axes by using an instrumented pointer, was then performed. This procedure also defined the anatomical reference frames for the femur and tibia, which provided target orientations for all relevant bone cuts.

Lower limb alignment, motion and ligament stability are calculated before bone resections (Fig. 9.2).

A medial parapatellar skin incision is used, directly over the medial femoral condyle, from the superomedial corner of the patella to the superomedial corner of the tibial tubercle to access easily the femoral condyle and medial tibial plateau. A mid-vastus approach could be suggested to obtain an adequate articular exposition and patellar lateralizing without the quadriceps tendon suffering.

Initially, a careful dissection of the capsule and deep fiber of the medial collateral ligament should be released from the proximal tibia. In this early stage, medial meniscectomy is performed and medial peripheral osteophytes are removed, especially those that may tight the medial collateral ligament. Moreover, medial osteophytes of the intercondylar notch should be removed to avoid an impingement with tibial component.

With 30° flexed knee, the patellofemoral joint and lateral compartment could be evaluated.

With the knee extended, a valgus stress allows one to evaluate the amount of the varus correction, and in this position, a contact line between anterior tibial edge and distal femur could be signed.

For a better exposition the fat pad could be partially removed and a K-wire could be placed 5 mm over intercondylar notch.

A freehand technique is used to fix the cutting jigs to the bone.

9.3.1 Tibial Preparation

With 90–100° flexed knee, the modified tibial cutting guide with tibial tracker is placed by observing the navigation system monitor to obtain an appropriate resection depth (usually 6 mm) and slope of the tibial plateau, and it is fixed with two pins (Fig. 9.3). The tibial slope is usually set on original posterior slope. In case of partial ACL deficiency (e.g., older patients or lower level activity), tibial slope could be set at 0° to minimize AP translation. In frontal plane, the tibial cut should not correct the preoperative deformity, but to fill the space created by passive correction of the deformity. After tibial guide positioning, a sagittal tibial cut is performed using a reciprocating saw, aligning with AP tibial axis, and avoiding carefully to undermine tibial spines. A transversal cut is then performed with oscillating saw, protecting accurately the medial collateral ligament. After bone removal, the tibial resection is verified using the navigation system (Fig. 9.4). An 8-mm spacer is introduced, and flexion-extension kinematics and articular stability are evaluated. If a well-balanced correction during flexion-extension arc is gained, no further resections are required, otherwise 2-mm plus resection could be necessary. The tibial trial of appropriate size could be selected, using a template in order to cover adequately the tibial surface.

9.3.2 Femoral Preparation

After tibial bone resection, the femoral tracker is fitted into the slot of modified femoral guide, which is fixed with two pins when a proper femoral orientation is achieved. The distal femoral resection is usually performed in complete extension, taking the mechanical axis of the leg to be 0° (Fig. 9.5). If the deformity is easily correctable, the amount of bone cut should be inferior (4.5 mm); otherwise if the correction of deformity obtained passively is not adequate, the bone cut should be greater (6.5 mm). After distal femoral cutting, a femoral trial component is placed upon femoral condyle and mediolateral coverage is evaluated. A corresponding sized femoral finishing guide is fixed with two/three pins, and posterior condyle and chamfer are then cut. When bone resection is performed, a femoral

Fig. 9.3 Freehand tibial resection guided by navigation tracker

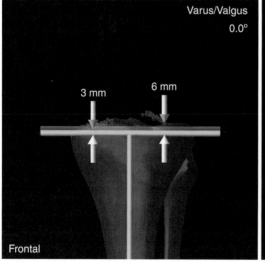
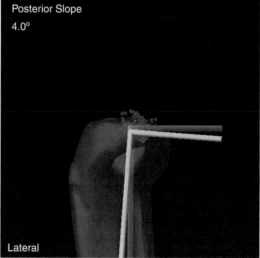

Fig. 9.4 Real-time checking of the amount of tibial bone resection

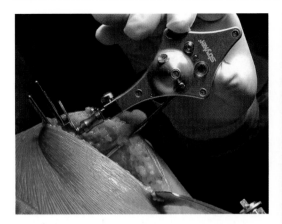

Fig. 9.5 Distal femur resection guided by navigation tracker

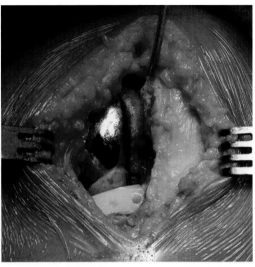

Fig. 9.6 Final implant

and tibial trial is inserted and kinematic patterns and articular stability are evaluated, following navigation system monitor.

Some instrumentations do not provide the traditional femoral distal and chamfer cut, and so it does not require the femoral alignment with navigation system. These afford to place a femoral component following kinematics patterns, tracking centrally on the tibial guide throughout the whole flexion-extension range.

9.3.3 Final Implant

Before the cementing, 2-mm holes in the sclerotic bones should be drilled in order to obtain an adequate cementing penetration. Pulsatile lavage allows one to remove residual bone, blood, and fat particles to maintain as clear as possible the trabecular bone.

The tibial component should be cemented first, putting a thin cement layer on the tibial surface and on the bottom of tibial component. When the tibial component is impacted, remove excess cement with an angulated instrument.

Usually, the femoral component is only cemented on the posterior surface (Fig. 9.6).

With the final components in place, lower limb mechanical axis and soft tissue balancing were evaluated following the navigation system (Fig. 9.7).

9.3.4 Advantages and Disadvantages

Unicompartmental knee arthroplasty permits one to intervene only on pathological tissue, sparing noninvolved compartments; this is particularly significant since analyzing a series of osteoarthritic knees, Brocklehurst et al. [8] found no significant difference in water content, glycosaminoglycan synthesis rates, and cell contents between intact cartilage in a osteoarthritic knee and cartilage from control joints, being instead quite different from the values of non-intact cartilage [8].

Being a bone-sparing procedure also lends UKA to easier revision procedures which can be often performed using primary TKA implants [7].

Other structures which are retained are the anterior and posterior cruciate ligaments; together they provide more physiological knee kinematics in respect to total knee replacement especially in medial compartment substitution, and they guarantee a significant improvement in proprioception [4], giving the patient the perception of a more natural knee.

Many studies also show that another great advantage of UKA is high range of motion (ROM) values, often higher than 120° [1, 28], reaching means above 130° such in the study by Lustig et al. who reported an average flexion of 133° on 144 all-polyethylene UKRs [30].

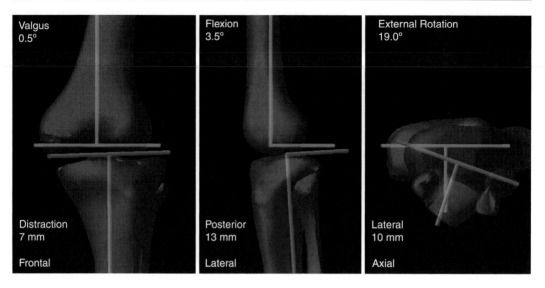

Fig. 9.7 Postoperative knee alignment is visualized on the navigation system screen

Another great advantage is low invasivity which leads to reduced blood loss, lower peri- and postoperative morbidity, and faster recovery time, further reduced by the introduction of minimally invasive techniques [34].

Reducing surgical approach produces a simultaneous increase of the technical difficulty of the intervention, already demanding because of the need for a correct soft tissue balancing [34].

The most important disadvantages bound to UKA have always been higher failure rate and earlier polyethylene wear if compared to TKA; in recent years, there have been many advances obtaining survival rates at 10 years higher than 90 %, e.g., 92 % with Miller-Galante arthroprosthesis [33], 95 % with Marmor arthroprosthesis [50], and even 97 % with Oxford arthroprosthesis [32], although it is important to remember that patient selection had a basic role in this progress, finding stricter indications but reducing the number of eligible patients.

Contralateral compartment osteoarthritis progression has often been indicated between the disadvantages of UKA, but this kind of complication is relatively rare and often related to an overload due to deformity overcorrection (Table 9.1).

Table 9.1 Main advantages and disadvantages of UKA

Advantages	Disadvantages
Bone sparing	Technically demanding
Cruciate retaining	Strict patient selection
Wider range of movement	Likely polyethylene wear
Better proprioception	Higher failure rate in respect to TKA
Physiological knee kinematics	Risk of contralateral osteoarthritis progression

9.4 Causes of Failure

The main causes of failure of a UKA may be classified in early and late, depending on the time of onset. Between the causes of early failure, infection is definitely the most formidable; however, infection rate is usually low (0.5–1 %) and generally lower than TKA. Other causes of early failure are pain, periprosthetic fractures, and components aseptic loosening (early cases are often caused by components' malpositioning). Aseptic loosening is also the main cause of late failure, while contralateral compartment osteoarthritis progression and polyethylene wear are less frequent [19].

Many of these elements can be related to technical errors, depending upon surgeon's ability and experience.

Frontal mechanical axis malalignment (often caused by an undercorrection or overcorrection of preoperative mechanical axis) may lead to an early progression of osteoarthritis in the contralateral compartment or to an abnormal stress over the tibial component, favoring polyethylene wear and aseptic loosening (Collier et al. have shown that for a medial UKR, the relative risk of revisions increases by 2 for every 8° of varus) [12].

Two values are very important in defining tibial component's alignment: posterior slope and Cartier's angle.

Posterior slope (P.S.) should be preserved equal to its anatomic value, although it would be recommended to avoid values over 7° since they determine an excessive increase of stress over the tibial component; even more attention must be kept in case of a damaged ACL since the joint lacks its stabilizing action [27].

Also, a component malalignment on the frontal plane may cause an increase in the risk of aseptic loosening; this fatigue failure is a result of excessive compressive stresses occurring at the bone-implant interface. Generally, the yielding area (%) increases as the position of the tibial component is rotated from valgus to varus. In the range from 6° valgus to 2° varus, the area increases by 15.4 %. Increasing the varus angle from 2° to 6° results in a substantial increase of 61.8 % [40].

All the factors that increase stress level over the tibial component may cause polyethylene wear, but, especially in the past years, these complications were related to intrinsic weaknesses such as the high amount of reactive oxygen species produced during gamma sterilization in air or the use of bearings of inadequate thickness (often lesser than 6 mm).

Aseptic loosening is supported by many factors, but they all generate the same reaction: a thin layer of fibrous tissue covering the bone whose presence generates implant micro-movements [44, 45].

The arthroprosthesis becomes consequently unstable, and its motion keeps favoring the bone resorption process that causes the loosening. At the present moment, there is no mean to stop this process unless revision of the arthroprosthesis.

9.5 Discussion

In the last decade, the orthopedic literature has reported excellent midterm and long-term results with both mobile- and fixed-bearing UKAs for the treatment of medial compartmental joint arthritis.

Several studies have indicated a lower incidence of infection, better range of motion, and higher patient preference when compared with total knee arthroplasties [18, 22, 25].

With such encouraging results, many orthopedic surgeons are led to perform this challenging technical procedure.

Furthermore, Repicci and Eberle in 1999 [35] reported excellent long-term results in more than 700 medial UKAs with a 3-in. incision, and now minimally invasive surgery (MIS) is preferred to conventional approach in UKAs as it reduces blood loss and disruption of soft tissue and it determines a quicker rehabilitation time for the patient.

Despite these undisputed advantages, some authors [17] reported that in MIS UKAs, the frequency of malalignment of the components was higher if compared to conventional open surgery group.

To avoid such events, the use of navigation system, yet introduced widely in TKA, could also provide to adequate component and limb alignment in UKAs.

Several studies [13, 23, 37, 42] reported more accurate insertion and satisfactory alignment of mechanical axis using navigation system, also in terms of femoral and tibial coronal inclinations and tibial sagittal inclination.

The use of navigation system in UKA allows to perform the tibial resection with the referee of lateral tibial plateau, considering the real amount of bone erosion. Furthermore, the surgeon could decide to implant UKA components respecting anatomical or mechanical varus, using different landmarks during bone-morphing, and it provides an adequate femoral component alignment following in real time the screen system.

Additional surgical time is required in unicompartmental knee arthroplasty using navigation system; however, some authors [42] reported no statistical differences in terms of surgical time, especially after an initial learning curve.

Stress fracture of the medial plateau is reported in the literature after UKA, especially in case of MIS UKA, probably due to pinhole of the tibia cutting guide, being too close of medial cortex of the proximal tibia.

Seon et al. [43] reported that two cases of medial plateau stress fracture occurred after UKA using navigation system, attributing to early weight bearing in osteoporotic and obese patients and stress effect of the guide pinholes but not due to the tracker pinholes of the navigation instrument.

The authors reported a case of diaphyseal tibia fracture following UKA with the use of navigation system. In this case, one of two tibial tracker pins is drilled into anterior crest of tibia, provoking a stress diaphyseal tibia fracture (Fig. 9.8). Six months after surgery, a complete bone healing is obtained without sequelae (Figs. 9.9 and 9.10, 9.11, and 9.12).

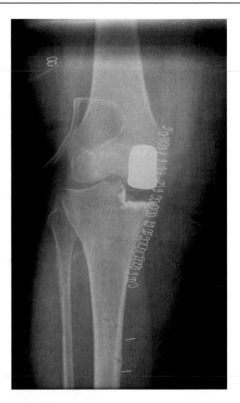

Fig. 9.8 Postoperative AP radiographs show an adequate component positioning. On diaphyseal middle third, two drilled holes on the tibial crest are visible

Figs. 9.9 and 9.10 Six months after surgery, AP and LL show a complete bone healing

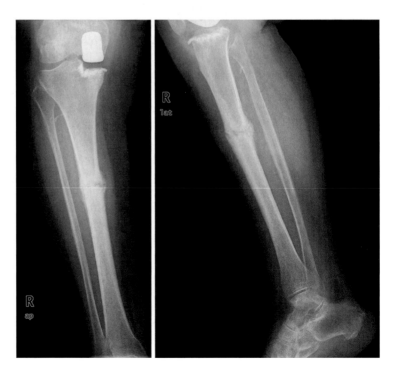

Figs. 9.11 and 9.12 MRI of the leg showing bone callus of the tibia

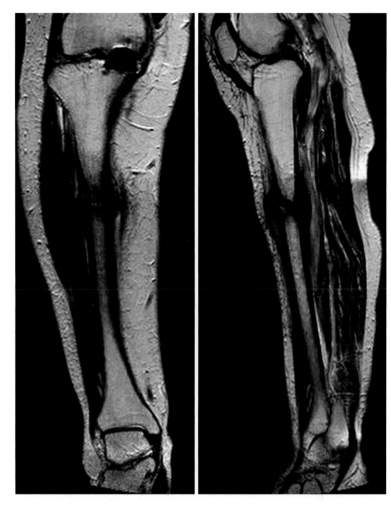

References

1. Ackroyd CE, Whitehouse SL, Newman JH, Joslin CC (2002) A comparative study of the medial St Georg sled and kinematic total knee arthroplasties. Ten-year survivorship. J Bone Joint Surg Br 84(5): 667–672
2. Argenson JN, Parratte S (2006) The unicompartmental knee: design and technical considerations in minimizing wear. Clin Orthop Relat Res 452: 137–142
3. Barnes CL, Mesko JW, Teeny SM, York SC (2006) Treatment of medial compartment arthritis of the knee: a survey of the American Association of Hip and Knee Surgeons. J Arthroplasty 21(7):950–956
4. Beard DJ, Pandit H, Gill HS (2007) The influence of the presence and severity of pre-existing patellofemoral degenerative changes on the outcome of the Oxford medial unicompartmental knee replacement. J Bone Joint Surg Br 89:1597–1601
5. Berger R, Della Valle C, Jacobs JJ, Sheinkop MB, Rosenberg AG, Galante JO (2006) The progression of patellofemoral arthrosis after medial unicompartmental replacement: results at 11 to 15 years. Clin Orthop Relat Res 452:285–286
6. Bert JM (1998) 10-year survivorship of metal-backed, unicompartmental arthroplasty. J Arthroplasty 13(8): 901–905
7. Böhm I, Landsiedl F (2000) Revision surgery after failed unicompartmental knee arthroplasty: a study of 35 cases. J Arthroplasty 15(8):982–989
8. Brocklehurst R, Bayliss MT, Maroudas A, Coysh HL, Freeman MA, Revell PA, Ali SY (1984) The composition of normal and osteoarthritic articular cartilage from human knee joints. With special reference to unicompartmental replacement and osteotomy of the knee. J Bone Joint Surg Am 66(1): 95–106
9. Buckup K, Linke LC, Hahne V (2007) Minimally invasive implantation and computer navigation for a unicondylar knee system. Orthopedics 30:66–69

10. Cartier P, Chaib S (1987) Unicondylar knee arthroplasty: 2–10 year follow-up evaluation. J Arthroplasty 2:157–162
11. Cartier P, Sanouiller JL, Grelsamer RP (1996) Unicompartmental knee arthroplasty surgery. 10-year minimum follow-up period. J Arthroplasty 11(7): 782–788
12. Collier MB, Eickmann TH, Sukezaki F, McAuley JP, Engh GA (2006) Patient, implant, and alignment factors associated with revision of medial compartment unicondylar arthroplasty. J Arthroplasty 21:108–115
13. Cossey AJ, Spriggins AJ (2005) The use of computer-assisted surgical navigation to prevent malalignment in unicompartmental knee arthroplasty. J Arthroplasty 20(1):29–34
14. Delp SL, Stulberg SD, Davies B, Picard F, Leitner F (1998) Computer assisted knee replacement. Clin Orthop Relat Res. Sep;(354):49–56
15. Engh GA (2002) Orthopaedic crossfire–can we justify unicondylar arthroplasty as a temporizing procedure? in the affirmative. J Arthroplasty 17(4 Suppl 1): 54–55
16. Ensini A, Catani F, Leardini A, Romagnoli M, Giannini S (2007) Alignments and clinical results in conventional and navigated total knee arthroplasty. Clin Orthop Relat Res 457:156–162
17. Fisher DA, Watts M, Davis KE (2003) Implant position in knee surgery: a comparison of minimally invasive, open unicompartmental, and total knee arthroplasty. J Arthroplasty 18:2–8
18. Foran JR, Mont MA, Rajadhyaksha AD, Jones LC, Etienne G, Hungerford DS (2004) Total knee arthroplasty in obese patients: a comparison with a matched control group. J Arthroplasty 19(7):817–824
19. Furnes O, Espehaug B, Lie SA, Vollset SE, Engesaeter LB, Havelin LI (2007) Failure mechanisms after unicompartmental and tricompartmental primary knee replacement with cement. J Bone Joint Surg Am 89(3):519–525
20. Haaker RG, Wojciechowski M, Patzer P, Willburger RE, Senkal M, Engelhardt M (2006) Minimally invasive unicondylar knee replacement with computer navigation. Orthopade 35(10):1073–1079
21. Hamilton WG, Collier MB, Tarabee E, McAuley JP, Engh CA Jr, Engh GA (2006) Incidence and reasons for reoperation after minimally invasive unicompartmental knee arthroplasty. J Arthroplasty 21:98–107
22. Harrysson OL, Robertsson O, Nayfeh JF (2004) Higher cumulative revision rate of knee arthroplasties in younger patients with osteoarthritis. Clin Orthop Relat Res. Apr;(421):162–168
23. Jenny JY, Boeri C (2003) Unicompartmental knee prosthesis implantation with a non-image-based navigation system: rationale, technique, case–control comparative study with a conventional instrumented implantation. Knee Surg Sports Traumatol Arthrosc 11(1):40–45
24. Jung KA, Kim SJ, Lee SC, Hwang SH, Ahn NK (2010) Accuracy of implantation during computer-assisted minimally invasive Oxford unicompartmental knee arthroplasty: a comparison with a conventional instrumented technique. Knee 17(6):387–391
25. Keene G, Simpson D, Kalairajah Y (2006) Limb alignment in computer-assisted minimally-invasive unicompartmental knee replacement. J Bone Joint Surg Br 88(1):44–48
26. Kort NP, van Raay JJ, Cheung J, Jolink C, Deutman R (2007) Analysis of Oxford medial unicompartmental knee replacement using the minimally invasive technique in patients aged 60 and above: an independent prospective series. Knee Surg Sports Traumatol Arthrosc 15(11):1331–1334
27. Krishnan SR, Randle R (2009) ACL reconstruction with unicondylar replacement in knee with functional instability and osteoarthritis. J Orthop Surg Res 4:43
28. Laurencin CT, Zelicof SB, Scott RD, Ewald FC (1991) Unicompartmental versus total knee arthroplasty in the same patient. A comparative study. Clin Orthop Relat Res. Dec;(273):151–156
29. Lindstrand A, Stenström A (1992) Polyethylene wear of the PCA unicompartmental knee. Prospective 5 (4–8) year study of 120 arthrosis knees. Acta Orthop Scand 63(3):260–262
30. Lustig S, Paillot JL, Servien E, Henry J, Ait Si Selmi T, Neyret P (2009) Cemented all polyethylene tibial insert unicompartmental knee arthroplasty: a long term follow-up study. Orthop Traumatol Surg Res 95(1):12–21
31. McAuley JP, Engh GA, Ammeen DJ (2001) Revision of failed unicompartmental knee arthroplasty. Clin Orthop Relat Res. Nov;(392):279–282
32. Murray DW, Goodfellow JW, O'Connor JJ (1998) The Oxford medial unicompartmental arthroplasty: a ten-year survival study. J Bone Joint Surg Br 80(6): 983–989
33. Pennington DW, Swienckowski JJ, Lutes WB, Drake GN (2003) Unicompartmental knee arthroplasty in patients sixty years of age or younger. J Bone Joint Surg Am 85-A(10):1968–1973
34. Price AJ, Webb J, Topf H, Dodd CA, Goodfellow JW, Murray DW, Oxford Hip and Knee Group (2001) Rapid recovery after oxford unicompartmental arthroplasty through a short incision. J Arthroplasty 16(8): 970–976
35. Repicci JA, Eberle RW (1999) Minimally invasive surgical technique for unicondylar knee arthroplasty. J South Orthop Assoc 8(1):20–27
36. Romanowski MR, Repicci JA (2002) Minimally invasive unicondylar arthroplasty: eight-year follow-up. Am J Knee Surg 15(1):17–22
37. Rosenberger RE, Fink C, Quirbach S, Attal R, Tecklenburg K, Hoser C (2008) The immediate effect of navigation on implant accuracy in primary mini-invasive unicompartmental knee arthroplasty. Knee Surg Sports Traumatol Arthrosc 16(12):1133–1140
38. Sanchis-Alfonso V (2007) Severe metallosis after unicompartmental knee arthroplasty. Knee Surg Sports Traumatol Arthrosc 15(4):361–364

39. Sanchis-Alfonso V, Alcacer-García J (2001) Extensive osteolytic cystlike area associated with polyethylene wear debris adjacent to an aseptic, stable, uncemented unicompartmental knee prosthesis: case report. Knee Surg Sports Traumatol Arthrosc 9(3):173–177

40. Sawatari T, Tsumura H, Iesaka K, Furushiro Y, Torisu T (2005) Three-dimensional finite element analysis of unicompartmental knee arthroplasty–the influence of tibial component inclination. J Orthop Res 23(3):549–554

41. Scott RD (2003) UniSpacer: insufficient data to support its widespread use. Clin Orthop Relat Res. Nov;(416):164–166

42. Seon JK, Song EK, Park SJ, Yoon TR, Lee KB, Jung ST (2009) Comparison of minimally invasive unicompartmental knee arthroplasty with or without a navigation system. J Arthroplasty 24(3):351–357

43. Seon JK, Song EK, Yoon TR, Seo HY, Cho SG (2007) Tibial plateau stress fracture after unicondylar knee arthroplasty using a navigation system: two case reports. Knee Surg Sports Traumatol Arthrosc 15(1): 67–70

44. Pilliar RM, Lee JM, Maniatopoulos C. (1986) Observations on the effect of movement on bone ingrowth into porous-surfaced implants. Clin Orthop Relat Res. Jul;(208):108–13.

45. Søballe K, Hansen ES, Brockstedt-Rasmussen H, Bünger C (1993) Hydroxyapatite coating converts fibrous tissue to bone around loaded implants. J Bone Joint Surg Br 75(2):270–278

46. Sparmann M, Wolke B, Czupalla H, Banzer D, Zink A (2003) Positioning of total knee arthroplasty with and without navigation support. A prospective, randomised study. J Bone Joint Surg Br 85(6): 830–835

47. Tabor OB Jr, Tabor OB (1998) Unicompartmental arthroplasty: a long-term follow-up study. J Arthroplasty 13(4):373–379

48. Thornhill TS (1986) Unicompartmental knee arthroplasty. Clin Orthop Relat Res. Apr;(205):121–131

49. Voss F, Sheinkop MB, Galante JO, Barden RM, Rosenberg AG (1995) Miller-Galante unicompartmental knee arthroplasty at 2- to 5-year follow-up evaluations. J Arthroplasty 10(6):764–771

50. Yang S, Hadlow S (2003) Unicompartmental knee arthroplasty: is it durable? N Z Med J 116(1183): U627

Unicompartmental Knee Arthroplasty: Robotics

10

Justin Cobb and Andrew Pearle

10.1 Surgical Technique

Orthopedics is a natural and fitting target for the application of recent advances in imaging technology. In an effort to achieve accurate implant placement with minimal invasiveness, many have utilized robotic navigation systems such as the MAKO RIO®.

The RIO® is used to implant medial and lateral unicompartmental knee arthroplasty (UKA) components and to perform patellofemoral arthroplasty. The platform facilitates the creation of a preoperative plan that can be adjusted mid-surgery. The robotic arm is surgeon directed and provides real-time, tactile feedback. This digital platform combines interactive robotics, computer-assisted guidance, and an intelligent bone-shaping tool, to minimize invasiveness.

J. Cobb, M.D. (✉)
Department of Orthopaedic Surgery,
Imperial College London, Charing Cross Hospital,
7th Floor, East Wing, Fulham Palace Road,
London W6 8RF, UK
e-mail: justinpetercobb@gmail.com

A. Pearle, M.D.
Orthopaedic Department, Hospital for Special Surgery,
New York, NY 10021, USA
e-mail: pearlea@hss.edu

10.1.1 Preoperative Imaging

All patients receive preoperative CT scans. Scans are taken with the patient lying supine, attached to a motion sensor on the affected leg. One-millimeter slices are taken at the knee joint, and 5-mm slices through the hip and ankle. Images are saved in digital imaging and communications in medicine (DICOM) format and transferred to the RIO® system. Sagittal slices of the distal and proximal femur are also segmented, defined, and recombined to form 3-dimensional (3-D) models. Implant representations are then positioned atop the digital models, resulting in a patient-specific CT-based plan (Fig. 10.1).

As cartilage cannot be visualized by CT, this preoperative approach is limited. Consequently, only bone alignment can be planned for, and the plan is usually modified intraoperatively to achieve gap balancing and long-leg alignment. Still, CT planning does permit an assessment of the subchondral bone bed, osteophyte and cystic formations, and regions of avascular necrosis.

10.1.2 Preoperative Planning

The preoperative plan is based on four parameters: 3-D visualization of implant position, metrics of component alignment, lower limb alignment, and intraoperative gap kinematics. Accurate implant

F. Catani, S. Zaffagnini (eds.), *Knee Surgery using Computer Assisted Surgery and Robotics*,
DOI 10.1007/978-3-642-31430-8_10, © ESSKA 2013

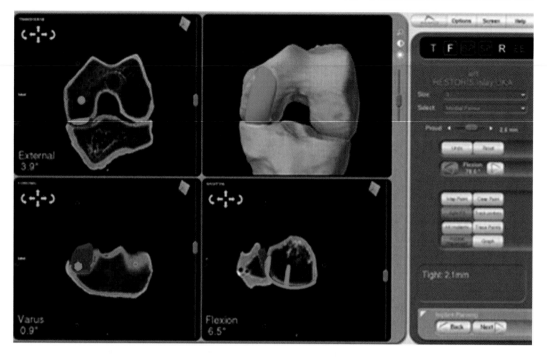

Fig. 10.1 CT-based patient-specific preoperative planning

positioning requires integrating the precise dimensions of the femoral and tibial prostheses with their target positions. The implant computer-assisted design (CAD) models are positioned atop the 3-D models of the patient's distal femur and proximal tibia, and alignment parameters are shown on the computer screen (note: as of now, planning and resection of the patellar implant is performed manually). During this step, the surgeon can visualize the predicted implant congruence and minimize areas of edge loading by adjusting the plan.

The RIO® platform also provides continuous visual feedback on bone alignment and anatomy (e.g., subchondral bone bed, cortical rim). Even though the implants are not patient-specific, implant orientation is unique and takes into account both bone and soft tissue anatomy. Resection volumes are automatically defined, and boundaries for the cutting instrument are set to prevent inadvertent harm.

The preliminary plan is based on alignment parameters and a 3-D visualization of implant position. During surgery, the plan is modified based on gap measurements throughout flexion and lower limb alignment values. Before surgery, the alignment parameters given by the robotic system (and recommended by MAKO) are used in combination with parameters cited in the literature. For example, the tibial slopes in the coronal and sagittal planes are carefully specified. In patients with medial compartment osteoarthritis, the medial tibial plateau is typically in varus with respect to the mechanical axis. Collier and colleagues [1] demonstrated that correction of this varus slope with the tibial implant improves survivorship. In addition, more than a 7° slope of the tibial component has been shown to increase the risk of ACL rupture. We recommend that the tibial components be in 2–4° of varus, without more than 7° of posterior slope. In patients with ACL deficiency, the posterior sagittal slope of the tibia is maintained between 2° and 5°.

Three-dimensional visualization of the implant position ensures proper sizing. For example, a 2-mm rim of bone surrounding the tibial inlay pocket is advocated. This rim can be planned for and measured on the 3-D model. On the femur, the prosthesis is sized such that coverage is robust and symmetric flexion and extension gaps are maintained. In addition, the depth of the tibial inlay pocket can be planned for (a start value of 3 mm is suggested). This resection depth can be modified accordingly based on intraoperative gap kinematics.

10.1.3 Setup

Before the patient arrives in the OR, the surgeon positions the RIO® to maximize accessibility of the knee being operated on. Once everything is in place, the surgeon secures the base with brakes. Then, he or she drapes the affected limb with sterile covering and begins instrument initialization of motion (ROMs).

Anatomical surface landmarks are registered before the surgeon incises the skin. The leg is put through a full ROM while the appropriate valgus load is applied on the joint. After skin incision, small articular accuracy checkpoint pins are inserted on the tibia and femur. Tibial and femoral bone surfaces are registered at these points, and the acquired data is matched to the CT models. Skin incisions can be made as short as 2.25 in. in some patients, which prevent needless strain on soft tissue.

10.1.4 Intraoperative Soft Tissue Balancing

After the surgeon registers the bone anatomy and sets the target implant position, he or she initiates soft tissue gap balancing. Virtual kinematic modeling and intraoperative tracking allow real-time adjustments to be made to obtain correct knee kinematics. Osteophytes that interfere with medial collateral ligament function are removed, and capsular adhesions interfering with knee function are relieved. Since some indications for UKA are correctable, removal of these impediments permits correct leg kinematics and tissue tension during passive manipulation throughout the full ROM. 3-D positions of the femur and tibia are captured throughout the ROM with the medial collateral ligament properly tensioned. This yields correct bone spacing (extension and flexion gaps) such that proper knee mechanics

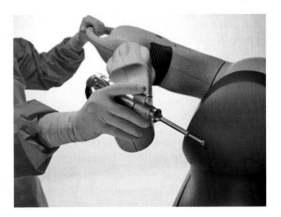

Fig. 10.2 Robot end effector and high-speed burr

will be restored after resection and component implantation. The articular surfaces of the implant components are adjusted to fill flexion and extension gaps. Once optimized, the plan incorporates alignment metrics, implant congruence, and gap kinematics in an individualized fashion.

As a final step, any varus deformity is manually corrected with application of a valgus force to the knee, while lower limb alignment is monitored by the navigation system. As the virtual components are optimized to fill the space necessary to correct this deformity, final lower limb alignment is predicted. Typically, we target a final lower limb alignment of approximately 2° of varus. Care is taken to avoid undercorrection (final alignment, <8° varus) and overcorrection (final alignment in valgus) of long-leg alignment [6].

10.1.5 Robotic Arm

The RIO® has three components: an optical camera, a computer, and a robotic arm. The optical camera is an infrared system, and the computer runs the software that operates the surgical plan. The end of the robotic arm has a full six degrees of freedom, and its movements are restricted to the incision site by 3-D boundaries preset at planning; intraoperative adjustments ensure correct soft tissue balancing. A high-speed burr is attached to the distal end of the robotic arm (Fig. 10.2). The surgeon moves the arm by guiding its tip within the preset boundaries. The robot gives the surgeon active tactile, visual, and auditory feedback while burring. While inside the resection volume, the arm operates without resisting. As the burr approaches the boundary, the devices give off a series of warning beep, and when it reaches the boundary, the arm resists motion outside the periphery altogether. In effect, the arm executes the preoperative plan with precision. In addition, excessive force at the limits of the cutting volume or rapid movement of patient anatomy immediately stops the cutting instrument to prevent unintentional resection.

Unlike other active and semi-active robot systems, the RIO® does not require rigid fixation of the robot to the patient. Rather, osseous reference markers track the position of the tibia and the femur. As the bones move during surgery, the haptic 3-D resection volume moves in sync. During resection, a leg holder is used to keep the limb stable to ensure optimal positioning of the knee and access to the targeted surfaces.

10.1.6 Bone Resection Burr

The resection burr is a hand-powered or foot-pedal high-speed device that operates at 80,000 rpm. Burrs of different sizes are available: a 6-mm-diameter spherical burr for the rapid removal of major bone material (to allow insertion of the femoral prosthesis post, for instance); a 2-mm-diameter spherical burr for fine finishing, including the edges and corners of the resection area; and a 2-mm or 1.4-mm router for keel canal preparation. All burring is visualized on a screen, which shows the 3-D models of the distal femur and proximal tibia. The models are color-coded and updated in real time based on resection progress (the resection area is colored different from the surrounding bone). If the robotic arm goes 0.5 mm outside the planned resection area (green), red appears on the display, and the arm stiffens progressively; if the user pushes the arm further outside the green area, the robot will resist (haptic feedback). The user will be warned, and the burr will immediately stop spinning. These

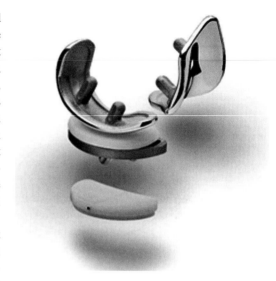

Fig. 10.3 UKA and PFA implants

features are intended to prevent the user from inadvertent cutting.

10.1.7 Prosthesis Selection

Implant choice depends on the surgeon's preference and the specific characteristics of the patient's osteoarthritis pattern. Current treatment options include isolated medial UKA, lateral UKA, and patellofemoral arthroplasty (PFA) (Fig. 10.3). In addition, bicompartmental arthroplasty may be performed, consisting of both a medial UKA and a PFA.

There are two tibial component implant choices: inlay and onlay designs. An inlay tibial prosthesis is an all-polyethylene design that utilizes the patient's formed tibial subchondral sclerotic bone bed to support the component (Fig. 10.4) [5, 9]. The implant cavity uses the intact tibial rim for rotational control. The angle of the tibial component is usually set within several degrees of varus to reproduce the patient's normal inclination. The patient's posterior slope is recreated with a deeper posterior pocket. Onlay tibial components utilize the patient's cortical rim for support (Fig. 10.5). The prosthesis is modular, with a metal backing. The tibial cut angle is usually 90° to the tibial mechanical axis.

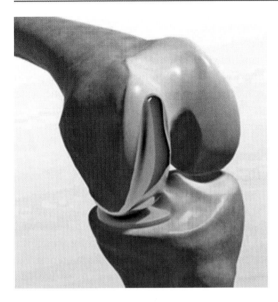

Fig. 10.4 Inlay UKA

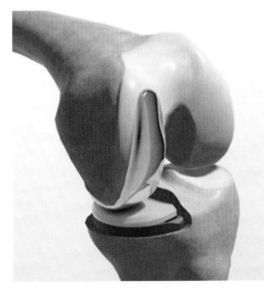

Fig. 10.5 Onlay UKA

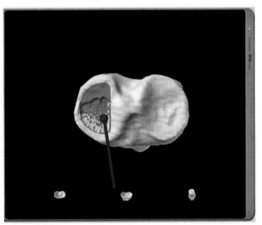

Fig. 10.6 Cavity milling process

10.1.8 Operative Technique

The robotic arm assists the surgeon with burring the tibial and femoral surfaces. The arm helps control depth, width, and length of burring, as the system provides real-time graphical feedback. It is recommended that the arm be used to prepare the tibial cavity before addressing the femoral surface so as to allow easier access to that surface, particularly its posterior side. The arm also allows intraoperative conversion to a metal-backed onlay implant.

With only the aid of soft tissue retractors, the surgeon burrs the tibial and femoral surfaces, including the femoral posthole, with a 6-mm sphere; he or she then fine-mills with a 2-mm burr and cuts the femoral keel slot with the 2-mm/1.4-mm fluted router. The navigation screen shows an overlay between the planned cavity and the burred result (Fig. 10.6). Once milling is completed (Fig. 10.7), the surgeon inserts the femoral and tibial components and maneuvers the leg through a complete flexion-extension arc. The computer monitor displays real-time long-leg alignment, so that the final alignment can be planned for. Once the surgeon is satisfied with implant position, both implant components are cemented and a final ROM of the knee joint is executed so that the original, trial, and final implant kinematics and knee alignment can be compared. Before closure, the surgeon removes the mini checkpoints and bone reference arrays.

10.1.9 Post-op Regimen

For UKA and PFA, patients can be discharged the same day if they are cleared by physical therapy (PT) and are medically stable. A 24-h

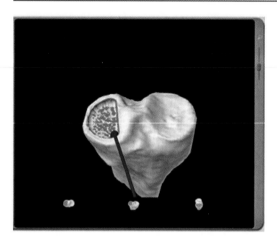

Fig. 10.7 Finished implant cavity

overnight stay for pain control, antibiotics, and anticoagulation is often prescribed. The patient can be mobilized the same day with PT, and continuous passive motion (CPM) is often administered to access comfort. Patients usually require minimal therapy over the next several weeks. Surgical teams should focus on quadriceps stability, and gait. Thereafter, range of motion returns rapidly. Squats or lunges should initially be avoided to minimize stress to the healing pin sites. Follow-ups can occur semiannually.

10.2   Clinical Experience

With the recent resurgence of unicompartmental knee arthroplasty (UKA), investigators have overcome difficulties related to implant design and patient selection while improving upon existing surgical techniques. Minimally invasive (MIS) UKA procedures that yield accurate component alignment have received significant attention; these procedures have resulted in significant clinical and financial benefits, including shorter hospital stays, faster recovery times, and reduced postoperative morbidity. Still, there are some drawbacks: technical challenges of conventional jig-based UKA techniques appear to be magnified through the MIS approach. Impaired ability to see the surgical space has resulted in inferior component alignment and a higher incidence of early implant failures. As a result, the goals of

proper implant alignment and minimal invasiveness have been difficult to achieve in tandem using manual instrumentation. In addition, there appears to be a significant learning curve with respect to the manual MIS UKA technique (a surgeon's initial cases may result in inferior outcomes as compared to subsequent ones).

10.2.1 Accuracy

In a study by Roche et al. [10], postoperative radiographs of 43 MAKOplasty® patients were examined for outliers, the criteria for which was defined by a panel of orthopedic surgeons. The radiographs (Fig. 10.8) show a typical pre- and postoperative series from a single patient. Of the 344 individual radiographic measurements, only 4 (1 %) were identified as outliers.

In a comparative study, Coon et al. [4] examined a cohort of 33 MAKOplasty® patients and 44 standard UKA patients. The coronal and sagittal alignments of the tibial components were measured on postoperative AP and lateral radiographs and compared to the preoperative plan. The RMS error of the tibial slope was 3.5° manually compared to 1.4° robotically. In addition, the variance using manual instruments was 2.8 times greater than the robotically guided implantations ($p < 0.0001$). In the coronal plane, the average error was $3.3° \pm 1.8°$ more varus using manual instruments compared to $0.1° \pm 2.4°$ when implanted robotically ($p < 0.0001$) (Fig. 10.9).

In a study of the first 20 MAKOplasty® patients at one institution, Sinha et al. [11] found that using the robotic arm resulted in extremely accurate and precise reconstruction of individual patient anatomy. Postoperatively, all femoral components matched their preoperative varus/valgus and flexion alignments. They also reported a change in the femoral joint line of only 0.4 ± 0.5 mm. On the tibial side, the bone preparation matched the preoperative alignment with respect to posterior slope and varus, but there was a slightly higher error rate in the final tibial component position, indicating that care must be taken such that pressurization and polymerization of polymethylmethacrylate

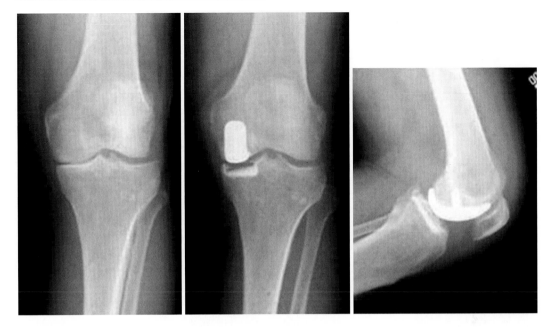

Fig. 10.8 Pre-op AP x-ray and post-op AP and lateral views

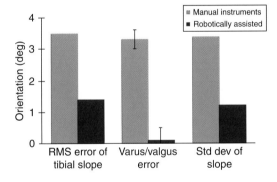

Fig. 10.9 Tibial slope error and variance in UKA using manual instrumentation versus robotically assisted UKA

does not change the component's position within the cavity.

10.2.2 Bone Preservation

In a study by Coon et al. [3] comparing MAKOplasty® inlay versus manual onlay implantations, the average depth of medial tibial plateau resection was significantly less with inlay tibial components (3.7 ± 0.8 mm) relative to onlay tibial components (6.5 ± 0.8 mm, $p < 0.0001$). In a separate study by Kreuzer et al.

[8], the depth of resection was compared between a group of 26 MAKOplasty® patients and 16 patients who received an all-poly manual "resurfacing" UKA implant. Average depth of bony medial plateau resection was significantly greater in the standard technique onlay design group (8.5 ± 2.26 mm) compared to the robotically assisted inlay group (4.4 ± 0.93 mm) ($p < 0.0001$). At conversion to a standard TKA, the proposed tibial osteotomy would require medial augmentation/revision components (insert thickness > 15 mm) in 75 % of the onlay group as compared to 4 % of the robotically assisted inlay group ($p < 0.0001$) (Fig. 10.10).

10.2.3 Clinical Outcomes

A study of 43 MAKOplasty® patients from Roche et al. [10] found that the average flexion significantly increased at 3 months postoperatively to $126° \pm 6°$ compared with $121° \pm 8°$ preoperatively ($p < 0.001$). Postoperative KSS and WOMAC total scores significantly improved from 95 ± 16 to 150 ± 27 ($p < 0.001$) and 41 ± 15 to 21 ± 17 ($p < 0.001$), respectively. Quality of life, as measured by the SF-12 physical summary, also

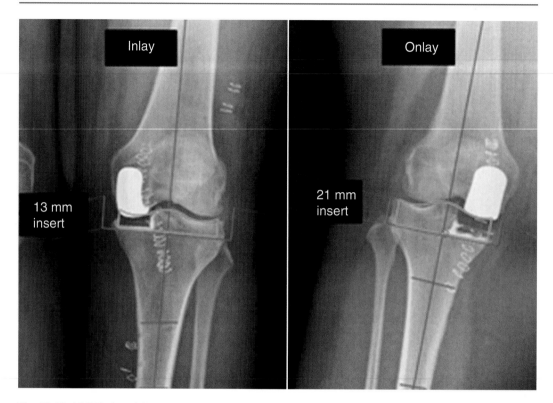

Fig. 10.10 MAKOplasty inlay and manual onlay implantations templated for a TKA with the predicted insert thicknesses as indicated

significantly improved from 30 ± 9 to 39 ± 12 ($p < 0.001$). Robot-guided UKA procedures improved every measured clinical outcome.

In a comparative study by Coon et al. [2], while the average length of hospital stays was the same for both onlay ($LOS = 1.0 \pm 0.2$ days) and inlay ($LOS = 0.9 \pm 0.5$ days) UKA procedures, a significantly higher percentage of inlay patients went home the day of surgery (18 % versus 2 %, $p < 0.0001$). There was no significant difference between the two groups in terms of average KSS, change in KSS, or Marmor rating, in any of the three follow-ups. At 12 weeks, the average increase in the combined KSS was 83.6 in the conventional group and 79.7 in the haptic-guided group ($p = 0.66$). Furthermore, there were no significant differences in the measures that comprise these scores, such as range of motion, pain, and use of assistive devices ($p > 0.05$) (Fig. 10.11).

We examined a cohort of 159 MAKOplasty® patients, consisting of 86 females and 73 males

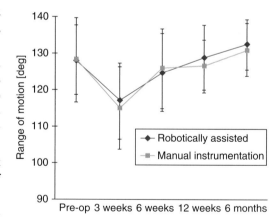

Fig. 10.11 Patient range of motion outcomes in UKA with manual instrumentation versus robotically assisted UKA. There was no significant difference between the two groups at any of the four follow-ups

with an average follow-up of 1 year (range: 6 weeks to 25 months). The average age at surgery was 69 years with an average BMI of 28.3 kg/m². The clinical outcomes of these

Functional metric	Pre-op	6 weeks	3 months	1 year
ROM	125 ± 12°	121 ± 14°	128 ± 8°	128 ± 12°
Knee society knee score	42 ± 10	85 ± 14	89 ± 12	89 ± 8
Knee society function score	55 ± 14	73 ± 23	80 ± 21	81 ± 17
SF-12 physical	33 ± 9	37 ± 10	43 ± 10	44 ± 8
WOMAC total	37 ± 14	22 ± 13	19 ± 14	22 ± 15
WOMAC pain	8 ± 4	5 ± 3	4 ± 3	4 ± 3
WOMAC stiffness	4 ± 2	3 ± 1	2 ± 1	3 ± 2
WOMAC physical function	26 ± 10	15 ± 9	13 ± 11	15 ± 11

Fig. 10.12 The first 73 (42 males, 31 females) patients (average age: 70 ± 10 years) to receive a robotically assisted UKA enrolled in an IRB-approved outcomes registry. The average follow-up was 30 months (range: 23–40 months). The tibial component for all patients was an all-poly inlay design. At 2-year follow-up, it was found

that the average range of motion significantly increased to 127.1 ± 1.8° compared with 124.6 ± 13.9° preoperatively ($p < 0.0001$, Fig. 10.2). Postoperative Knee Society Knee and Functional scores also increased from 48.2 ± 10.4 to 85.8 ± 3.8 ($p < 0.0001$) and from 60.5 ± 10.1 to 80.6 ± 6.8 ($p < 0.0001$), respectively

patients were measured preoperatively and at follow-ups of 6 weeks, 3 months, and 1 year. MAKOplasty® significantly improved all measured clinical outcomes (Figs. 10.12, 10.13, and 10.14).

10.2.4 Learning Curve

Integrating new technology into the operating room can be a long and significant learning process, one that introduces inefficiencies into a surgeon's work flow. Jinnah et al. [7] examined the surgical times of 781 MAKOplasty® patients, as performed by 11 different surgeons. Each surgeon had performed at least 40 surgeries with the new technology prior to the study. The average surgical time for all surgeries across all surgeons was 55 ± 19 min (range: 22–165 min). The surgeon with the shortest steady state surgical time averaged 38 ± 9 min, and the surgeon with the longest steady state surgical time averaged 64 ± 16 min. The average number of surgeries required to have three surgeries completed within the 95 % confidence interval of the steady state surgical time was 14 ± 8 (range: 5–29) (Fig. 10.15).

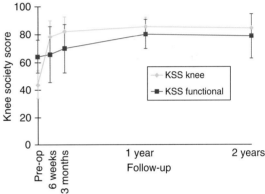

Fig. 10.13 KSS Knee and Functional Scores for first 73 MAKOplasty patients

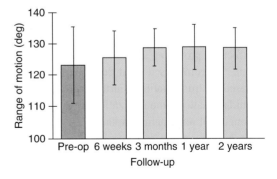

Fig. 10.14 Range of motion for the first 73 MAKOplasty patients

Conclusions

This robot-assisted UKA allows for comprehensive, 3-D planning of UKA components, including soft tissue balancing, followed by accurate resection of the femur and tibia. We

have shown that this preparation yields more accurate, less variable alignment of implant components as compared to manual, jig-based instrumentation. We have also shown that,

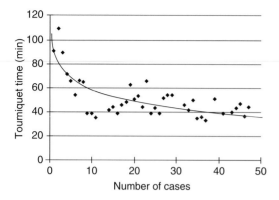

Fig. 10.15 A typical MAKOplasty learning curve

when appropriate, resurfacing inlay components require less bone resection and lead to a
quicker recovery than standard onlay UKA
components. These bone preserving, resurfacing inlay implants preserve the option of conversion to an onlay UKA or a standard TKA
without bone augmentation should prosthesis
failure occur. All patients showed significant
improvement in every measure of postoperative function. The clinical result of this initial
series of UKAs is comparable to that of procedures utilizing more established techniques,
thus alleviating concerns regarding the acquisition of new skills that result in inferior outcomes. Furthermore, the learning curve has
been shown to be manageable. The procedure
has low complication and revision rates. The
use of robot guidance for unicompartmental
knee arthroplasty has proved to be safe and
effective, providing a more precise and accurate "instrument set" than that of manual jig-
based instrumentation. Furthermore, robotic
guidance allows the realization of the clinical
benefits of resurfacing implants.

References

1. Collier MB, Eickmann TH, Sukezaki F et al (2006)
Patient, implant, and alignment factors associated with
revision of medial compartment unicondylar arthroplasty. J Arthroplasty 21(6 Suppl 2):108–115
2. Coon T, Driscoll M, Conditt MA (2008a) Early clinical success of novel tactile guided UKA technique. In:
Proceedings of the 21st annual congress of the
international society of technology in arthroplasty,
International Society for Technology in Arthroplasty,
Sacramento, p 141
3. Coon T, Driscoll M, Conditt MA (2008b) Does less
medial tibial plateau resection make a difference in
UKA? In: Proceedings of the 21st annual congress of
the international society of technology in arthroplasty,
International Society for Technology in Arthroplasty,
Sacramento, p 274
4. Coon T, Driscoll M, Conditt MA (2008c) Robotically
assisted UKA is more accurate than manually instrumented UKA. In: Proceedings of the 21st annual congress of the international society of technology in
arthroplasty, International Society for Technology in
Arthroplasty, Sacramento, p 274
5. DeHaven KE (2003) Repicci II unicompartmental
knee arthroplasty. Arthroscopy 19(Suppl 1):117–119
6. Hernigou P, Deschamps G (2004) Alignment
influences wear in the knee after medial unicompartmental arthroplasty. Clin Orthop Relat Res
423:161–165
7. Jinnah R, Horowitz S, Lippincott CJ et al (2009) The
learning curve of robotic-assisted UKA. Submitted to
the Institute of Mechanical Engineers, knee arthroplasty: from early intervention to revision, Institute of
Mechanical Engineers, London
8. Kreuzer S, Driscoll M, Conditt MA (2008) Does conversion of a UKA to a TKA require medial augmentation? In: Proceedings of the 21st annual congress of
the international society of technology in arthroplasty,
International Society for Technology in Arthroplasty,
Sacramento, p 274
9. Romanowski MR, Repicci JA (2002) Minimally invasive unicondylar arthroplasty: eight-year follow-up.
J Knee Surg 15(1):17–22
10. Roche M, Augustin D, Conditt MA (2008) Accuracy
of robotically assisted UKA. In: Proceedings of the
21st annual congress of the international society of
technology in arthroplasty, International Society for
Technology in Arthroplasty, Sacramento, p 175
11. Sinha RK, Plush R, Weems VJ (2008) Unicompartmental
arthroplasty using a tactile guided system. In: Proceedings
of the 21st annual congress of the international society of
technology in arthroplasty, International Society for
Technology in Arthroplasty, Sacramento, p 276

Bicompartmental Knee Reconstruction Computer Assisted: Bi-UKR and UKR + PFA

11

Norberto Confalonieri and A. Manzotti

11.1 Introduction

Since the beginning of this century, a new idea for less invasive reconstructive surgery has been growing in the orthopaedic world. Minimally invasive total knee replacement is growing in popularity because of faster recoveries, theoretical reduced blood loss and reduced economical costs [12, 18, 20]. Nevertheless, less invasive surgery has often been identified both by surgeons and manufacturers as shorter surgical approaches to implant the same prostheses used with traditional approaches, performing so-called keyhole surgery even with new potential risks (malalignment, avulsions and local wound problems). More recently, different authors recommend caution towards these mini-incision techniques in total joint replacement [3, 8].

It has been hypothesized that real mini-invasive surgery should not be identified with shorter skin incisions but both with a new respect for all the tissues and with preserved joint kinematics using new tools and smaller implants, redefined as tissue sparing surgery [6].

Unicompartmental knee replacement (UKR) is a well-accepted surgical procedure for the treatment of knee arthritis aiming to replace only the damaged compartment while preserving physiological kinematics [1, 2, 10, 31]. In the literature, good results support this increased popularity among orthopaedic surgeons to offer a relatively less invasive as well as a more physiological approach to the arthritic knee [7, 9, 23, 29].

In modern practice, more and more orthopaedic surgeons have to manage young patients with the tibiofemoral joint affected by osteoarthritis and with a healthy PF compartment and ACL often following posttraumatic events or high-impact sports ("knee abuser"). For several years, a few surgeons in the world have been experimenting with different small implants to achieve a real patient-customized procedure, but there are few in the literature with long-term results [11, 19, 26, 28]. Parratte et al. in 2010 published 17-year follow-up results of both bi-UKRs and UKR + PFR with, respectively, a 78 and 54 % survivorship [25]. All the authors underline how this high-demand procedure based on a customized approach to knee arthritis should be reserved for selected patients and performed in a specifically trained centre [19, 22, 30].

Computer-assisted surgery has been developed to help surgeons performing reconstructive procedures improve implant alignment and performance. In the literature, authors have already demonstrated its efficacy in traditional knee replacement surgery despite different systems that are available achieving better aligned implants despite longer surgical time [13, 16, 17, 24, 32].

N. Confalonieri (✉) • A. Manzotti
Department of Orthopaedics and Traumatology,
Istituti Clinici di Perfezionamento,
Centro Traumatologico Ortopedico,
Via Bignami 1, Milan 20100, Italy
e-mail: norberto.confalonieri@icp.mi.it;
alf.manzotti@libero.it

F. Catani, S. Zaffagnini (eds.), *Knee Surgery using Computer Assisted Surgery and Robotics*,
DOI 10.1007/978-3-642-31430-8_11, © ESSKA 2013

Very few studies have analysed the application of navigation in small implants, mainly in UKR, demonstrating results similar to TKR with a superior final implant alignment even in these implants [5, 14, 15, 21].

Computer-/robotic-assisted surgery could offer further advantages in high-demand surgeries: It could help surgeons to achieve a restored joint line and slope, and the surgeon is always aware of the amount of bone cuts according to the limb alignment and soft tissue balancing; this could be more evident when using small implants [21, 27].

On the basis of their positive experience in computer-assisted TKR with over 1,000 implants, the adoption of new improved dedicated software, the authors explored its applications even for bicompartmental implants (bi-UKR and UKR + PFR) to reproduce easier this high-demand surgery [21].

The authors present their experiences in bi-UKR together with their own interpretation of less invasive surgery in knee reconstruction through an analysis of these "customized implants", their performance and the potential advantages of their association to the computer-assisted surgery.

11.2 Bi-unicompartmental Knee Replacement

Bicruciate ligament retention in TKR has been evaluated since the earliest nonhinged implants in the late 1960s. In gait studies by Andriacchi et al., the knees in which both cruciate ligaments were retained were the only arthroplasties that had normal flexion [1]. Stiehl et al. demonstrated that bicruciate-retaining TKR typically experienced a physiological posterior femoral rollback during a deep knee bend with limited anterior–posterior translation and remained posterior to the midsagittal line in all positions [4].

Despite these biomechanical studies, the first results in the literature were quite poor with the first designs having a higher rate of failure in respect to the traditional implants. In 1986, Goodfellow et al. reported a low revision rate (4.8 %) in 125 bicompartmental implants followed for 2–6 years [23]. In 1992, Stewart et al.

presented a long-term follow-up with the Manchester knee with a cumulative success rate of 73 % at 10 years [26]. Lewallen et al. reported in a 10-year follow-up study of polycentric TKR only 66 % survivorship [26]. Morrison recently reported on early adverse results in a 2-year study compared to a TKR prospective study but showing better early stiffness [22].

New designs with modified surgical techniques have been introduced. Cloutier et al. in 1991 reported a 96 % success rate in a 9- to 11-year follow-up study with bicruciate-retaining implants [4].

Surgeons around the world have been using an even less invasive implant than the above-mentioned bicruciate-retaining TKR using two unicompartmental knee replacements to address the two tibiofemoral compartments simultaneously. The benefits of this approach when compared to TKR include greater tissue sparing, reduced surgical morbidity and easier revision surgery. In addition, a recent study has demonstrated that bi-UKR more closely resembles the biomechanics of an intact knee than a TKR [1, 2, 10]. Fuchs et al. reported that implants preserving both the cruciate ligaments can achieve functional results at least similar to TKR without any arthritis progression [10]. Current patient's expectations following knee replacement surgery include a knee that resembles normal and allows an unrestricted active life, and the superior biomechanical resemblance of the bi-UKR to a normal knee might better match these expectations.

11.3 Preoperative Planning

Even for navigated implants, our basic principle always starts from "The thickness of the prosthesis should correct the joint deformity and approach firstly the most damaged compartment". From these principles, we should estimate how much the deviation angle of the lower limb and the minimum thickness of the prosthetic components (femoral component + tibial component + polyethylene or polyethylene and metal back) size.

For this purpose preoperatively a long-standing x-ray of the lower limbs in full weight-bearing and both patellae and ankles pointing forward should be taken. Calculate the axial deviation angle in varus or valgus and subtract it from the minimum thickness, expressed in millimetres, of the prosthesis.

This expresses the rule that the minimum tibial bone cut is equal to the minimum unicompartmental prosthesis cut:

The thickness of the prosthesis – axial deviation angle = tibial bone resection (mm), e.g., with a valgus arthrosis of 8°, a prosthesis thickness of 11 mm and 11 − 8 = 3 mm of lateral tibial bone resection.

The guidance of the navigation system permits us to know how much tibial bone to cut, bringing the femoral–tibial axis back to 180°. The bone resection of the other compartment will be judged during the operation, once the trial components have been applied on the basis of the ligament balance and of the joint space.

11.4   Surgical Technique

Since 2001 in our department, a CT less computer-assisted navigation system (Orthopilot, Aesculap, Tuttlingen, Germany, version 2.0 and 4.0) has been used in more than 360 joint replacements (knee and hip).

Step 1: Prepare the surgical field as you would for a total prosthesis. The patient should be in the supine position, at the bottom of the bed with the feet outside leaving the knee flexed at 90°. Place a support by the side of the thigh to keep the lower limb in position, with the knee flexed. In this way, the surgeon operates in front of the patient and can therefore check the mechanical axis constantly.

Step 2: We always position a metal locator in the centre of the hip as further limb alignment reference during the surgery in order to keep a constant check on axial adjustment and on the correct positioning of the prosthetic femoral component (an x-ray of the hip should give you the position of the metal locator).

Step 3: Under anaesthesia, the surgeon should evaluate clinically the deformity and how much can be corrected.

Step 4: The skin incision with the limb flexed at 90° should not exceed 11/12 cm, in a median or paramedian medial direction. The patella should only be retracted and not dislocated.

Step 5: Approach the most damaged compartment with two options for arthrotomy: a single anteromedial parapatellar with lateralization of the patella or medial arthrotomy for the medial implant and a simultaneous lateral arthrotomy for the lateral implant. Remove the meniscus but leave the posterior wall intact.

Step 6: Position the support screws for the IR reflecting diodes (LED) of the computer scanner with tiny skin incision of 1 cm. Locate one on the femur and one on the tibia both 10 cm away from the joint line. A third diode will be applied to the foot clipping it to an external metal support fixed by an elastic band. Proceed with the data acquisition of the inferior limb using the computer. By moving the limb and using mathematical models, the navigator determines the axis which goes through the centre of the femoral head, the centre of the knee and ankle. With a mobile pointer, acquire the deepest point in the more damaged tibial plateau, than the deepest point of the other tibial compartment, the centre of the tibial plateau, both the posterior femoral condyles, the superior femoral cortex and medial and lateral epicondyles, always following the indications on the screen step by step.

Step 7: With the data reported on the screen, the surgeon can recalculate the deformity and how much can be corrected. Data processing empowers the system to produce on-screen information related to the mechanical in frontal and lateral projection within the entire given range of movement (Fig. 11.1). Furthermore, it suggests implant size, amount of bone according to the deformity and tridimensional implant alignment.

Step 8: The deformity should always be reducible, but in case it is not, the surgeon should proceed with a slight release of the ligaments under the direct control of the system.

Step 9: Position the tibial cut guide and connect with a mobile diode to the computer (Figs. 11.2 and 11.3). The height of the resection is based on preoperation planning calculations, its orientation (varus–valgus), guided and checked

Fig. 11.1 Data processing empowers the system to produce on-screen information related to the mechanical in frontal and lateral projection within the entire given range of movement

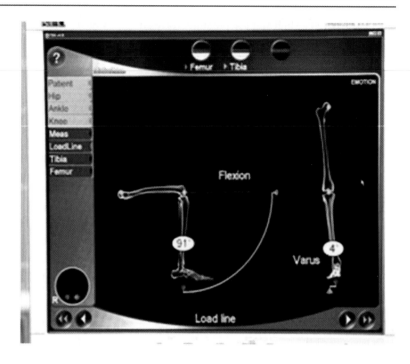

on the display. The slope will be almost normal, about 5°. In a knee with intact ACL, the articular space is reduced in flexion; therefore, it has to be enhanced by the slope and the cut of the posterior femoral condyle. After fixing the guide, continue using an oscillating horizontal blade for the vertical cut, near the ACL insertion point, moving in an anterior–posterior direction. Then change to a "lamellate" blade for the horizontal bone cut.

Step 10: After the removal of the bone block, insert the tibial trial component. The size of the component should be equal to the amount of the resected bone, and the height depends on the deviation axis correction either in flexion or in extension. The computer permits one to check correct alignment during a full range of motion.

With the knee extended, mark the front edge of the tibial trial component on the femoral condyle, to check the size of the femoral component.

Step 11: On the femoral condyle, a cutting guide has to be used. It must be positioned parallel to the tibial component and perpendicular to the mechanical femoral axis just to the largest contact surface between the components for the whole knee range of motion. Remove the femoral–condylar cartilage, and prepare the holes for the pegs of the femoral implant.

Step 12: Position the trial components and check the mechanical axis and the ligament balance, always reading the values and the morphology of the inferior limb in motion on the computer screen.

Step 13: Achieve a correct alignment without ligament tension; the other femorotibial compartment should be approached under the control of the navigation system. Choose the height of the cut on the basis of space (in terms of flexion and extension). In any case, it must be less than 11 mm (prosthesis thickness – deviation angle – articular space = minimum cut).

The latest version (4.0) of our navigation system provides distractors which tense the ligaments and open the articular space according to values expressed in mm. This is particularly helpful in flexion where the joint space is reduced and we have to act both upon the posterior slope and the osseous resection of the posterior femoral condyle (Figs. 11.4 and 11.5).

Figs. 11.2 and 11.3 Position the tibial cut guide and connect with a mobile diode to the computer. The height of the resection is based on preoperation planning calculations, its orientation (varus–valgus), guided and checked on the display

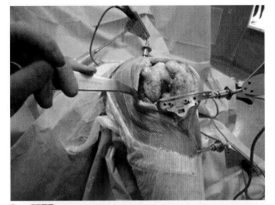

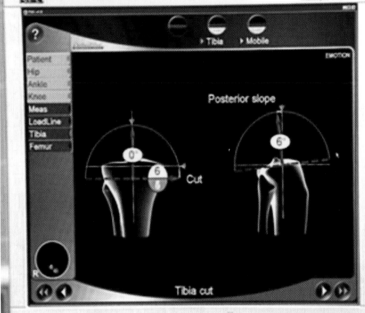

Step 14: Position the femoral trial components and decide on the definitive tibial thickness, basing your decision on the optimum ligament balance in terms of extension and flexion and the mechanical axis, almost to 180°, without procurvatum or recurvatum. Everything is shown on computer by numeric values and visualized by a scheme of the inferior limb.

Step 15: We first implant the two tibial components and then the femoral one; the limb should be extended and compressed securely against the chest of the operator to complete the operation (Figs. 11.6 and 11.7). Finalize recording of data for the personal computerized file card of the patient.

11.5   Personal Experience in Bi-UKR

We have been performing bi-unicompartmental knee replacement since 1999 in very selected cases (less than 5 % of our volume of knee replacement for year). In our indications, all the patients undergoing bi-UKR should have an asymptomatic patellofemoral joint with arthritis less than or equal to Älback grade II. Contraindications include obesity, osteopenia, history of systematic articular disease, significant ligamentous laxity and limb deformity greater than 10°. In our experience, the main aetiology of knee arthritis is posttraumatic mainly in patients younger than 70 years old.

Figs. 11.4 and 11.5 The
latest version of our
navigation system provides
distractors which tense the
ligaments and open the
articular space according to
values expressed in mm

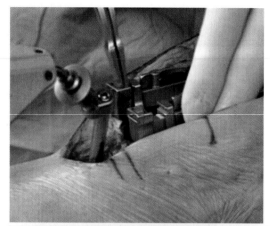

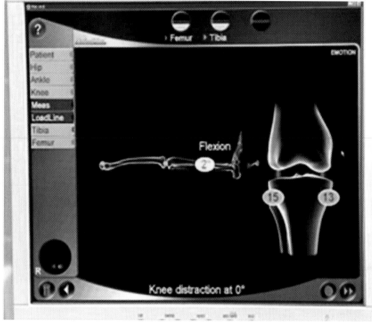

In 2006, we have reviewed, at a minimum follow-up of 3 years (mean: 57.8 months), our experience with these implants in 23 patients enrolled prospectively for a bi-unicompartmental knee replacement [19]. Preoperatively, patients were evaluated with both the WOMAC osteoarthritis index and the Knee Society score. At latest follow-up, the mean WOMAC index was 4 for pain, 1.5 for stiffness and 7.7 for function. The mean Knee Society score was 84.6, a mean functional score of 86.3 was recorded and a mean UKR dedicated outcome score (GIUM) was 78.1 with no abnormal results. All the patients were satisfied with the outcome and would undergo the same procedure again. No implant has required revision. The most common complication occurred intra-operatively. In three cases (12.5 %), an intra-operative fracture of the tibial spines during implantation of the prosthesis possibly related to excessive tension on the anterior cruciate ligament. All fractures were managed successfully with intra-operative internal fixation. This fracture did not adversely affect the final result.

In an attempt to overcome this complication, a more precise computer-assisted technique for bi-UKR has been introduced since 2003 [21] to achieve a well-balanced implant both in extension

Figs. 11.6 and 11.7 Final result with a good alignment of the implants in different planes

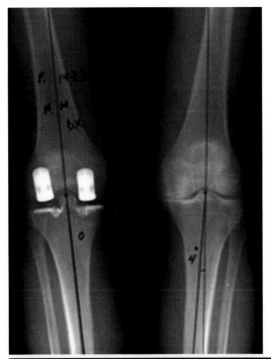

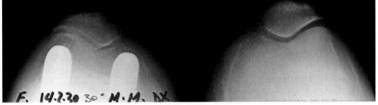

and flexion and with no tension on the ACL tibial insertion.

In 2009, we reviewed, at a minimum follow-up of 2 years (mean: 31.1 months), our experience in navigated bi-unicompartmental knee replacement assessing 16 implants [7]. Every single patient was matched to a similar patient affected by bicompartmental tibiofemoral arthritis who had undergone a computer-assisted TKR between August 2003 and September 2007. There were no statistical significant differences in the surgical time, while the hospital stay was statistically longer in the TKR group. No statistically significant difference was seen in the limb alignment, Knee Society, Functional and GIUM scores between the two groups. Statistically significant better WOMAC function and stiffness indexes were registered for the navigated bi-UKR group. In both the groups, all the implants were positioned within 4° of an ideal hip-knee-ankle (HKA) angle of 180°. No particular complication occurred in both groups even in relation to the navigation, and we did not experience any intraoperative fractures of the tibial spines during implantation of navigated bi-UKRs.

Conclusion

The shifting demographics of patients with localized knee arthritis, including younger, more active patients, is a major impetus for growing interest in conservative surgical alternatives such as UKR and bi-UKRs [22, 30].

The role of minimally invasive techniques for the treatment of knee arthritis continues to evolve towards a concept of "tissue sparing surgery" [6]. The early enthusiasm towards shorter surgical approaches has been mitigated by no permanent advantages together with new complications. Small implants and preserved joint biomechanics could represent a new development in reconstructive surgery, and the approach described in this chapter could be a very attractive approach [2, 6, 10]. Using computer assistance may help the surgeon in reproducing this highly demanding surgery in a standardized technique. The authors strongly believe that this "personalized on time treatment" for each patient according to the severity of the disease using different implant options in association with computer assistance could be one of the most new and interesting improvements in the next years.

References

1. Andriacchi TP, Andersson GB, Fermier RW et al (1980) A study of lower-limb mechanics during stair-climbing. J Bone Joint Surg Am 62(5):749–757
2. Banks SA, Frely BJ, Boniforti F et al (2005) Comparing in vivo kinematics of unicondylar and bi-unicondylar knee replacement. Knee Surg Sports Traumatol Arthrosc 13:551–556
3. Berend KR, Lombardi AV Jr (2005) Avoiding the potential pitfalls of minimally invasive total knee surgery. Orthopedics 28(11):1326–1330
4. Cloutier JM, Sabouret P, Deghrar A (1999) Total knee arthroplasty with retention of both cruciate ligaments. A nine to eleven-year follow-up study. J Bone Joint Surg Am 81(5):697–702
5. Confalonieri N, Manzotti A (2005) Computer assisted bi-unicompartmental knee replacement. Int J Med Robot Comput Assist Surg 1(4):1–6
6. Confalonieri N, Manzotti A (2006) Tissue-sparing surgery with the bi-unicompartmental knee prosthesis: retrospective study with minimum follow-up of 36 months. J Orthop Traumatol 7:108–112
7. Confalonieri N, Manzotti A, Cerveri P et al (2009) Bi-unicompartmental versus total knee arthroplasty: a matched paired study with early clinical results. Arch Orthop Trauma Surg 129(9):1157–1163
8. Dalury DF, Dennis DA (2005) Mini-incision total knee arthroplasty can increase risk of component malalignment. Clin Orthop Relat Res 440:77–81
9. Eickmann TH, Collier MB, Sukezaki F et al (2006) Survival of medial unicondylar arthroplasties placed by one surgeon 1984–1998. Clin Orthop Relat Res 17:167–175
10. Fuchs S, Tibesku CO, Frisse D et al (2005) Clinical and functional of uni-and bicondylar sledge prostheses. Knee Surg Sports Traumatol Arthrosc 13:197–202
11. Goodfellow JW, O'Connor J (1986) Clinical results of the Oxford knee. Surface arthroplasty of the tibiofem-oral joint with a meniscal bearing prosthesis. Clin Orthop Relat Res (205):21–42
12. Haas SB, Cook S, Beksac B (2004) Minimally invasive total knee replacement through a mini midvastus approach: a comparative study. Clin Orthop Relat Res (428):68-73
13. Huang TW, Hsu WH, Peng KT et al (2011) Total knee arthroplasty with use of computer-assisted navigation compared with conventional guiding systems in the same patient: radiographic results in Asian patients. J Bone Joint Surg Am 93(13):1197–1202
14. Jenny JY (2005) Navigated unicompartmental knee replacement. Orthopedics 28(10 Suppl):s1263–s1267
15. Jung KA, Kim SJ, Lee SC et al (2010) Accuracy of implantation during computer-assisted minimally invasive Oxford unicompartmental knee arthroplasty: a comparison with a conventional instrumented technique. Knee 17(6):387–391
16. Khan MM, Khan MW, Al-Harbi HH et al (2011) Assessing short-term functional outcomes and knee alignment of computer-assisted navigated total knee arthroplasty. J Arthroplasty 27(2):271–277
17. Konyves A, Willis-Owen CA, Spriggins AJ (2010) The long-term benefit of computer-assisted surgical navigation in unicompartmental knee arthroplasty. J Orthop Surg Res 5:94
18. Laskin RS (2005) Minimally invasive total knee arthroplasty: the results justify its use. Clin Orthop Relat Res 440:54–59
19. Lewallen DG, Bryan RS, Peterson LF (1984) Polycentric total knee arthroplasty. A ten-year follow-up study. J Bone Joint Surg Am 66(8):1211–1218
20. Lonner JH (2006) Minimally invasive approaches to total knee arthroplasty: results. Am J Orthop 35(7 Suppl):27–33
21. Lonner JH (2009) Modular bicompartmental knee arthroplasty with robotic arm assistance. Am J Orthop (Belle Mead NJ) 38(2 Suppl):28–31
22. Morrison TA, Nyce JD, Macaulay WB et al (2011) Early adverse results with bicompartmental knee arthroplasty a prospective cohort comparison to total knee arthroplasty. J Arthroplasty 26(6 Suppl):35–39
23. O'Rourke MR, Gardner JJ, Callaghan JJ et al (2005) The John Insall Award: unicompartmental knee replacement: a minimum twenty-one-year follow-up, end-result study. Clin Orthop Relat Res 440:27–37
24. Pang HN, Yeo SJ, Chong HC et al (2011) Computer-assisted gap balancing technique improves outcome in total knee arthroplasty, compared with conventional measured resection technique. Knee Surg Sports Traumatol Arthrosc 19(9):1496–1503
25. Parratte S, Pauly V, Aubaniac JM et al (2010) Survival of bicompartmental knee arthroplasty at 5 to 23 years. Clin Orthop Relat Res 468(1):64–72
26. Stewart HD, Newton G (1992) Long-term results of the Manchester knee. Surface arthroplasty of the tibiofemoral joint. Clin Orthop Relat Res (278):138–146

27. Stiehl JB, Komistek RD, Cloutier JM et al (2000) The cruciate ligaments in total knee arthroplasty: a kinematic analysis of 2 total knee arthroplasties. J Arthroplasty 15(5):545–550
28. Swanson AB, Swanson GD, Powers T et al (1985) Unicompartmental and bicompartmental arthroplasty of the knee with a finned metal tibial-plateau implant. J Bone Joint Surg Am 67(8):1175–1182
29. Swienckowski JJ, Pennington DW (2004) Unicompartmental knee arthroplasty in patients sixty years of age or younger. J Bone Joint Surg Am 86-A(Suppl 1 (Pt 2)):131–142
30. Tria AJ Jr (2010) Bicompartmental arthroplasty of the knee. Instr Course Lect 59:61–73
31. Weale AE, Halabi OA, Jones PW et al (2001) Perceptions of out-comes after unicompartmental and total knee replacements. Clin Orthop 382: 143–153
32. Zhang GQ, Chen JY, Chai W et al (2011) Comparison between computer-assisted-navigation and conventional total knee arthroplasties in patients undergoing simultaneous bilateral procedures: a randomized clinical trial. J Bone Joint Surg Am 93(13): 1190–1196

Cruciate Ligament Reconstruction: Kinematic Evaluation

12

Stefano Zaffagnini, Simone Bignozzi,
Nicola Lopomo, F. Iacono, M.P. Neri, Alberto Grassi,
T. Roberti Di Sarsina, and Maurilio Marcacci

12.1 Introduction

CAS in anterior cruciate ligament (ACL) reconstruction has now completed over 15 years of research. The first publications started in the second half of the 1990s [34]. The main goal

S. Zaffagnini (✉) • F. Iacono • M. Marcacci
Laboratorio di Biomeccanica e Innovazione Tecnologica,
Istituto Ortopedico Rizzoli, via di Barbiano 1/10,
Bologna, 40136, Italy

Clinica Ortopedica e Traumatologica III,
Istituto Ortopedico Rizzoli, via di Barbiano 1/10,
Bologna, 40136, Italy
e-mail: s.zaffagnini@biomec.ior.it;
m.marcacci@biomec.ior.it

S. Bignozzi
Laboratorio di Biomeccanica e Innovazione Tecnologica,
Istituto Ortopedico Rizzoli,
via di Barbiano 1/10, Bologna, 40136, Italy

Orthokey LLC, Lewes, DE, USA
e-mail: s.bignozzi@biomec.ior.it

N. Lopomo
Laboratorio di Biomeccanica e Innovazione Tecnologica,
Istituto Ortopedico Rizzoli, via di Barbiano 1/10,
Bologna, 40136, Italy

Laboratorio di NanoBiotecnologie – NaBi,
Istituto Ortopedico Rizzoli, Bologna, Italy
e-mail: n.lopomo@biomec.ior.it

M.P. Neri • A. Grassi • T.R. Di Sarsina
Laboratorio di Biomeccanica e Innovazione Tecnologica,
Istituto Ortopedico Rizzoli,
via di Barbiano 1/10, Bologna, 40136, Italy

of the navigated procedures was to improve the correct position of the graft, using anatomical references and graft isometry during the range of motion, considering that 70–80 % of the complications were due to malpositioned tunnels [10].

The purpose of these first systems was to augment the information given to the surgeon, in order to better identify the anatomical landmarks that were difficult to recognize in an arthroscopic setup. The efficacy of this enhanced information given by computer-based ACL reconstruction was evaluated in clinical use by Dessenne et al. [1, 10] who demonstrated the feasibility of navigation in routine clinical setup.

More recently, thanks to more surgeon-friendly systems and to the evolution of software for computer-based ACL surgery, there has been an increased interest in this field. This development includes the possibility of performing stability testing, including rotational and translational measurements or decomposition of complex clinical tests such as the pivot shift [4], allowing better evaluation of the effect of different surgical procedures on the stability of the knee and to better describe patients' specific laxity [27]. The augmented performance of navigation systems allows one to use this methodology to assess the performance of new and more complex reconstructive surgical techniques, like double bundle. In fact, starting in 2005, there has been a big number of articles on navigated ACL as well as on anatomical double-bundle reconstruction techniques.

F. Catani, S. Zaffagnini (eds.), *Knee Surgery using Computer Assisted Surgery and Robotics*,
DOI 10.1007/978-3-642-31430-8_12, © ESSKA 2013

The usefulness of navigation for the kinematic evaluation of ACL reconstruction can be clearly expressed by the words of Lord Kelvin Thompson: "I often say that when you can measure what you are speaking about, and express it in numbers, you know something about it; but when you cannot measure it, when you cannot express it in numbers, your knowledge is of a meagre and unsatisfactory kind" [35] which can be summarized in "If it can be measured, it can be improved." This philosophy fully adapts to the concept of computer-assisted surgery (CAS). With the help of this technology over the last few years, the knowledge about anatomy and kinematics of the anterior cruciate ligament (ACL) has improved dramatically.

At present, instrumental evaluation during surgery, with the use of navigation systems, remains the more accurate procedure; therefore, several clinical studies have evaluated the effect of different surgical techniques to joint kinematics at time zero.

12.2   Kinematic Evaluation Using CAS

The use of navigation for kinematic evaluation has been evaluated since 2000, but interest in this feature of navigation grew after 2005 in conjunction with the evaluation of double-bundle technique. In vitro and in vivo studies confirmed its repeatability [23, 24, 25, 36] and reliability [28]. Correlation with kinematic acquisition and clinical classification of complex tests like the pivot shift was also demonstrated [2, 5, 9, 18].

Pearle et al. [28] on a controlled laboratory setup, with the help of a robotic system, demonstrated the reliability of an image-free navigation system. They concluded that surgical navigation is a precise intraoperative tool to quantify knee stability examination and may help delineate pathologic multiplanar or coupled knee motions, particularly in the setting of complex rotatory instability patterns. The repeatability of load application during clinical stability testing remains problematic.

The same results were found by Kendoff et al. [16] on a cadaver setup with intact and dissected ACL reconstruction. In addition to a comparison between KT1000 and navigation, they also compared a mechanical goniometer with navigated measurements for tibial rotation, finding no differences in the two methodologies.

While in a laboratory setup, navigation technology has been demonstrated to be reliable, understanding the usability of instrumented CAS manual test in the operating room remained fundamental to comprehending the usability of navigation technology in assessing knee laxity intraoperatively. In fact in vivo results of navigated kinematic tests during surgery are not affected only by the nominal accuracy of localizing technology or the experimental setup but also by other external factors, such as surgeon-subjective and manually applied loads, limb positioning during testing, and patients' specific laxity.

Our first research works were aimed in characterizing the intraoperative acquisition protocol [24, 25, 36], in order to be aware of all possible pitfalls and errors that could jeopardize the results of kinematic studies; therefore, a more accurate evaluation of the in vivo kinematic evaluation was performed. We assessed the reliability of navigation technology to quantify knee laxity in in vivo setup, evaluating intraobserver reliability and interobserver repeatability and correlation with manual instrumental evaluation, where possible, as used in clinical routine.

The first clinical application of kinematic ACL evaluation was performed in our institute in 2005 [36]. The purpose of our research was to optimize the intraoperative setup for the kinematic evaluation of the knee at time zero, trying to define a system that could be used routinely and that could give a global description of the joint laxities. The study was performed on 15 patients in order to analyze the capability of this new CAS procedure. The capability of the protocol was studied, by analyzing the accuracy and repeatability of the tests, ergonomics of the setup, time taken, and interaction with the surgical steps.

The repeatability of laxity computed from manual tests at maximum forces showed an average standard deviation of 0.78° for varus–valgus (VV) rotation, 1.83° for internal–external (IE) rotation, and 0.88 mm for anteroposterior (AP) translation. Repeatability tests of the neutral position used during kinematic tests were lower than 1 mm for all flexion angles. Average standard deviation in the tibia orientation was lower than 3° for tests at 0° and 30° of flexion and lower than 4° for tests at 90° of flexion. Navigation was practicable and reliable, also in clinical setup and for kinematic evaluation of ACL reconstruction.

12.3 Pivot Shift

While the primary control in the AP direction of the native ACL and of the reconstructed graft has been demonstrated to be effective, the controversial results obtained with IE rotation may be related to the fact that the ACL has a secondary control for this laxity or that other structures of the knee joint may be involved in the definition of the constitutional laxity of the patient. Results shown by Steckel et al. [33] on the contribution of AM and PL bundles in vitro, of native ACL in controlling tibial translation and rotation, highlight that current clinical knee laxity measurements may not be suited for detecting subtle changes such as PL bundle deficiency in the ACL anatomy.

Recently, Bull et al. [4] reported that these specific clinical procedures allow assessing two different types of joint instability: static and dynamic instability. The static measurement is in general associated with uniplanar laxity tests. On the other hand, the dynamic instability of the knee is commonly presented as symptoms, thus clinical tests try to mimic these symptoms by controlling loads/movements of the joint. For this reason several authors have recently focused on the analysis of the pivot-shift test, trying to quantify and describe the dynamic laxity of the joint.

Amis et al. [5], Colombet et al. [9], and Ishibashi et al. [14] described the envelope of passive motion of the tibia during a pivot-shift test before and after anterior cruciate ligament reconstruction, finding consistent reductions

during the pivot shift as a combination of external tibial rotation and posterior tibial translation.

Hoshino et al. [13], in an office setup, and Lane et al. [18], intraoperatively, found that the increase of tibial anterior translation and acceleration of subsequent posterior translation could be detected in knees with a positive pivot-shift result, and this increase was correlated to clinical grading. Similar experiences with the electromagnetic tracking system were reported by Kubo et al. [17].

12.4 Description of Navigated Surgery

The computer-assisted operation is performed with a standard approach and equipment; typically, surgery is performed under general or spinal anesthesia, with the patient placed in a supine position on the operating table. Arthroscopic portals are created, and evaluation of the ACL lesion can be performed.

At this point tibial and femoral navigated references can be fixed with surgical wires. There is no indication for the positioning of the reference tools; they can be inserted within the skin incision or percutaneously. Care must be taken in order to allow complete visibility of the tools during the navigated steps of surgery without interfering with the surgical procedure. Typically, the tibial reference array is fixed in the approach for tendon harvesting or on the distal tibia, oriented distally with respect to the knee, while the femoral array is inserted above the end of medial condyle, distally oriented with respect to the knee (Fig. 12.1).

After reference fixation the registration of the patient's anatomy is performed with a navigated pointer. The registration phase consists of the acquisition of anatomical landmarks, percutaneously and arthroscopically, in order to identify anatomical coordinate systems. Typically, on the tibia, the following points are digitized: medial and lateral malleoli, most medial and lateral points on the plateaus, external tunnel exit holes, percutaneously; internal tunnel holes, ACL

Fig. 12.1 Execution of drawer preoperative test with a navigation system. Tibial and femoral reference arrays are positioned medially, far from the surgical area

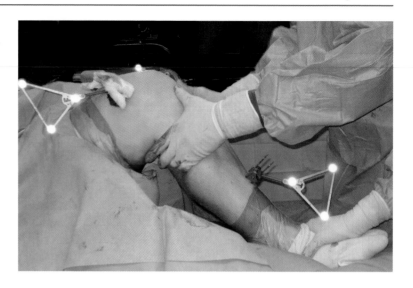

insertions, and the most distal points on medial and lateral plateaus, arthroscopically. On the femur the following points are digitized: femoral head, by leg pivoting; medial and lateral epicondyles and lateral tunnel exit hole, percutaneously; and most distal points on medial and lateral condyles, ACL insertions, and internal tunnel exit hole, arthroscopically.

After registration it is possible to perform the preoperative kinematic tests. During tests the leg is flexed with the foot laid on the operating table; the thigh is held during tests by an assistant. Kinematic acquisitions are performed according to clinical practice and may include passive range of motion (PROM), VV rotation at 0° and 30° of flexion, at maximum force; IE rotation at 30° and 90° of flexion, at maximum force; AP 18° and 90° of flexion at maximum force; and pivot-shift test.

12.5   Our Clinical Experience

To evaluate the joint laxity and kinematics, we used an optical navigation system (BLU-IGS, Orthokey, Delaware) with software focused in kinematic acquisitions (KLEE, Orthokey, Delaware). This system applied in the OR allowed us to perform different studies. Nearly 200 cases have been performed since 2004, with different reconstructive techniques.

Clinical studies included the evaluation of knee laxity before and after ACL reconstruction with two different surgical techniques utilized at our institute: the first technique is a hamstring double bundle with one tibial tunnel, over-the-top passage for the PL bundle and femoral tunnel passage for the AM bundle [20, 22] (Fig. 12.2a). The second technique is an intra-articular hamstring single bundle with over-the-top passage and additional extra-articular lateral plasty [21] (Fig. 12.2b).

Comparison of AP, VV, and IE laxities between the two techniques was performed, and we found no statistical difference ($P>0.05$) for all laxity tests (Fig. 12.3).

12.6   Antero-Medial Instabilities

More interesting results were obtained evaluating patients operated on with both techniques, with different preoperative conditions. We wondered whether it was possible to identify some residual laxity in patients with combined chronic ACL and MCL lesions, compared to patients with pure ACL lesion [37]. Patients were prospectively classified in two groups: patients with an isolated ACL lesion were used as control group, (group I) and patients with grade II injury of the medial collateral ligament combined with ACL lesion were used as a study group (group II).

Fig. 12.2 Double-bundle over-the-top hamstring reconstruction (**a**) and single-bundle over-the-top plus extra-articular plasty (**b**)

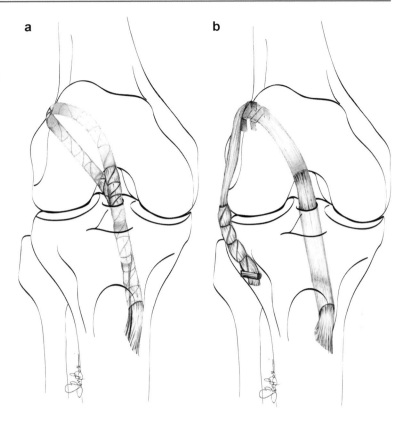

Fig. 12.3 Results of laxity tests for hamstring over-the-top double-bundle and single-bundle plus lateral plasty

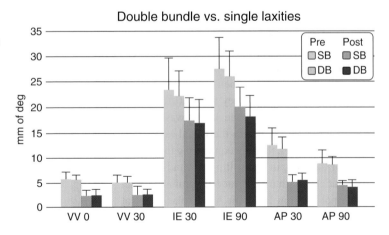

Clinical evaluation was performed using the International Knee Documentation Committee (IKDC) knee ligament standard evaluation form. Fifty seven patients were included in the study, 37 patients were put in group I, and 20 patients in group II. Age, gender distribution, and time from injury to surgery were similar in the two groups. Preoperative laxities were different in both groups for VV and AP tests (Fig. 12.4).

Postoperative AP comparison has shown that, at 90° of flexion, some residual laxity remained in patients with combined injuries with respect to patients with isolated ACL lesion. On the other hand, at 30° of flexion the postoperative laxities were not statistically different.

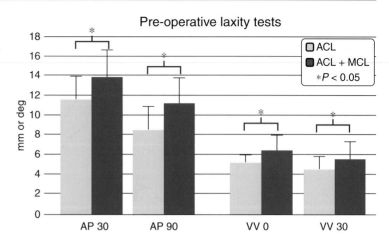

Fig. 12.4 Preoperative laxities in patients with pure ACL lesion and patients with combined ACL and MCL strain

Our findings agree with those of Sakane et al. [30] and Shapiro et al. [32] who reported in vitro that the role of the MCL during AP loading was minimal toward extension but became clinically more important when the knee was flexed.

Similar patterns of results were found for VV tests: residual laxity remained for patients with an ACL lesion with MCL sprain, compared with patients with pure ACL lesions, at 30° of flexion, while in extension the graft was able to control the rotation since no statistical difference between the two groups was found. Our results agree with the findings of Seering et al. [31] who reported that in vitro the MCL created a larger resistive moment when the specimens were at 30° of flexion than it did when they were at full extension. The reduction of knee laxity was slightly greater for group II, where the initial laxity was statistically higher, thereby confirming the importance of the ACL in controlling AP and VV laxities. Patients with MCL grade II sprains have an additional 1.3-mm laxity in AP displacement at 90° of flexion and 1° in VV rotation at 30° in comparison with patients with ACL injury only, which was detectable with the navigated kinematic evaluation.

12.7 Extra-Articular Lateral Plasty

Navigation is not only able to evaluate with high accuracy uniplanar laxities, like AP translations or VV and IE rotations, but it can be used for more detailed kinematic analyses like the evaluation of AP translation in medial and lateral compartments or the decomposition of rotations and translations during the pivot-shift test. Evaluation of translation in the two tibial compartments resulted in the useful evaluation of the effect of the extra-articular lateral plasty in controlling joint laxity [3]. In in vivo and in vitro studies, there was no general consensus about the effect of the additional extra-articular procedure to knee laxity. These studies were in agreement only in indicating that there was a load sharing between the intra and extra-articular portions and, in particular, that the load on the ACL graft diminished with knee extension [6, 11, 12, 19, 26]. The effect of this load sharing remains a matter of debate.

We wanted to measure the effect of an additional extra-articular procedure, adding a single-bundle hamstring over-the-top ACL reconstruction, evaluating coupled tibial translation during the Lachman and drawer test. We evaluated 28 patients with a computer-assisted kinematic evaluation protocol, excluding from the study patients with associated ligament tears or meniscal damages.

After tibial bone tunnel drilling, but before graft insertion, the operating surgeon performed standard clinical tests at maximum force to evaluate the AP joint laxities, during Lachman and drawer tests, in the ACL-deficient knee. A single-bundle (SB) graft was inserted into the tibial tunnel, fixed with two staples on the femur in the over-the-top position, and the laxity tests were

Fig. 12.5 Tibia displacement during Lachman and drawer tests, in medial central and lateral compartments, for ACL deficient (PRE), single-bundle reconstruction (SB), and after extra-articular procedure (SB + EA)

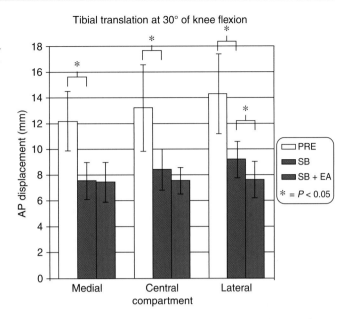

repeated. After this step the additional extra-articular (EA) procedure was executed, passing the remaining part of the graft under the fascia lata to reach Gerdy's tubercle where it was fixed with another staple. Laxity tests were repeated again.

In order to quantify the effect of the SB graft and of the EA procedure, we compared the knee laxity of the ACL-deficient knee with laxity obtained after SB fixation and EA fixation, respectively (Fig. 12.5).

At 30° of flexion the SB graft reduced tibial displacement in both compartments (5 mm). Laxity on the medial plateau was not reduced using the EA procedure ($P = 0.741$), while on the lateral plateau, the reduction was of about 2 mm ($P = 0.015$).

At 90° of flexion laxity on the medial plateau was slightly reduced by SB graft (2 mm), while on the lateral plateau, the reduction greater (5 mm). The additional extra-articular procedure causes a further significant reduction of knee laxity of about 1 mm ($P < 0.05$) in both compartments. Significant reduction was also noted for varus–valgus laxity, while the extra-articular procedure was not able to control rotational laxity (Fig. 12.6).

We have found that, despite the SB, hamstring graft has a primary role in reducing the knee laxity; an extra-articular procedure, added to the graft, is effective in further controlling the laxity: near extension, the SB graft reduces AP translation while the extra-articular procedure controls internal rotation, reducing by 1.6 mm the translation of lateral tibial compartment. This result shows that the coupled tibial translation, which is not controlled by SB graft, is reduced by the EA procedure. In contrast, in flexion, the SB graft reduces coupled AP translation in both compartments, while the extra-articular procedure contributes to controlling tibial translation, reducing laxity by 1 mm in both compartments.

Our results confirm the in vitro studies of Engebresten et al. [12] about subluxation of lateral plateaus prevention performed by the EA procedure. Moreover, the control of the lateral compartment at 30° may explain the reduction of "giving way" sensation reported by Jensen et al.[15] and the good clinical outcome, observed in clinical studies, using this combined procedure[20, 22].

12.8 Anatomical Double Bundle

Between September 2007 and April 2008, 18 patients, with isolated anterior cruciate ligament injury, were operated on with an anatomical

Fig. 12.6 Tibial rotations (varus–valgus and internal–external) for ACL deficient (PRE), single-bundle reconstruction (SB), and after extra-articular procedure (SB+EA)

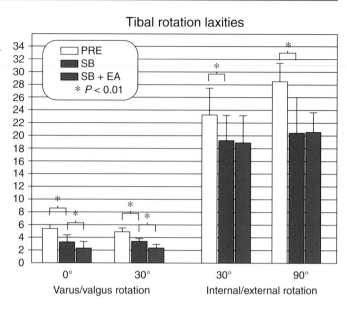

double-bundle hamstring technique as described by Chhabra et al. [7];11 patients had a preoperative IKDC C score and 7 had a D score.

The operating surgeon performed manually clinical tests at maximum force, before and after the reconstruction. Tests consisted of VV stress at 0° and 30° of flexion, IE stress at 30° and 90° of flexion, Lachman test (AP 30), drawer test (AP 90), and pivot-shift test.

For the pivot-shift test, we analyzed laxity of the joint as the decomposition of two different parameters with respect to flexion angle: AP translation and IE rotation. For each decomposition, we evaluated the areas included by the curves obtained during the test (the "hysteresis" of the joint due to positive pivot shift) as dynamic joint laxity. Within those curves we also identified the highest or lowest peaks obtained and recorded at which angle they occur, to describe static laxity during test. A typical result of pivot-shift kinematic decomposition in AP translation, with BLU-IGS software, is shown in Fig. 12.7.

All laxities were significantly reduced by the reconstruction. In particular, anterior laxity showed a great reduction, which was highly significant ($P<0.0001$) during Lachman and

drawer tests. VV rotation showed a highly significant reduction ($P<0.0001$) both in extension and at 30° of flexion. The reduction of IE rotation even if significant ($P<0.01$) was less compared to the other tests (Fig. 12.8).

These results are in agreement with results reported by Bull et al. [4] and Colombet et al. [8] which indicate this test as more discriminating of the effect of the two bundles in controlling the dynamic instability of the knee. Peak analysis showed that maximum laxity is always reached, between 20° and 30° of flexion. Both AP translations and IE rotation peaks were significantly reduced ($P<0.0001$, Fig. 12.9).

The comparison between preoperative and postoperative laxity areas (Fig. 12.10) highlighted a huge recovery of the dynamic stability of the joint. Both AP and IE areas showed a high reduction ($P<0.0001$). In our results pivot-shift AP and IE areas not only showed a high statistical difference between preoperative and postoperative laxities but also correlated with the preoperative IKDC score, as reported by Hoshino et al. [13] with a large number of patients. In patients with IKDC grade C, the area during pivot shift was significantly larger, in ACL deficient knees, compared to patients graded D

Fig. 12.7 Result of pivot-shift test with BLU-IGS system (Orthokey, Lewes, Delaware). Screen shows anteroposterior translation during pivot-shift maneuver. On the left it is possible to read the value of laxity peak around 30° (15.5 pre-op and 4.0 post-op); in the graph it is possible to evaluate the envelope of passive motion of tibia (*red pre-op, green post-op*)

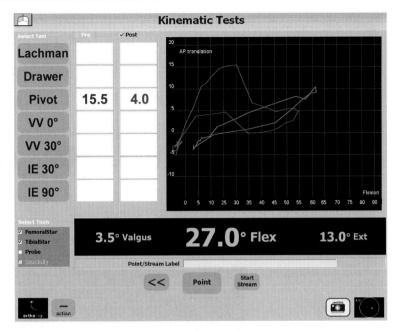

Fig. 12.8 Results of static laxity test before and after reconstruction for anatomical double-bundle reconstruction

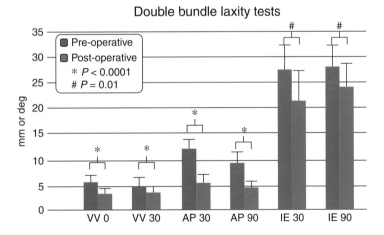

(Fig. 12.11). This difference was not found after reconstruction.

This type of measurement can reflect the feeling reported by the surgeon during manual clinical test, quantifying and summarizing joint laxity in all ranges of flexion during pivot shift, and therefore it can be used to clinically quantify associated or constitutional rotatory instabilities of the knee.

We found no correlation between the laxities obtained during static tests and pivot-shift test. This may explain the contradictory results found in the literature analyzing joint laxity with different methods. Primary or coupled IE rotations may be not sufficient in describing the effect of two grafts in reducing knee laxity.

From an anatomical point of view, the evaluation of graft positioning, shown in Fig. 12.12, clearly illustrates how reconstructive grafts, if correctly positioned, have similar position patterns as the native ACL bundles as defined in

Fig. 12.9 Average peaks of laxity during pivot-shift test

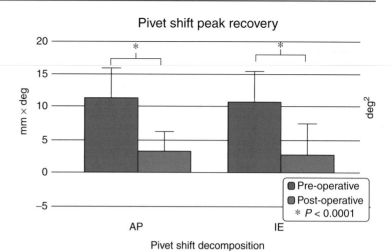

Fig. 12.10 Description of area obtained from the anteroposterior tibial translation during the pivot-shift test

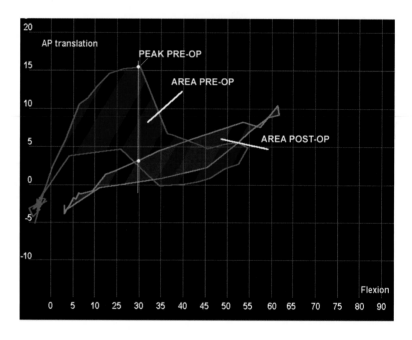

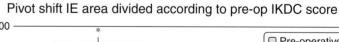

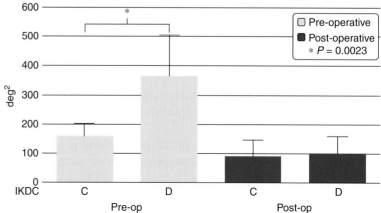

Fig. 12.11 Area of dynamic laxity in anteroposterior direction during pivot-shift test, in patients divided according to IKDC score (mean ± standard error)

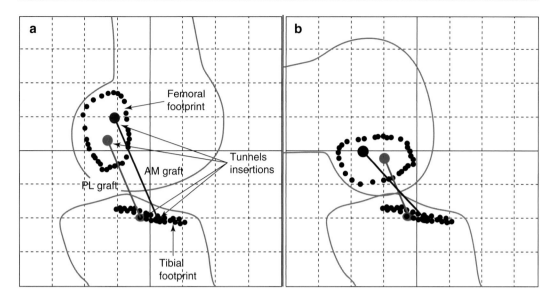

Fig. 12.12 Acquired points on ACL insertions showed on sagittal view, with leg in extension (**a**) and in flexion (**b**). Dots represent the acquisitions done on patient. Tibial and femoral shapes have been superimposed for clarification

Fig. 12.13 AM bundle and PL bundle elongations during passive range of motion

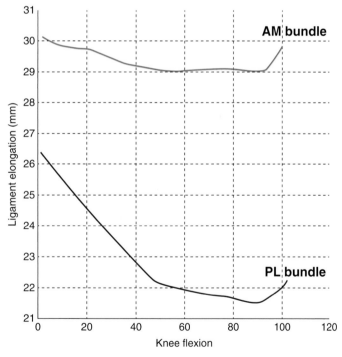

previous anatomical studies [7, 29, 38], being parallel in extension and crossed in flexion. The analysis of bundle elongation during PROM has shown that there are little variations in AM bundle length, while PL bundles shortened during flexion (Fig. 12.13).

Conclusions

With the help of less invasive and image-free systems in the last 15 years, the knowledge about anatomy and kinematics of the ACL has improved dramatically. The possibility to describe with high precision insertion areas of the different bundles of the ACL and to measure correct tunnel positioning intraoperatively can lead to reduced numbers of outliers during surgery, improving the final surgical outcome.

However, the use of surgical navigation for tunnel placement remains limited because the targets and tolerances for this optimal graft positioning are still poorly understood. With the introduction of kinematic evaluation, it becomes possible to quantify at time zero the effect of the surgery in controlling knee laxity.

Initial navigated knee-stability measurements included standard uniplanar tests such as the Lachman test, the anterior drawer test, and the maximal internal and external rotation at various flexion angles. More recent iterations of the navigated stability examination have included more complex pathologic movements, such as those that occur in the pivot-shift phenomenon, leading to a complete quantification of clinical laxity.

These data begin to define surgical parameters for various ACL reconstruction techniques. With this information available intraoperatively, it is now possible to think about the "on demand" surgery, where quantitative data can help to refine the surgical outcome. The principles for the on-demand surgery require description of the pathology that needs to move outside the operating room. More recently, some efforts have been made in order to quantify, in an office setup, joint laxity [13].

References

1. Bernsmann K, Rosenthal A, Sati M et al (2001) Using the cas (computer-assisted surgery) system in arthroscopic cruciate ligament surgery–adaptation and application in clinical practice. Z Orthop Ihre Grenzgeb 139:346–351
2. Bignozzi S, Zaffagnini S, Lopomo N et al (2009) Clinical relevance of static and dynamic tests after anatomical double-bundle ACL reconstruction. Knee Surg Sports Traumatol Arthrosc 18:37–42
3. Bignozzi S, Zaffagnini S, Lopomo N et al (2009) Does a lateral plasty control coupled translation during antero-posterior stress in single-bundle ACL reconstruction? an in vivo study. Knee Surg Sports Traumatol Arthrosc 17:65–70
4. Bull AM, Andersen HN, Basso O et al (1999) Incidence and mechanism of the pivot shift. An in vitro study. Clin Orthop Relat Res 363:219–231
5. Bull AMJ, Earnshaw PH, Smith A et al (2002) Intraoperative measurement of knee kinematics in reconstruction of the anterior cruciate ligament. J Bone Joint Surg Br 84:1075–1081
6. Carson WGJ (1988) The role of lateral extra-articular procedures for anterolateral rotatory instability. Clin Sports Med 7:751–772
7. Chhabra A, Starman JS, Ferretti M et al (2006) Anatomic, radiographic, biomechanical, and kinematic evaluation of the anterior cruciate ligament and its two functional bundles. J Bone Joint Surg Am 88(Suppl 4):2–10
8. Colombet PD, Robinson JR (2008) Computer-assisted, anatomic, double-bundle anterior cruciate ligament reconstruction. Arthroscopy 24:1152–1160
9. Colombet P, Robinson J, Christel P et al (2007) Using navigation to measure rotation kinematics during ACL reconstruction. Clin Orthop Relat Res 454:59–65
10. Dessenne V, Lavallée S, Julliard R et al (1995) Computer-assisted knee anterior cruciate ligament reconstruction: first clinical tests. J Image Guid Surg 1:59–64
11. Draganich LF, Reider B, Ling M et al (1990) An in vitro study of an intraarticular and extraarticular reconstruction in the anterior cruciate ligament deficient knee. Am J Sports Med 18:262–266
12. Engebretsen L, Lew WD, Lewis JL et al (1990) The effect of an iliotibial tenodesis on intraarticular graft forces and knee joint motion. Am J Sports Med 18:169–176
13. Hoshino Y, Kuroda R, Nagamune K et al (2007) In vivo measurement of the pivot-shift test in the anterior cruciate ligament-deficient knee using an electromagnetic device. Am J Sports Med 35:1098–1104
14. Ishibashi Y, Tsuda E, Yamamoto Y et al (2009) Navigation evaluation of the pivot-shift phenomenon during double-bundle anterior cruciate ligament reconstruction: is the posterolateral bundle more important? Arthroscopy 25:488–495
15. Jensen JE, Slocum DB, Larson RL et al (1983) Reconstruction procedures for anterior cruciate ligament insufficiency: a computer analysis of clinical results. Am J Sports Med 11:240–248
16. Kendoff D, Meller R, Citak M et al (2007) Navigation in ACL reconstruction – comparison with conventional measurement tools. Technol Health Care 15:221–230
17. Kubo S, Muratsu H, Yoshiya S et al (2007) Reliability and usefulness of a new in vivo measurement system of the pivot shift. Clin Orthop Relat Res 454:54–58

18. Lane CG, Warren RF, Stanford FC et al (2008) In vivo analysis of the pivot shift phenomenon during computer navigated ACL reconstruction. Knee Surg Sports Traumatol Arthrosc 16:487–492
19. Lobenhoffer P, Posel P, Witt S et al (1987) Distal femoral fixation of the iliotibial tract. Arch Orthop Trauma Surg 106:285–290
20. Marcacci M, Molgora AP, Zaffagnini S et al (2003) Anatomic double-bundle anterior cruciate ligament reconstruction with hamstrings. Arthroscopy 19: 540–546
21. Marcacci M, Zaffagnini S, Iacono F et al (1998) Arthroscopic intra- and extra-articular anterior cruciate ligament reconstruction with gracilis and semitendinosus tendons. Knee Surg Sports Traumatol Arthrosc 6:68–75
22. Marcacci M, Zaffagnini S, Iacono F et al (2003) Intra- and extra-articular anterior cruciate ligament reconstruction utilizing autogeneous semitendinosus and gracilis tendons: 5-year clinical results. Knee Surg Sports Traumatol Arthrosc 11:2–8
23. Martelli S, Zaffagnini S, Bignozzi S et al (2006) Validation of a new protocol for computer-assisted evaluation of kinematics of double-bundle ACL reconstruction. Clin Biomech (Bristol, Avon) 21:279–287
24. Martelli S, Zaffagnini S, Bignozzi S et al (2007) Description and validation of a navigation system for intra-operative evaluation of knee laxity. Comput Aided Surg 12:181–188
25. Martelli S, Zaffagnini S, Bignozzi S et al (2007) KIN-Nav navigation system for kinematic assessment in anterior cruciate ligament reconstruction: features, use, and perspectives. Proc Inst Mech Eng H 221: 725–737
26. O'Brien SJ, Warren RF, Wickiewicz TL et al (1991) The iliotibial band lateral sling procedure and its effect on the results of anterior cruciate ligament reconstruction. Am J Sports Med 19:21–24; discussion 24–25
27. Pearle AD, Kendoff D, Musahl V et al (2009) The pivot-shift phenomenon during computer-assisted anterior cruciate ligament reconstruction. J Bone Joint Surg Am 91(Suppl 1):115–118
28. Pearle AD, Solomon DJ, Wanich T et al (2007) Reliability of navigated knee stability examination: a cadaveric evaluation. Am J Sports Med 35: 1315–1320
29. Robinson J, Stanford FC, Kendoff D et al (2009) Replication of the range of native anterior cruciate ligament fiber length change behavior achieved by different grafts: measurement using computer-assisted navigation. Am J Sports Med 37:1406–1411
30. Sakane M, Livesay GA, Fox RJ et al (1999) Relative contribution of the ACL, MCL, and bony contact to the anterior stability of the knee. Knee Surg Sports Traumatol Arthrosc 7:93–97
31. Seering WP, Piziali RL, Nagel DA et al (1980) The function of the primary ligaments of the knee in varus-valgus and axial rotation. J Biomech 13: 785–794
32. Shapiro MS, Markolf KL, Finerman GA et al (1991) The effect of section of the medial collateral ligament on force generated in the anterior cruciate ligament. J Bone Joint Surg Am 73:248–256
33. Steckel H, Murtha PE, Costic RS et al (2007) Computer evaluation of kinematics of anterior cruciate ligament reconstructions. Clin Orthop Relat Res 463:37–42
34. Wetzler M, Bartolozzi A, Gillespie M et al (1996) Revision anterior cruciate ligament reconstruction. Operat Tech Orthop 6:181–189
35. William TS (1889) Popular lectures and addresses. Macmillan and Co., London
36. Zaffagnini S, Bignozzi S, Martelli S et al (2006) New intraoperative protocol for kinematic evaluation of ACL reconstruction: preliminary results. Knee Surg Sports Traumatol Arthrosc 14:811–816
37. Zaffagnini S, Bignozzi S, Martelli S et al (2007) Does ACL reconstruction restore knee stability in combined lesions?: an in vivo study. Clin Orthop Relat Res 454: 95–99
38. Zelle BA, Vidal AF, Brucker PU et al (2007) Double-bundle reconstruction of the anterior cruciate ligament: anatomic and biomechanical rationale. J Am Acad Orthop Surg 15:87–96

Anterior Cruciate Ligament Reconstruction: Isometric Positioning

13

Philippe Colombet

13.1 Introduction

The normal knee kinematics is provided by articular surface shape and a complex ligament and tendon system [21]. The stability is controlled by ligaments, and the anterior cruciate ligament (ACL) is the primary restraint ligament [1]. The ACL controls part of the anteroposterior translation and rotation during flexion/extension. We will consider in this chapter only anteroposterior translation control. A lot of studies were published on natural ACL behavior; the goal of these studies was how to better place a graft during ACL reconstruction [3, 6, 11, 22, 31]. From all of these papers, a concept of isometry was formed. The goal of this chapter is to describe this concept of ACL isometry and to see how to assess it. To avoid confusion, we will use a surgical nomenclature (deep-shallow and superior-inferior) as recommended by ESSKA.

13.2 Definition of Isometry

The geometric definition is a transformation with length conservation, and when this condition is not respected, we will talk about non-isometry. In reference to ACL ligament reconstruction, it was described by Amis [3] as meaning that the dis-

tance between the femoral and tibial attachments of the reconstruction remains constant as the knee is moved in flexion/extension.

13.3 ACL and Isometry

Given that during the flexion/extension motion the femur rolls and sleeps [21], it can be inferred that there is not a single axis of rotation on the femur. So there are several axes of femoral rotation. Each axis tallies with an arc of flexion and a group of ACL fibers tightened. During the flexion/extension motion, some groups of fibers strain and others become slack. The length variations depend on the femoral and tibial fiber attachment position from these axes. The ACL ligament is composed of collagen fibers attached on the bone over a pretty large area. This is the reason why different authors described an isometric area [5, 11, 15]. Among these papers, some of them showed that the isometric areas were not superimposed to the natural ACL footprint. Amis [2] used a mechanical measurement with sutures on cadaver knees and reported the behavior of three groups of fibers, anterior, intermediate, and posterior (Fig. 13.1); the most isometric was the anterior group. Many other studies provided similar results [18, 26]. Friederich [10] reported a study on 38 cadaver knees, with the same method. He showed that the fibers inserted at the shallow part of the tibial foot print combined with fibers inserted superior shallow of the femoral foot print were the most isometric. The maximum length

P. Colombet, M.D.
Department of Knee Surgery,
Orthopaedic and Sports Medicine Center,
9 rue Jean Moulin, Bordeaux-Merignac 33700, France
e-mail: philippe.colombet5@wanadoo.fr

F. Catani, S. Zaffagnini (eds.), *Knee Surgery using Computer Assisted Surgery and Robotics*,
DOI 10.1007/978-3-642-31430-8_13, © ESSKA 2013

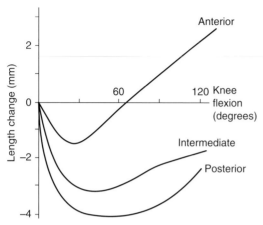

Fig. 13.1 Length variation of different anterior, intermediate, and posterior ACL group fibers reported from several studies. All the fibers appear slacked around 30–40° flexion (Amis the knee [3])

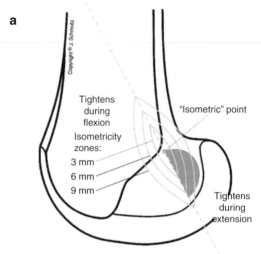

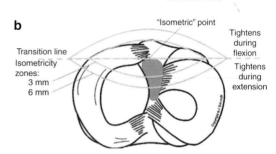

Fig. 13.2 Isometric map, isometricity zones, and transition line: (**a**) on the femur, notice that the native ACL insertion in orange is completely situated posteriorly to the transition line. (**b**) On the tibia the whole implantation of ACL is also posterior to the transition line [10]

difference was less than 1 mm (0.2±0.1 mm) between −5° and 135° of flexion. He provided transition lines and an isometric map (Fig. 13.2). Every point located deeply from the transition line led to length increasing during knee extension, and conversely every point shallow to this line led to length increasing during knee flexion. The whole natural ACL foot print on the tibia and on the femur is situated deeply from this line with fiber length augmentation during knee extension. The center of the anatomic ACL insertion is located in an area with 6 mm length variation. He showed, as Hefzy reported, [14] that when you put the tibial point deeply from the transition line, the femoral transition line and the isometric map turn shallow.

The complex structure of the ACL allows perfect control of knee stability and a continuous absorption of constraints. In ACL reconstruction, we are unable to reproduce this complex anatomy and we need to accept a compromise. If there is much length difference between flexion and extension, the graft will become slack, regardless of the flexion angle chosen for the graft fixation. If we fix the graft in the short length position, the graft will be stretched at the opposite extreme flexion angle and will be slack when returned to the initial position. Moreover, in this situation, if the graft is very stiff, the cartilage will be over constrained. This situation will provide a stiff

knee and osteoarthritis. If we fix the graft in the long-length position, the graft will become slack immediately with the change of flexion angle and the reconstruction will be ineffective.

Many different authors [2, 20, 23] have shown that a graft elongation more than 14–27 % leads to graft damage and failure, and in terms of length, stretching more than 7 mm should provide a rupture. So graft placement and isometry is very important for laxity control, stiff knee, cartilage damage, or graft rupture. We saw that isometry depends on tunnel placement, and each patient has his own knee architecture; in consequence, during ACL reconstruction the most difficult thing will be to find the optimum position. We can use either bony references or specific tools to measure the length difference during flexion/extension motion. We are going to describe these two situations.

13.4 Graft Placement and Isometry

13.4.1 Conventional Procedure

Most actual procedures use arthroscopy to perform ACL reconstruction, and the surgeon sees the landmarks. On the tibial side, in primary reconstruction, we clearly see the remnant fibers of the different bundles of the native ACL. To get a better view, the knee can be placed at 20° of flexion, and the arthroscopic portal must be placed close to the patella to get a "sky view" on the tibia. In this situation, it is quite easy to find a good location for the graft and to drill the tibial tunnel. In single-bundle ACL reconstruction (view the previous data), the placement in the anterior ACL fiber attachment seems to be the best choice because they are the most isometric fibers. In double-bundle reconstruction, the placement of each tunnel will be in the center of posterolateral (PL) and anteromedial (AM) bundle attachments. If we refer to the isometric map and transition line, mediolateral change will have a small impact on isometry; however, a medial situation is recommended to avoid impingement with the lateral condyle medial edge especially in the case of a narrowing intercondylar notch or osteophyte [12]. In case of revision when there is no native ACL remnant, arthroscopic landmarks are required. The perfect area is limited by the posterior horn of the lateral meniscus posteriorly, the anterior horn of the lateral meniscus laterally, the intermeniscal ligament anteriorly, and the limit of cartilage of the medial plateau medially [16].

On the femoral side, it is completely different. Because of the lateral arthroscopic portal, the posterior cruciate ligament, the remnant ACL fibers, and the different knee flexion angle, it is not always easy to find the optimum placement. It is well known that femoral placement error is the most common reason for ACL reconstruction

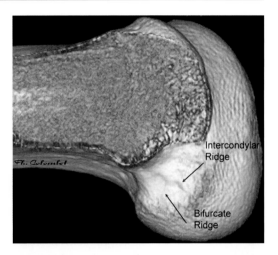

Fig. 13.3 3D CT scan reconstruction: the intercondylar ridge (resident's ridge) which is the anterior limit of the femoral insertion. The bifurcate ridge representing the separation between AM bundle (superior part) and PL bundle (inferior part)

failure. Two different methods can be used to place the femoral tunnel: the conventional method using vision and anatomic references and the radiology method. Under arthroscopy the classic bony references are represented by the ridges (Fig. 13.3): the lateral intercondylar ridge and the lateral bifurcate ridge [9, 28]. These ridges determine the two areas of AM and PL bundles. It is recommended at this step to place the scope through the anteromedial portal to improve the quality of vision on the lateral condyle. In single-bundle reconstruction, we have seen that the top of this area is the best point. However, it is not always easy to find these ridges, and most surgeons use the clock face positioning situated at 11 or 1 for the AM bundle [29]. A cadaveric study reported that this method is dependent on knee flexion and is a source of error [4]. A radiologic method has been developed to achieve the ideal location [17]. In all these methods, the isometry is inferred from work which showed that anterior fiber's femoral attachment is the aim, but no assessment or real length measurements are done. A more precise method is needed to perfectly locate the best femoral point and achieve the optimal isometric positioning.

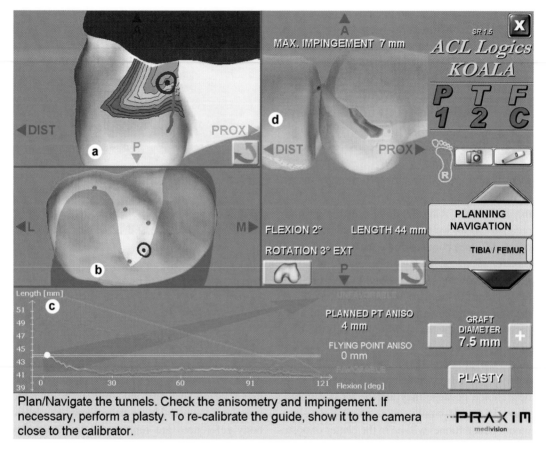

Fig. 13.4 Screen view of planning navigation window: (a) the colored isometric map (*green* is 2 mm, *purple* is 10-mm length difference between flexion and extension of the knee), the blue circle represents the femoral selected point. (b) Tibial plateau, the *pink zone* is the projection of the notch on the tibia and the *blue circle* represents the tibial selected point. (c) Graph of the length difference between the femoral and tibial selected points during the flexion/extension motion. (d) Lateral view, the virtual graft *pink* and the potential impingement with the roof of the notch in *red*

13.4.2 Navigated Procedure

This method uses computer assistance. It was developed in 1995 [8] and is a three-dimensional system. During the first step, a digitalization of the lateral part of the notch and tibial pre-spine surface is performed using a probe equipped with captors. Then a full flexion extension of the knee is registered. Once these data are collected, the surgeon selects a point on the tibia, and then the computer calculates the length difference between the full extension and the full flexion. This calculation is repeated from each point of the digitalized femoral area and produces a map with different colored isometric zones (Fig. 13.4).

If the placement seems to be incorrect or the length difference too important, another tibial point should be selected and a new map is provided. Then a femoral point is selected, and a graphic is shown with maximum length difference and distance between the tibial and femoral selected points all along the flexion. Two different situations should exist: a favorable case with reduction of length during the flexion, the graft will be tight only close to extension, and an unfavorable case in which the graft will be stretched during the flexion and will return to slack in extension. This second situation is unfavorable because it is preferable that the graft should be tight instead of slack close to the extension. Giving way mostly occurs when the knee is in the first 20° of flexion. The computer provides graft impingement zone which can be helpful to prevent graft damage and change of selected points before drilling. We have registered 45 navigated ACL reconstructions; we have selected on the tibia the center of native AM bundle from the ACL remnant and checked different o'clock positions on the femur (9–10–11 o'clock), 4 mm far from the posterior edge of the lateral condyle. For the 9 h–15 h position, we found 9.31 mm±2.81 of length difference; for 10–14 h position, it was 6.60 mm±2.28; and for 11–13 h, 4 mm±1.7. It appeared clearly that the most favorable femoral position was the 11 or 13 o'clock (Fig. 13.5), even though this situation is not ideal to control the rotational laxity. On planned graphic the mean of isometry was 3.6 mm±1.8. At the end of reconstruction, we have checked the final isometry; we have selected using the probe the anterior fibers of the graft. We have noticed a better result on isometry with a mean of 1.87 mm±1.31. That final measurement was close to the data reported in the studies on intact knees [18]. From these data by navigated procedure, we selected the femoral point at the posterior part of the most isometric zone (green zone <2 mm of isometry) (Fig. 13.6) to place the anterior part of the femoral tunnel in the center of this optimal isometric zone after drilling. On cadaver knee, Plaweski compared conventional and navigating technique and reported a mean of 3.3 mm±0.7 of length difference in navigated knee and 5.4 mm±1.2 in conventional technique and concluded that navigation was the perfect tool to place the graft in the anatomic area [25]. The same author showed, in a clinical randomized study of 60 patients, that the navigated group had significantly better result in terms of residual laxity [24]. Hart reported a comparative, prospective, randomized double-blind study on functional results after single-bundle ACL reconstruction by use of computer-assisted system (CAS) or a manual targeting technique. The follow-up was a minimum of 24 months; he did not find any statistical difference in terms of clinical results. The only difference between the

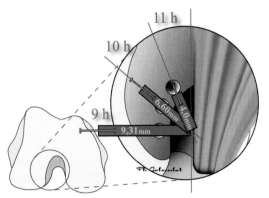

Fig. 13.5 View of the notch: different clock face positions and the length variation for the same tibial selected point. Eleven o'clock position is the most favorable placement

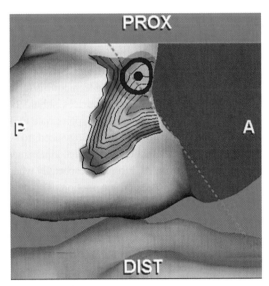

Fig. 13.6 Lateral view of the intercondylar notch: optimal placement of the graft (*blue circle*) to get after drilling the anterior part of the graft in the best isometric situation

two groups was in radiographic tunnel position measurement and especially on the femoral side [13]. Other studies recognized CAS as beneficial to reduce surgical error [7, 27]. Zaffagnini explored 15 years of literature on computer-assisted ACL reconstruction and noticed an increasing interest in CAS since 2006. He reported a quotation from Lord Kelvin in the nineteenth century, "If you cannot measure it, you cannot improve it." This philosophy fully adapts to the concept of navigation. He concluded that navigation provides information available during surgery and allows the surgeon to move to "on-demand" individualized surgery level [30].

13.5 Discussion

Some surgeons think that with experience femoral tunnel placement is not an issue. However, a recent study compared experienced and non-experienced surgeons using isometry and fluoroscopy technique and showed that in both categories the surgeon changed in the same ratio, the position of femoral tunnel after isometry and fluoroscopy assessment. It is demonstrated that experience does not provide enough security in tunnel placement [19]. Isometry is required in single-bundle ACL reconstruction to improve the graft behavior, prevent elongation, and graft failure. Each patient is different in terms of morphotype and laxity; a personalized technique is mandatory. Isometric measurement devices should be helpful; navigation seems to be the appropriate tool. However, minimally invasive technology needs to be developed. We need to know the normal kinematics on the knee before the ACL rupture, especially when we record the flexion/extension motion. This is a remaining issue, and new noninvasive technology should be able to collect these data on the normal knee to apply this normal kinematics to the injured knee. Isometry is related to the strategy of reconstruction, single bundle, double bundle, or more. The concept of multi-bundles reconstruction has been validated at time zero, but to date there is no consensus on its effect on clinical results. In double-bundle reconstruction, the graft placement is based on anatomy, and isometry is not the main goal because each bundle is supposed to be isometric during a part of flexion/extension motion; one bundle is tightened, while the other is slack and reciprocal. Most of the ACL reconstructions in the world are single-bundle reconstructions, and in this situation the quest for isometry has to be the main surgeon worry. Isometry is a quid of Graal, and studies of graft placement are academic; new technologies are coming; 3D imaging in the operating room combined with augmented reality should provide optimum operating conditions

to better place our single- or multi-bundles grafts. We have considered in this chapter only the relationship between isometry and control of translation, but instability is a 3D motion, consisting of translation and rotation. Basic science studies and clinical experiences will be needed to improve the knowledge about ACL reconstruction.

References

1. Amis A, Bull AM, McDermott ID (2004) Mechanical properties of knee ligament and meniscus. In: Landreau P, Christel P, Djian P (eds) Mechanical properties of knee ligament and meniscus. Springer, Paris
2. Amis AA, Dawkins GP (1991) Functional anatomy of the anterior cruciate ligament. Fibre bundle actions related to ligament replacements and injuries. J Bone Joint Surg Br 2:260–267
3. Amis A, Zavras TD (1995) Isometricity and graft placement during anterior cruciate ligament reconstruction. The Knee 3:5–17
4. Basdekis G, Abisafi C, Christel P (2009) Effect of knee flexion angle on length and orientation of posterolateral femoral tunnel drilled through anteromedial portal during anatomic double-bundle anterior cruciate ligament reconstruction. Arthroscopy 10:1108–1114
5. Bradley J, FitzPatrick D, Daniel D et al (1988) Orientation of the cruciate ligament in the sagittal plane. A method of predicting its length-change with flexion. J Bone Joint Surg Br 1:94–99
6. Cooper DE, Urrea L, Small J (1998) Factors affecting isometry of endoscopic anterior cruciate ligament reconstruction: the effect of guide offset and rotation. Arthroscopy 2:164–170
7. Degenhart M (2004) Computer-navigated ACL reconstruction with the OrthoPilot. Surg Technol Int 12:245–251
8. Dessenne V, Lavallee S, Julliard R et al (1995) Computer-assisted knee anterior cruciate ligament reconstruction: first clinical tests. J Image Guid Surg 1:59–64
9. Ferretti M, Ekdahl M, Shen W et al (2007) Osseous landmarks of the femoral attachment of the anterior cruciate ligament: an anatomic study. Arthroscopy 11: 1218–1225
10. Friederich NF (2004) Anatomie fonctionnelle du pivot central du genou. In: Landreau P, Christel P, Djian P (eds) Anatomie fonctionnelle du pivot central du genou. Springer, Paris, pp 1–44
11. Good L, Gillquist J (1993) The value of intraoperative isometry measurements in anterior cruciate ligament reconstruction: an in vivo correlation between substitute tension and length change. Arthroscopy 5: 525–532
12. Good L, Odensten M, Gillquist J (1991) Intercondylar notch measurements with special reference to anterior cruciate ligament surgery. Clin Orthop 263:185–189

13. Hart R, Krejzla J, Svab P et al (2008) Outcomes after conventional versus computer-navigated anterior cruciate ligament reconstruction. Arthroscopy 5: 569–578

14. Hefzy MS, Grood ES (1986) Sensitivity of insertion locations on length patterns of anterior cruciate ligament fibers. J Biomech Eng 1:73–82

15. Hefzy MS, Grood ES, Noyes FR (1989) Factors affecting the region of most isometric femoral attachments. Part II: The anterior cruciate ligament. Am J Sports Med 2:208–216

16. Jackson DW, Gasser SI (1994) Tibial tunnel placement in ACL reconstruction. Arthroscopy 2:124–131

17. Klos TV, Harman MK, Habets RJ et al (2000) Locating femoral graft placement from lateral radiographs in anterior cruciate ligament reconstruction: a comparison of 3 methods of measuring radiographic images. Arthroscopy 5:499–504

18. Kurosawa H, Yamakoshi K, Yasuda K et al (1991) Simultaneous measurement of changes in length of the cruciate ligaments during knee motion. Clin Orthop Relat Res 265:233–240

19. Mehta VM, Paxton EW, Fithian DC (2009) Does the use of fluoroscopy and isometry during anterior cruciate ligament reconstruction affect surgical decision making? Clin J Sport Med 1:46–48

20. Melhorn JM, Henning CE (1987) The relationship of the femoral attachment site to the isometric tracking of the anterior cruciate ligament graft. Am J Sports Med 6:539–542

21. Müller W (1994) Kinematics. In: Müller W (ed) Kinematics. Springer, Berlin/Heidelberg, pp 8–75

22. Musahl V, Plakseychuk A, VanScyoc A et al (2005) Varying femoral tunnels between the anatomical footprint and isometric positions: effect on kinematics of the anterior cruciate ligament-reconstructed knee. Am J Sports Med 5:712–718

23. Penner DA, Daniel DM, Wood P et al (1988) An in vitro study of anterior cruciate ligament graft placement and isometry. Am J Sports Med 3:238–243

24. Plaweski S, Cazal J, Rosell P et al (2006) Anterior cruciate ligament reconstruction using navigation: a comparative study on 60 patients. Am J Sports Med 4:542–552

25. Plaweski S, Rossi J, Merloz P et al (2011) Analysis of anatomic positioning in computer-assisted and conventional anterior cruciate ligament reconstruction. Orthop Traumatol Surg Res 6(Suppl):S80–S85

26. Sapega AA, Moyer RA, Schneck C et al (1990) Testing for isometry during reconstruction of the anterior cruciate ligament. Anatomical and biomechanical considerations. J Bone Joint Surg Am 2:259–267

27. Sati M, Staubli H, Bourquin Y et al (2002) Real-time computerized in situ guidance system for ACL graft placement. Comput Aided Surg 1:25–40

28. Shino K, Suzuki T, Iwahashi T et al (2010) The resident's ridge as an arthroscopic landmark for anatomical femoral tunnel drilling in ACL reconstruction. Knee Surg Sports Traumatol Arthrosc 9:1164–1168

29. Siebold R, Ellert T, Metz S et al (2008) Femoral insertions of the anteromedial and posterolateral bundles of the anterior cruciate ligament: morphometry and arthroscopic orientation models for double-bundle bone tunnel placement – a cadaver study. Arthroscopy 5:585–592

30. Zaffagnini S, Klos TV, Bignozzi S (2010) Computer-assisted anterior cruciate ligament reconstruction: an evidence-based approach of the first 15 years. Arthroscopy 4:546–554

31. Zavras TD, Race A, Bull AM et al (2001) A comparative study of 'isometric' points for anterior cruciate ligament graft attachment. Knee Surg Sports Traumatol Arthrosc 1:28–33

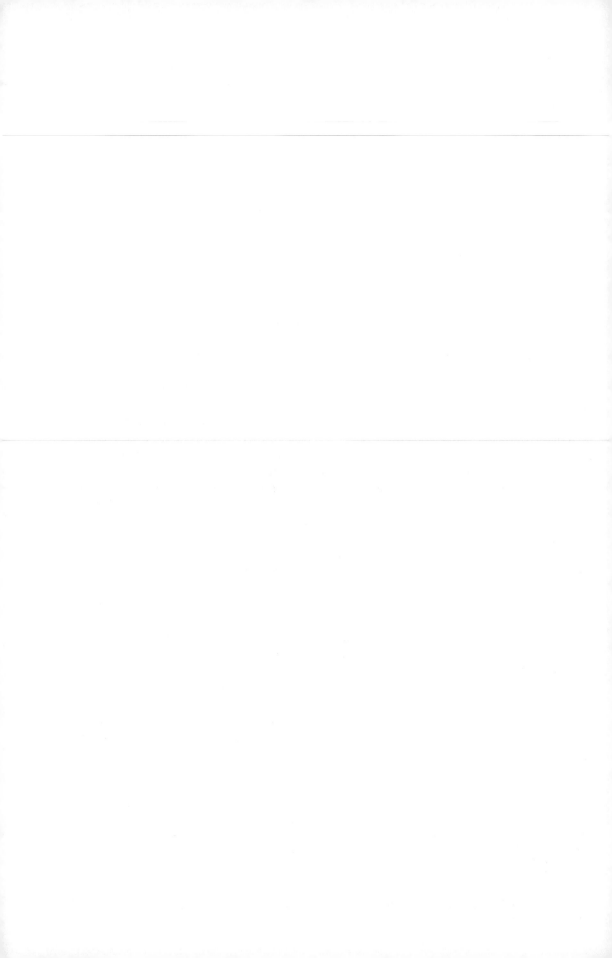

Arthroscopic-Assisted, Navigated Triplane Osteotomies of the Lower Extremity

Francisco Maculé and Luis Lozano

14.1 Background

The osteotomy procedure has always relied on a visual approach that lacks scientific rigour. During surgery, the complex mathematical and empirical formulae which may be used when planning the intervention give way to a rough reckoning based on a line running from the centre of the femoral head to the second toe.

Having demonstrated its exactitude in the context of knee arthroplasty, surgical navigation has gone on to be used in knee osteotomies. Conventional radiology shows minimal precision when measuring angular deformities [4, 11]. Furthermore, it is difficult to evaluate rotational changes and, above all, to carry out a dynamic assessment prior to performing an osteotomy and, more importantly, to determine how a correction in one plane might alter the deformity as a whole. The conclusions to be drawn from this are, firstly, that the human eye is unable to calculate the deformity in the different planes and, secondly, that deformities which are shown by preoperative planning to require a considerable corrective wedge are minimized by derotational and, especially, translational osteotomy, although neither can be performed as part of conventional surgery without the help of navigation.

14.2 Introduction

The aim of osteotomy is to restore a physiological mechanical axis of the limb, with a margin of ±2°. However, the corrections obtained by means of osteotomy are always approximate, and they depend on the experience of the surgeon. Several retrospective studies have indicated that the principal cause of osteotomy failure is the variability of the achieved correction [13, 19].

One of the reasons for the error in obtaining the desired correction is the difficulty of preoperative planning. Conventional radiology is imprecise because the rotation of the limb can lead to important measurement errors [4]. Its precision is therefore limited to the evaluation of angular deformities and to the measurement of the rotational component of a deformity, and similarly it does not provide dynamic information about the behaviour of the deformity with movements of the hip, knee or ankle [9, 19]. In the past, surgeons have had to solve these problems by using their personal experience, and this has often led to over- or underestimation of the size of the osteotomy wedge required for the correction. Furthermore, there have been no reliable intra-operative methods for evaluating the size of the wedge, the orientation of the osteotomy or the axial alignment obtained [14]. Consequently, neither reproducible nor comparable results could be obtained.

In recent years, navigation has become widely used for prosthetic surgery on the knee. In a previous paper [18], we proposed using the same

F. Maculé (✉) • L. Lozano
Department of Orthopaedic Surgery,
Knee Surgery Unit, University of Barcelona,
Barcelona, Spain
e-mail: f.macule@clinic.ub.es; llozano@clinic.ub.es

F. Catani, S. Zaffagnini (eds.), *Knee Surgery using Computer Assisted Surgery and Robotics*,
DOI 10.1007/978-3-642-31430-8_14, © ESSKA 2013

navigation software that is used in prosthetic surgery, but in combination with arthroscopy, to improve the precision of measurements and the outcome of osteotomies in complex deformities. The value of navigation in this context is that it enables the deformity to be precisely evaluated in three spatial planes, as well as allowing precise intra-operative and real-time control of the axes obtained with the correction [6, 9, 19].

14.3 Indications and Contraindications of the Technique

The technique is indicated in all femoral and tibial deformities that have not severely altered the anatomy of the knee [3, 7, 12, 15, 17]. However, it is contraindicated for knee joint deformities that have caused an oblique interline or ligament instability, as well as in cases of osteoporosis or in obese patients in whom it is difficult to locate the epicondyles [18]. Some authors [13, 19] currently treat acute or chronic ligament instability in a combined or sequential way by means of tibial osteotomy and associated ligament reconstruction. In these cases, it is important to avoid altering the posterior slope of the tibia, and in this regard navigation proves highly useful.

14.4 Surgical Technique

Traditional preoperative planning is based on telemetry of the lower limbs under load whereby ankles must be joined and neutral rotation of lower extremities is required. It is necessary to ensure that the image intensifier, the arthroscopy equipment, and the surgical navigator are all available in the operating theatre. Having initiated the surgical intervention, we then put the navigation sensors in place and identify the centre of rotation of the hip and of the surface points of the knee and ankle. In order to avoid arthrotomy of the knee, arthroscopy can be used to take intra-articular references (centre of the tibial surface, anteroposterior axis of the tibia, femoral

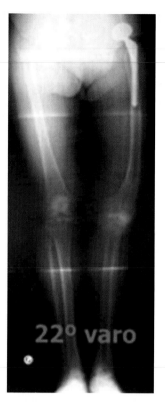

Fig. 14.1 Radiology telemetry with the deformity of the extremity

condyles and tibial plateau surface) (Fig. 14.1). We also use arthroscopy to document the state of the cartilage and to perform necessary procedures on other intra-articular structures. When this process is complete, the navigator provides a precise report of the deformity in three spatial planes, as well as in relation to movement of the limb. We perform osteotomy with fluoroscopic control and, prior to its definitive fixation, verify in real time the quality of the correction obtained and make any modifications necessary to achieve a physiological mechanical axis of the limb. Finally, the navigator creates a record containing all the pre- and postoperative information regarding the corrected deformity.

In our experience, consolidation of the osteotomy is observed within 12 weeks, without local complications and without loss of reduction, the final physiological axes being between 1° and 1.5° of valgus.

14.4.1 Definition of the True Deformity

1. Navigation (first part) (Figs. 14.1 and 14.2)
   (a) Place sensors on either side of the deformity. Check stability.
   (b) Calibrate instruments and take references from the centre of rotation of the hip and epicondyles (percutaneously).
2. Arthroscopy (Fig. 14.3)
   (a) Access the joint through lateral and medial infrapatellar portals, take references of the femoral and tibial centre and map the femoral condyles and tibial plateau.
   (b) Create accessory portal through the quadricipital tendon and take a reference from the bottom of the sulcus or Whiteside's line.
3. Navigation (second part)
   (a) Take references from the malleoli.
   At this point, the navigator informs the surgeon of the true deformity, taking into account the following aspects: varus/valgus, flexion/extension and internal/external rotation.

14.4.2 Osteotomy with Radiology

1. Radiology
   (a) Locate the apex of the deformity.
   (b) Mark out the osteotomy line with data from the navigator.
   (c) Bicortical osteotomy (Figs. 14.4 and 14.5).
2. Navigation
   (a) Progressive correction by means of opening or closing wedges, in accordance with the plan derived from the navigation data (Fig. 14.6)
At this point, the surgeon has only the navigator as a reference for controlling the osteotomy correction.
1. Osteosynthesis
   (a) Provisional navigation-guided fixation with Kirchner's wires.
   (b) Monitor transverse displacement (Fig. 14.7).
   (c) Option for either a one- or two-plate strategy.
   (d) Definitive navigation-guided fixation (Fig. 14.8).

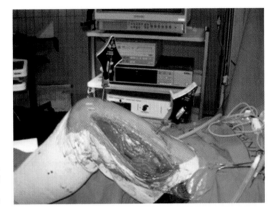
Fig. 14.2 Navigator sensors on either side of the deformity

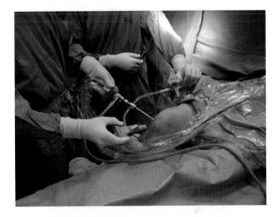
Fig. 14.3 Taking anatomical references with the navigator and arthroscopic view

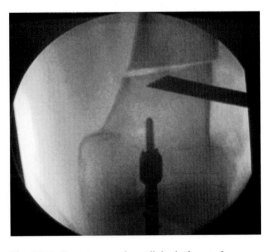
Fig. 14.4 Osteotomy under radiological control

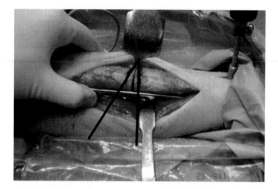

Fig. 14.5 Marking out the corrective osteotomy line at the apex of the deformity

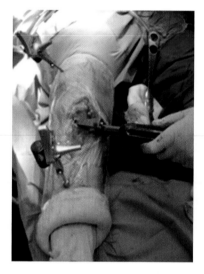

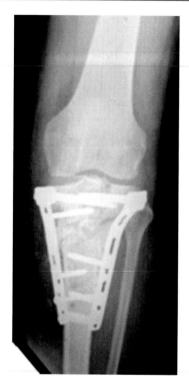

Fig. 14.8 Definitive fixation of two osteosynthesis plates and an autologous graft

Fig. 14.6 Progressive correction by means of opening wedges

14.4.3 Details and Recommendations

1. Navigation
   (a) No special software is required as that used for knee arthroplasty is suitable.
   (b) Take into account the correction of the deformity so as to facilitate the post-osteotomy sensor readings.
2. Radiology
   (a) Avoid and/or control any translation of bone parts and incorporate them into the correction of the deformity (Fig. 14.7).
   (b) Take the anatomical plane of greatest deformity as the reference for the osteotomy.
3. Arthroscopy
   (a) Take readings of the condylar groove in a semi-flexed position to avoid interference with the femoral sensor.
4. Osteosynthesis
   (a) Ensure permanent control of navigation while the plate is being fixed.

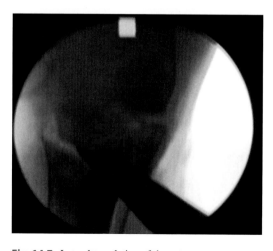

Fig. 14.7 Lateral translation of the osteotomy

(b) When using two plates, first fix the one that maintains the correction and then the neutralization plate.

(c) The use of single-plate systems is recommended.

14.5 Discussion

The knee is one of the joints most commonly affected by arthritis, which appears in 1 % of the population under 65 years of age and in 2–6 % of those over 65 [14]. The study by Odenbring in 1991 described the progression of unicompartmental arthritis over a 16-year follow-up. This risk of progression multiplies by four in the case of genu varus and by five in the case of genu valgus in comparison to a well-articulated knee, which is why the correction of deformities in adulthood can delay the appearance of arthritis in this joint. Long-term tibial osteotomy studies show survival rates of about 75 % after 10 years and of about 60 % after 15 years [17]. However, with classical osteotomy techniques, it is very difficult to achieve exactly the defined preoperative objective (correct result in only 50 % of cases, according to published studies; [10, 19]). Some surgeons use guides for a precise cut [2], while others consider that precise measurement methods do not exist, and therefore they perform osteotomies without preoperative planning [7]. At all events, osteotomy results (i.e. the correction achieved) vary considerably, and several authors believe this to be the principal cause of the technique's failure, which has led many surgeons to limit its indications [7].

The degree of correction needed is that which shifts the weight-bearing axis to the outer two-thirds of the external tibial plateau [1]. Authors vary with regards to the system they use to calculate the degree of opening required by internal addition osteotomy or the height of the wedge to be resected in the case of closing osteotomy, although the majority base their approach on complex trigonometric calculations [1] that are difficult to reproduce during surgery and which can be imprecise in radiographic studies [18]. Consequently, surgical navigators are increasingly being used in our setting to determine the correct intra-operative alignment. Navigators enable the deformity to be precisely evaluated in three spatial planes and allow intra-operative and real-time monitoring of the axes obtained with the correction. Controlling the three planes of correction is essential with regards to the correct orientation of the osteotomy [5, 6, 8, 16–19].

Several authors have reported excellent results with navigation assistance in valgus osteotomies of the tibia in genu varus, with specific computer programs being used to evaluate, plan and execute the procedure [7]. Recent studies have confirmed the utility of navigation without previous scanning as a way of improving the precision of valgus osteotomies of the tibia [5, 6, 8, 16–19] as well as of double osteotomies of the femur and tibia for the treatment of gonarthrosis in genu varus [14, 16]. In valgus osteotomies of the tibia for genu varus, navigation allows 86–96 % reproducibility with regards to the objective of obtaining a final axis of $184° \pm 2°$, compared with the 23–71 % reproducibility offered by the conventional technique [6, 17]. Navigation also enables instantaneous perioperative goniometry, which is an excellent way of improving precision when performing complex osteotomies. Another advantage is that navigation systems allow continuous visualization of the three axes and can detect undesired changes in the tibial slope during the correction procedure, changes which would influence knee kinematics and stability [6, 10]. Iorio et al. [6] reported 100 % modification of the posterior tibial slope between $-2°$ and $+2°$ with computer-assisted open-wedge high tibial osteotomy, whereas this goal was only achieved in 24 % of cases with conventional high tibial osteotomy.

The disadvantages of navigated osteotomies are the additional time required for the operative procedure (10–23 min), the extra wounds required in the femur and tibia for fixing the navigation system and the additional cost. Furthermore, implantation of pins can cause pin tract infection or fractures. During the procedure, mechanical or software malfunctions, as well as registration errors, may also occur [5, 19].

In our practice, the computer-assisted surgical software used is the same as that for the implant of total knee prostheses, although we also use arthroscopy to obtain the necessary intra-articular references. It is worth noting that the arthroscopy serves at the same time to evaluate, and to treat if necessary, possible intra-articular injuries (e.g. meniscal) that can be associated with severe misalignment of the lower limb. The use of navigation enables precise measurement of the flexum and recurvatum, at the same time as evaluating the varus/valgus deformity and the rotation, and, moreover, does so intra-operatively, in real time and in relation to articular movements [9, 18]. As a working tool, it is therefore considered to be highly superior to the use of classical equipment and preoperative planning based on radiology or scanning and the surgeon's experience. Note also that the use of the scanner has important disadvantages such as its high cost and the irradiation it produces. By contrast, kinematic acquisition of the centre of rotation of the hip, the knee and the ankle makes preoperative scanning unnecessary. Furthermore, the use of arthroscopy for the precise acquisition of the intraarticular points avoids arthrotomy and minimizes surgical complications [8, 18]. In conclusion, although the arthroscopy-assisted navigationguided technique requires increased surgical time to obtain the reference points, the final outcomes and the absence of complications justify its use.

Conflict of Interests The authors state that they have no conflict of interests and nor have they received any funding for the work reported in this chapter.

References

1. Aryee S, Imhoff AB, Rose T et al (2008) Do we need synthetic osteotomy augmentation materials for opening-wedge high tibial osteotomy? Biomaterials 29(26):3497–3502
2. Billings A, Scott DF, Camargo MP et al (2000) High tibial osteotomy with a calibrated osteotomy guide, rigid internal fixation, and early motion. Long-term follow-up. J Bone Joint Surg Am 82:70–79
3. Dobbe JG, du Pré KJ, Kloen P et al (2011) Computer-assisted and patient-specific 3-D planning and evaluation of a single-cut rotational osteotomy for complex long-bone deformities. Med Biol Eng Comput 49(12):1363–1370
4. Ellis RE, Tso CY, Rudan JF et al (1999) A surgical planning and guidance system for high tibial osteotomy. Comp Aided Surg 4:264–274
5. Gebhard F, Krettek C, Hüfner T et al (2011) Reliability of computer-assisted surgery as an intraoperative ruler in navigated high tibial osteotomy. Arch Orthop Trauma Surg 131(3):297–302
6. Iorio R, Pagnottelli M, Vadalà A et al (2011) Open-wedge high tibial osteotomy: comparison between manual and computer-assisted techniques. Knee Surg Sports Traumatol Arthrosc. 2011 Nov 24. [Epub ahead of print]
7. Keppler P, Gebhard GPA et al (2004) Computer aided high tibial open wedge osteotomy. Injury 35:68–78
8. Lo WN, Cheung KW, Yung SH et al (2009) Arthroscopy-assisted computer navigation in high tibial osteotomy for varus knee deformity. J Orthop Surg (Hong Kong) 17(1):51–55
9. Maculé-Beneyto F, Hernández-Vaquero D, Segur-Vilalta JM et al (2006) Navigation in total knee arthroplasty. A multicenter study. Int Orthop 30: 536–540
10. Marti CB, Gautier E, Wachtl SW et al (2004) Accuracy of frontal and sagittal plane correction in open-wedge high tibial osteotomy. Arthroscopy 20:366–372
11. Moreland Bassett LW, Hanker GJ (1987) Radiographic analysis of the axial alignment of the lower extremity. J Bone Joint Surg Am 69(A):745–749
12. Murphy SB (1994) Tibial osteotomy for genu varum. Indications, preoperative planning and technique. Orthop Clin North Am 25:477–482
13. Noyes FR, Barber-Westin SD, Hewett TE (2000) High tibial osteotomy and ligament reconstruction for varus angulated anterior cruciate ligament-deficient knees. Am J Sports Med 28:282–296
14. Phillips MJ, Krackow KA (1998) High tibial osteotomy and distal femoral osteotomy for valgus or varus deformity around the knee. Instr Course Lect 47:429–436
15. Rudan JF, Simurda MA (1991) Valgus high tibial osteotomy. A long-term follow-up study. Clin Orthop Relat Res 54:157–160
16. Saragaglia D, Blaysat M, Mercier N, Grimaldi M (2011) Results of forty two computer-assisted double level osteotomies for severe genu varum deformity. Int Orthop 36(5):999–1003
17. Saragaglia D, Roberts J (2005) Navigated osteotomies around the knee in 170 patients with osteoarthrosis secondary to genu varum. Orthopaedics 28(10): s1269–s1274
18. Sastre S, Torner P, Maculé F (2007) Knee osteotomy: navigation guided and arthroscopy assisted. Knee Surg Sports Traumatol Arthrosc 15: 1215–1218
19. Song EK, Seon JK, Park SJ, Seo HY (2008) Navigated open wedge high tibial osteotomy. Sports Med Arthrosc 16(2):84–90

The Use of Computer-Assisted Surgery During Patellofemoral Arthroplasty

15

Robin K. Strachan and Andrew A. Amis

15.1 Introduction

During total knee arthroplasty (TKA), the patellofemoral joint (PFJ) has a tendency to be considered as an afterthought despite the fact that the patella and trochlea of the femur are frequently involved in certain patterns of knee osteoarthritis and deformity. Indeed, the PFJ in arthroplasty is a well-documented source of complications including subluxations, dislocations, tilts and impingements which are associated with pain and poor function [8, 30]. Such issues should therefore not be dismissed lightly (Fig. 15.1). Archibeck et al. [3] found that patellar tilt or subluxation occurred in 45 % of primary TKAs. Baldini et al. [4] reported high rates of pain and fracture when patellar issues were ignored.

Of course, with a TKA, tibiofemoral and patellofemoral dynamics are very closely related. In valgus deformities and also where excessive tibial external rotation is present, the patella is subject to large lateralising forces. On the other hand, correction of varus during medial unicompartmental replacement tends to reduce pressure on the medial side of the PFJ and improve patellar tracking.

Poor tibiofemoral component positioning and sizing is often correctly blamed for patellofemoral problems. However, the fundamental understanding has to be that problems with the PFJ can exist in isolation. This may simply present as patellofemoral osteoarthritis associated only with modest patellar tilt and minimal subluxation (Fig. 15.2). However, a small percentage of patients with so-called isolated patellofemoral osteoarthritis have a high incidence of 'primary' structural problems with the PFJ. These include morphological abnormalities of the knee often associated with patellar tracking problems such as trochlear dysplasia, torsional abnormalities and limb malalignment. Such knees have to be treated with careful consideration of these abnormalities during any attempts to insert an arthroplasty.

Chronic patellar subluxations and dislocations may lead on to contractures of the lateral part of the extensor mechanism and laxity of the medial retinacular structures. Indeed, experienced patellofemoral arthroplasty surgeons often describe the operation as primarily a 'soft tissue procedure'. Descriptions of the mechanical consequences of poor patellar tracking, such as described by Verlinden et al. [37], lead to the understanding that any abnormal forces operating on the patella cannot only cause

R.K. Strachan, FRCS (✉)
Consultant Orthopaedic Surgeon
and Honorary Senior Lecturer,
Imperial College NHS Trust, Charing Cross Hospital,
W6 8RF, Fulham Palace Road, London, UK
e-mail: strachanrk@yahoo.com

A.A. Amis, Ph.D., D.Sc.(Eng)
Department of Mechanical Engineering
and Musculoskeletal Surgery Group,
Imperial College London, London, SW7 2AZ, UK
e-mail: a.amis@imperial.ac.uk

F. Catani, S. Zaffagnini (eds.), *Knee Surgery using Computer Assisted Surgery and Robotics*,
DOI 10.1007/978-3-642-31430-8_15, © ESSKA 2013

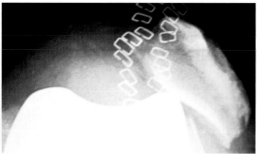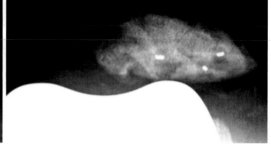

Fig. 15.1 Consequences of poor patellofemoral technique

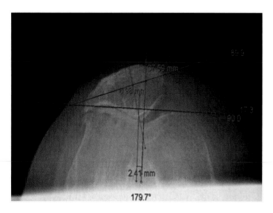

Fig. 15.2 Patellofemoral osteoarthritis with moderate lateral patellar tilt

severe erosions of polyethylene components but are also likely to have been previously responsible for erosion of cartilage and bone. The end stage of this process is usually bony collapse and tight lateral patellar retinacular structures (Fig. 15.3). It is often within this difficult mechanical environment that patellofemoral arthroplasty has to be performed. Accuracy of component positioning then becomes extremely important, with proper soft tissue balancing of the patellofemoral joint being an absolute necessity. Set against this background, computer-assisted navigation can assist the surgeon by providing precise intraoperative alignment and tracking information. Special tools, techniques and software are, however, needed to perform such surgery.

15.2 Biomechanics of the Native and Prosthetic Patellofemoral Joint

15.2.1 Patellofemoral Joint Kinematics and Articular Geometry

The kinematics of the patella during knee flexion-extension is controlled by a combination of factors, which include the articular geometry and passive soft tissue restraints locally, then the magnitudes and directions of the muscle tensions and finally the overall limb alignment, the body posture and their related effects on further muscle actions, such as around the hip. It will be assumed in this chapter related to joint replacement surgery that the patellar tracking is not affected by abnormalities away from the knee and that the partial or total knee arthroplasty procedure will be addressing only problems local to the knee, which may include misalignment caused by erosion of articular cartilage and underlying bone.

Although the most common pattern of articular damage in the tibiofemoral joint is predominantly in the medial compartment, leading to progressive varus deformity, the opposite occurs at the patellofemoral joint, with erosion of the lateral facets of the patella and trochlea. The loss of joint space allows some slackening of the retinacular restraints, and so the arthritis causes progressive lateral patellar tilting (in which, by definition, the lateral edge of the patella approaches the underlying trochlea while the

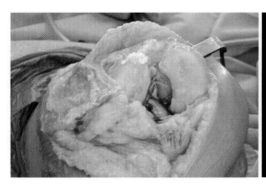 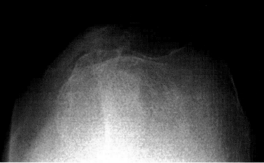

Fig. 15.3 End-stage patellofemoral osteoarthritis with dislocation and bone collapse

medial edge does not), accompanied by lateral maltracking, in which the path of motion is translated further lateral than it should be in the normal knee. This combination of lateral translation plus rotation means that there will be a stress concentration caused by the prominent lateral edge of the trochlea pressing into the centre of the lateral articular facet of the patella, while the medial facet is unloaded, and so a vicious circle of lateral facet articular stress and erosion may be set up. This leads eventually to the lateral facet of the patella being hollowed out, leaving a thin remnant which is prolonged laterally by a large osteophyte that follows the path of the lateral retinaculum. The sequence of cause and effect may be debateable, but one consequence of the patella being loaded with a lateral bias in these knees is that, at the commencement of knee flexion from full extension, the distal-lateral aspect of the patella will collide with the lateral-proximal aspect of the trochlea, and that may be a mechanism which initiates the osteoarthritic changes.

A further point, which follows from the lateral maltracking, is that the medial retinacular restraints suffer chronic stretching. Although several retinacular bands have been identified, only the medial patellofemoral ligament (MPFL) has a sufficient role to be worthy of reconstruction during surgery. It is the principal medial passive restraint to patellar lateral maltracking, contributing 50–60 % of the total restraint [12, 14].

The course of the MPFL is from the femoral attachment midway between the medial epicondyle and the adductor tubercle, passing to the medial edge of the patella [5, 7], and so it is near to having a transverse orientation and so is the most efficiently orientated of the medial retinacula to restrain patellar lateral translation. There have been several studies of the length change pattern of the MPFL, and the consensus is that it is approximately isometric across the range of knee flexion-extension but that it tightens during the last 20° of knee extension [15, 16]. Work in vitro which complements this observation has shown that the MPFL is the single structure which is dominant in controlling patellar lateral translation when the knee is between full extension and 20° flexion [33]. These findings mean that the principal function of the MPFL is to guide the patella into the trochlear groove when the knee starts to flex, after which the articular geometry should ensure patellar stability, if the sulcus has normal geometry.

If the kinematics of the patellofemoral joint is to be understood, then the guiding function of the articular geometry of the joint must be known. In the normal knee, the patella is relatively disengaged from the trochlea in extension and then articulates congruently in mid-flexion. In deep knee flexion, the patella moves onto the distal aspect of the femur, and so it leaves the trochlea and rests on the two femoral condyles, bridging over the intercondylar notch.

It is only recently that there has been much work on three-dimensional (3D) reconstruction of the articular geometry from medical images. In summary, the articular geometry of the trochlea has been found to correspond approximately to two (medial and lateral) part-spherical surfaces, which are joined by a concave blending radius at the base of the trochlear groove. Thus, the 3D geometry is akin to a bobbin or pulley, which has a central axis passing medially-laterally through the centres of the two spheres. The lateral sphere has a larger radius than the medial, and this results in the lateral edge of the trochlea being more prominent where it meets the anterior surface of the femur. The trochlear axis has been found to be parallel to the femoral condylar axis, which is also defined as joining the centres of medial and lateral condylar spheres, this time matching the posterior-distal parts of the femoral condyles [19, 20]. The condylar axis is perpendicular to the mechanical axis of the femur, and so it follows that the trochlear axis is, too. This means that the groove of the trochlea is aligned with the femoral mechanical axis. This work also defined the proximal and anterior offsets of the trochlear axis from the condylar axis, and this information should allow the position and orientation of the trochlea to be defined in relation to the femoral condyles.

There have been many studies of patellar kinematics, both in vivo and in vitro, showing many differing results for the path of motion during knee flexion-extension [23]. However, most studies agree that the patella is relatively lateral when the knee is in full extension, and that corresponds to the elongation of the MPFL. In early knee flexion, when the patella meets the proximal aspect of the lateral facet of the trochlea, it is guided into the trochlear groove, and so it moves medially during the first 15–20° degrees of knee flexion. Beyond that point, the patellar tracks in a stable manner along the groove, and so this path of motion will be parallel to the mechanical axis of the femur [19, 20]. Some studies have used the shaft of the femur, the femoral anatomical axis, as their datum, and that deviates approximately 6° or 7° from the mechanical axis. Thus, when the kinematics are displayed in femoral anatomical axes, the data show the patella moving progressively lateral beyond 20° knee flexion [1]; mathematical reprocessing shows that that is the same as the patella moving parallel to the mechanical axis. A full three-dimensional analysis shows that the central point of the patella actually moves in a circular path around the distal femur, from anterior to distal, when the knee flexes, apart from the small lateral deviation near to full extension [19, 20] (Fig. 15.4). This description is relatively easy to define and to navigate.

Kinematic studies have also examined patellar tilting during knee flexion-extension. When the motion of the patella is reviewed in relation to the trochlear axis, it is seen that there is very little patellar tilting in the normal knee [1]: the line joining the most medial and lateral points of the patella in a 'skyline' view remains close to horizontal, parallel to the trochlear axis.

15.2.2 Patellar Kinematics After TKA

During TKA, the path of the patella is determined partly by the muscle and retinacular tensions, but also by the new trochlear geometry, and how the surgeon places the femoral component. This is the case whether the patella itself is resurfaced or left intact: they are both pulled into the trochlear articulation if the soft tissue tensions have been balanced. Many TKA systems include a procedure which places the femoral component into 3° of external rotation, in relation to the transepicondylar axis. This has become normal practice because it was found to reduce the prevalence of lateral retinacular releases. If the femoral component is placed into external rotation, then that causes the patella to be translated laterally near knee extension and also to be tilted laterally, as it remains congruent on the flange of the trochlea [31]. A side effect of that manoeuvre is that the slope of the lateral facet of the trochlea will be reduced by 3°, thus reducing patellar lateral stability [33].

There have been many studies examining the accuracy of positioning the components of TKA, and those have shown clearly that there can be a large variability when the internal–external rotational position of the femoral component is defined by digitising the epicondyles to define

Fig. 15.4 The patella follows a circular path around the distal femur. The plane of the circle is aligned with the femoral mechanical axis in the coronal plane. There is a lateral deviation in the last 15–20° of knee extension

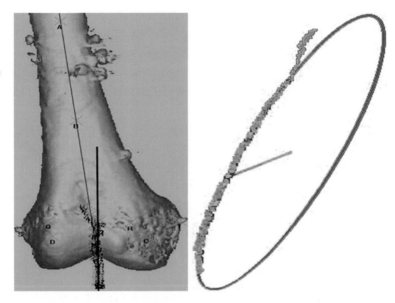

the transverse axis: Jerosch [22] found that the medial epicondyle was digitised over an area 22 mm wide and the lateral 14 mm, leading to a range of transepicondylar axis orientations of 23°. Similarly, Jenny and Boeri [21] found a mean intra-observer difference of 6° and mean interobserver error of 9°. Although it is recognised that the femoral lateral condyle may be hypoplastic in the valgus knee, it has been found that it is more accurate to define femoral rotation from the most posterior points of the medial and lateral femoral condyles (known as the posterior condylar axis) than to use the transepicondylar axis. Yoshino et al. [39] found a mean interobserver error of 1°. It is clear that inaccuracy when positioning the femoral component in internal–external rotation may have a large effect on the kinematics of the patella and that the posterior condylar axis is more precise than use of the transepicondylar axis.

femoral cut (AFC) based upon registration of the anterior cortex of the femur. Currently, the sizing of the femoral PFJR component is simply based upon assessment of anterior femoral coverage and not the navigation software. Axial alignment is then monitored and compared with the transepicondylar axis (TEA), posterior condylar line (PCL) and flexion/extension axis (FEA) (Fig. 15.5). In the example shown, some 3° of internal rotation of the cut is noted in relation to the TEA but with 1° external to the PCL. It is the author's preference to then adjust the cut to match the TEA rather than the PCL. Slope in the sagittal plane seems best to be around 2–3° of flexion as shown in Fig. 15.5. Rotation in the coronal plane is firstly determined by lining up the femoral reaming jig with the mechanical axis of the femur (Fig. 15.6). The trochlear groove of the femoral trial can then be used to check and then fine-tune the final alignment of the femoral component if necessary.

15.3   Navigation Technique for the Femoral Component in PFJR

Correct placement of the femoral component in patellofemoral joint replacement (PFJR) is best carried out after routine registration has been carried out and any steps to cut the distal femur bypassed. Standard TKA software can then give a precise indication of the height of the anterior

15.4   Preparation of the Patella

A vital step towards successful function in PFJR is the thickness, shape and configuration of the final patellar construct. Work by Iranpour et al. [18] has shown that the thickness of the patella should be approximately half the transverse diameter, and so that is a useful guide for

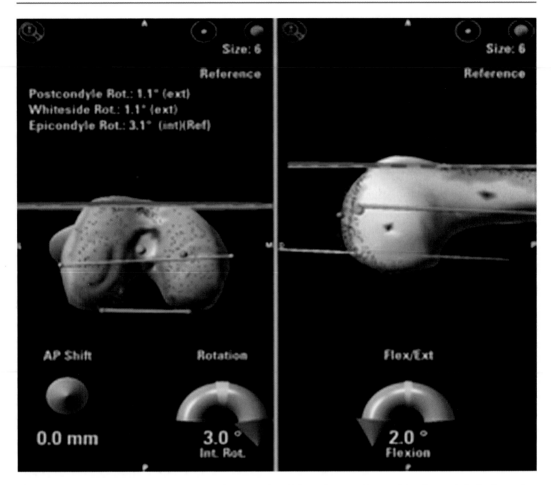

Size: 6

Reference

Postcondyle Rot.: 1.1° (ext)
Whiteside Rot.: 1.1° (ext)
Epicondyle Rot.: 3.1° (int)(Ref)

Size: 6

Reference

AP Shift

0.0 mm

Rotation

3.0 °
Int. Rot.

Flex/Ext

2.0 °
Flexion

Fig. 15.5 Verified anterior cut in relation to the transepicondylar axis, posterior condylar line and flexion/extension axis

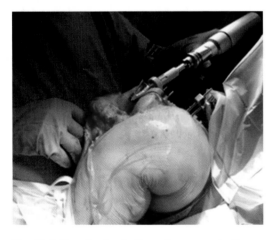

Fig. 15.6 Reaming for the femoral component with coronal alignment based upon the mechanical axis of the femur

restoration of the correct thickness in cases with deep erosion. Also, the effect of overstuffing the patella seems more likely to stretch the medial patellofemoral ligament than the lateral patellar retinaculum [15, 16]. The authors' preference is to make the initial bone cut parallel to the plane of the quadriceps and patellar tendons, leaving the cut approximately 2 mm proud of this plane. Marginal osteophytes are removed and the edges of the patella bevelled to create an oval shape as shown in Fig. 15.7. This shape facilitates smooth entry onto the femoral component and variable patellar tilt angles throughout the flexion/extension cycle. Use of a recessed biconvex patella facilitates this method. Variable reaming depth then permits adjustment of the final patellar thickness. In order to avoid

Fig. 15.7 Suggested patellar preparation technique

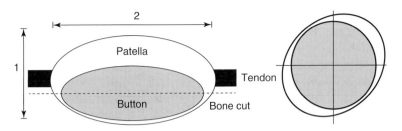

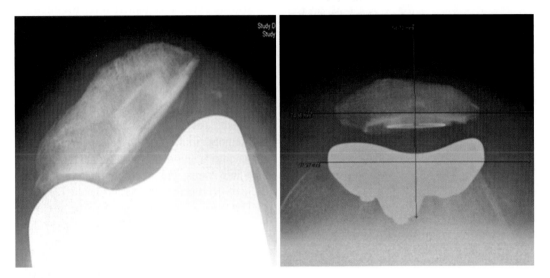

Fig. 15.8 An unsatisfactory and a satisfactory final situation

'overstuffing' of the anterior compartment, this thickness is calculated by the equation '0.5 × diameter minus 1 mm'. Button position is best centred on the intersection of mid-longitudinal and mid-transverse lines as shown. An unsatisfactory and a satisfactory final situation is shown in Fig. 15.8.

15.5 Preparation to Assess Patellar Tracking

The first steps in the assessment of patellar tracking involve attaching a marker array (Fig. 15.9). This is easily accomplished with a single cortical screw.

Then the patella is registered as shown, followed by registration of a line running along the lowest portions of the trochlea which is used to reference all patellar motion in the coronal plane (Fig. 15.10).

The 'no-thumb test' is useless for such navigation, and despite arrays themselves becoming lighter, they still cause tilting moments. Such moments must be countered by use of a '2-stitch technique', one at the level of the VMO and the other at the centre of the medial retinaculum (Fig. 15.9). This temporary repair of capsule and medial retinaculum is carried out with all trial components in place and is less likely to cause tears of the retinaculum than use of a towel clip. This manoeuvre provides highly reproducible results during the intraoperative assessment of both tibiofemoral and patellofemoral motion. Also, erratic motion of the patella is reduced, and the range of patellar tilt angles minimised. However, increased lateral retinacular tension is often then seen to be associated with large residual amounts of lateral patellar shift. This tends to lift the patella out of the trochlear groove and up onto the lateral flange of the femoral component.

This then provides the rationale for observing the distance between the patella and the epicondylar axis during the dynamic tracking studies to be described in the section below on tracking values.

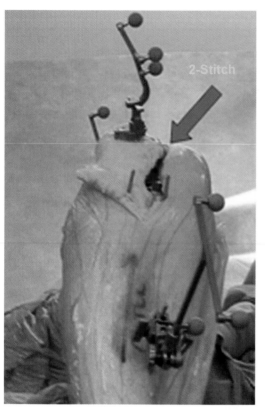

Fig. 15.9 The '2-stitch' wound closure technique and the patellar tracking optical marker array

15.6 Assessment of Patellar Tracking

Study of patellar tracking must involve dynamic assessment. Indeed, patellar motion is dependent upon not only tibial and femoral component positions but also tibiofemoral relative motion. Valgus and varus alignments are of course important but so also are external and internal relative motions between tibia and femur (Fig. 15.11).

In order to quantify the maximum possible effect that such relative motions might have, the joint should have its trial components in place and 2-stitch temporary capsular closure effected. The joint should now be stressed to test the stability of the patellofemoral joint as well as the tibiofemoral joint. The knee can be moved as shown into valgus and external tibial rotation and then into varus and internal rotation during a cycle of flexion and extension (Fig. 15.12).

The relative motions can then be stored as tracking curves to be carefully considered before any further adjustments are made. Care must be taken to use only enough force to tension the capsule and ligament to its 'end point' and not to a point where significant tension, stretching or tearing, might occur. This technique is, therefore, no different from routine 'surgical feel' of knee stability assessed during non-navigated surgery.

The basic patella tracking screen shown below shows a knee at 62° of flexion with a satisfactory situation. The patella is lying in a position of minimal lateral shift, zero patellar rotation and optimal patellar tilt at 5° (Fig. 15.13). The patella

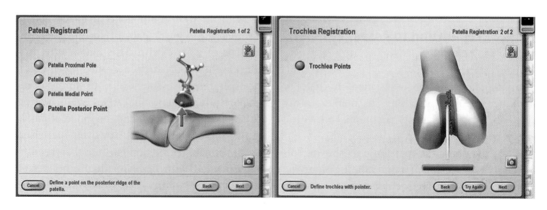

Fig. 15.10 Registration of patella and trochlea

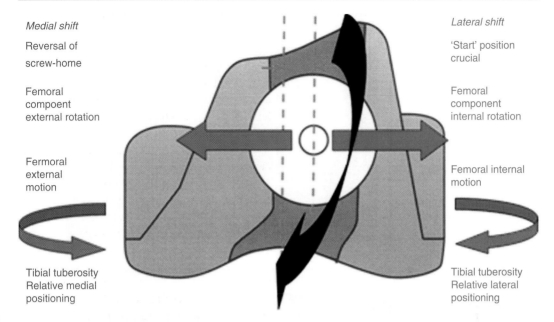

Medial shift

Reversal of
screw-home

Femoral
compoent
external rotation

Fermoral
external
motion

Tibial tuberosity
Relative medial
positioning

Lateral shift

'Start' position
crucial

Femoral
component
internal rotation

Femoral internal
motion

Tibial tuberosity
Relative lateral
positioning

Fig. 15.11 Dynamic relations between femur, tibia and patella

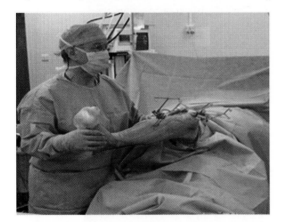

Fig. 15.12 Dynamic assessment of patellar tracking: application of valgus and tibial external rotation

is also seen to lie on the trochlear line on the sagittal view, indicating that the patella is indeed well seated in the trochlea; no adjustments are required in this case.

15.7 Soft Tissue Balancing and Tracking Values

The first panel on the screen below shows an example of patellar maltracking where the registered trochlea is the green line and lateral shift as

a red line, monitoring patellar positioning throughout flexion and extension. Patellar tilt is shown in the second panel, and in the third panel, the patella (blue line) is seen to be further away from the transepicondylar axis than the registered trochlea (green line) (Fig. 15.14a).

The next screen (Fig. 15.14b) shows the situation after soft tissue balancing of the patellofemoral joint including a lateral release of the patellar retinaculum. The patella has moved medially, tilt is reduced and the patella has now moved down into the trochlea.

15.8 Lateral Release Technique

There are several techniques available to release a tight lateral retinaculum, including both inside-to-out and outside-to-in types. Division of tissues can be localised particularly to the centre of the retinacular structure by cutting from the inside or 'peeling' the retinaculum for the patella [34]. Meshing of the ligament from the outside can also be a successful way of lengthening the structure without destroying its continuity [17]. The authors' preferred method is to start proximally from outside-to-in and release the retinaculum in stages as shown below (Fig. 15.15).

Fig. 15.13 'Patella tracking' screen showing satisfactory patellar positioning in mid-flexion

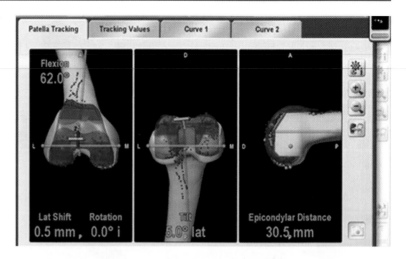

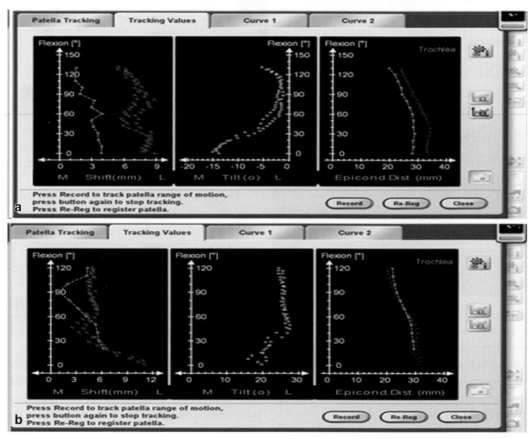

Fig. 15.14 **a** Patellar tracking parameters: the *left-hand* graph shows patellar lateral shift away from the trochlear groove. **b** Correction of patellar tracking resulting from lateral retinacular release

With care, the capsule can be preserved and therefore keeps the knee cavity closed and the deep lateral patellofemoral and patellomeniscal (capsular) ligaments intact. It also facilitates direct observation and preservation of the superior lateral geniculate vessels. Incremental release

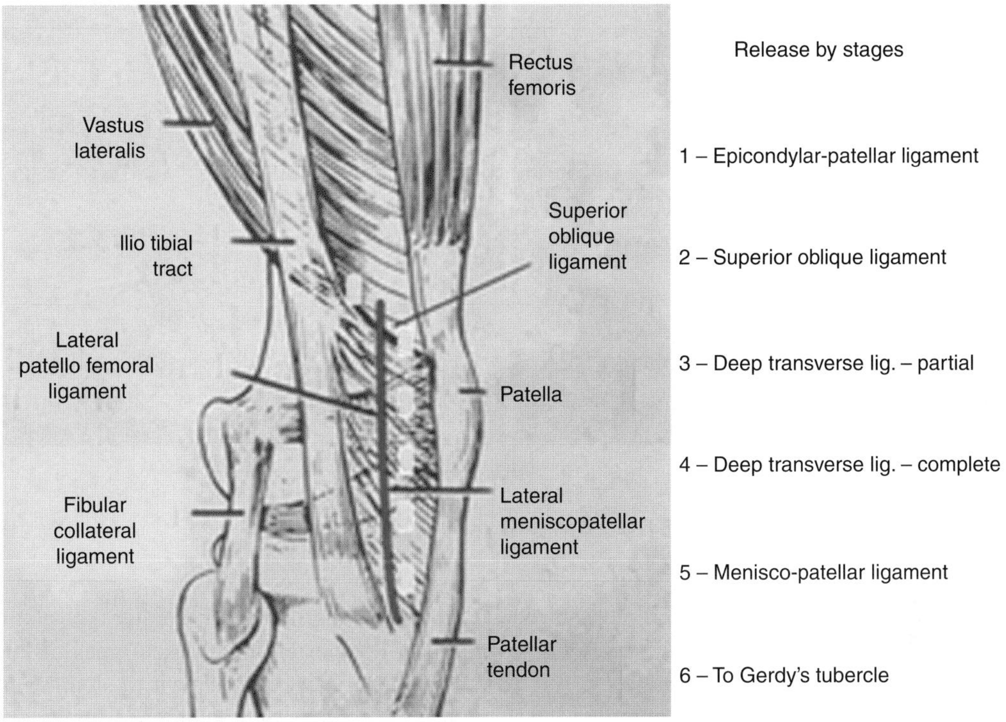

Fig. 15.15 Staged lateral release of patella [36]

then results in a gradual and controlled adjustment of tracking [36].

However, lateral release is not an altogether benign event, and 'all-or-nothing' techniques may result in erratic patellar motion and reduction of lateral stability [11]. However, the negative consequences of lateral release have been described as minimal by some authors [38]. The release also need not compromise the clinical outcomes or complication rates of primary total knee arthroplasty [25], but that implies that retinacular release has been used only in appropriate biomechanical situations, with contracted structures, and not indiscriminantly. The effect of a staged lateral release is clear in Fig. 15.16, where after a stage 4 release, the patellar array is now in an upright position even with knee flexion. The efficacy of the release is demonstrated by the way that the gap in the lateral retinaculum opens during knee flexion. The closed nature of the release reduces the risk of a subcutaneous haematoma.

15.9 Discussion

Many factors influence success in patellofemoral arthroplasty. These include variation in morphology of the patella, femur and tibia, iatrogenic factors, implant design, tibiofemoral dynamics, deformity and contracture. Tibiofemoral and patellofemoral motions are highly interdependent, and patellar tracking is a complex function of the proper assessment of morphology, component positioning, tibiofemoral dynamics and soft tissue balance of the tibiofemoral compartment, as well as the extensor mechanism. Historically, there has been much evidence for poor patellar performance with tilts, shifts, impingements, subluxations and dislocations being primarily the consequence of surgical error and in particular femoral component rotation [24, 31, 35]. Variability in the various femoral and tibial axes means that each knee is best treated on an individual basis. The shape and position of the patella also has an effects, with limb alignment, torsions

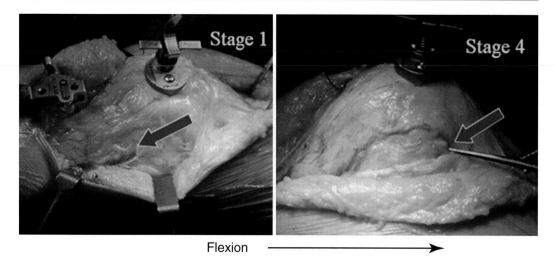

Fig. 15.16 Before and after staged lateral release of patella during TKA

and prior damage to the extensor mechanism being other potentially significant factors in terms of treating every knee as a special case.

Iatrogenic factors are also important and include component positions, limb alignment and gap balancing. The patellar preparation can also be a significant source of error, including the obliquity of the bone cut, the thickness of the bone remnant and of the patellar component and the positioning of the component on the resection surface. The positionings of the femoral component, including mediolateral translation, proximal-distal height in relation to the joint line and internal–external rotation, are all potential sources of error. Implant design is also important, including component contour, constraint and congruence. Two philosophies seem to exist where, firstly, high levels of patellofemoral component constraint seem a safer option and, secondly, a flatter and less constrained trochlear profile allows freer motion in terms of tilt and mediolateral motion. Both design types seem to have reasonable clinical success, but the price for increased stability may be increased loading and shear forces on the devices, particularly if soft tissue balance is suboptimal.

There has been much interest in how different types of knee arthroplasty might affect patellar tracking. However, neither the rotating platform nor posterior stabilised types of knee replacements have been shown to significantly reduce the prevalence of lateral release [26, 32]. Minimally invasive surgery has not been shown to increase rates of lateral retinacular release [13]. Use of the 'no-thumb' technique has, however, been shown to cause a significant increase in rates of release in comparison with a 'towel-clip' technique which provides some medial restraint [10], as does the '2-stitch' method described above.

Deformity and contracture have the potential to cause poor results. The saying that 'I never do a lateral patellar release these days' is still heard from the podium at meetings. Of course, the days of patellar release rates of up to 50 % are long gone, but the release rates in series of standard total knee arthroplasties still seem to be of the order of 6 % [10, 26, 27]. Evidence also exists for an increased rate of lateral patellar release in knees with valgus alignment [35], and the rate of release in any clinical series must always be dependent on the number of complex primary cases within that series that have significant deformities. Some series therefore report rates as low as 3 % [28].

Soft tissue balancing associated with chronic patellar maltracking problems will always

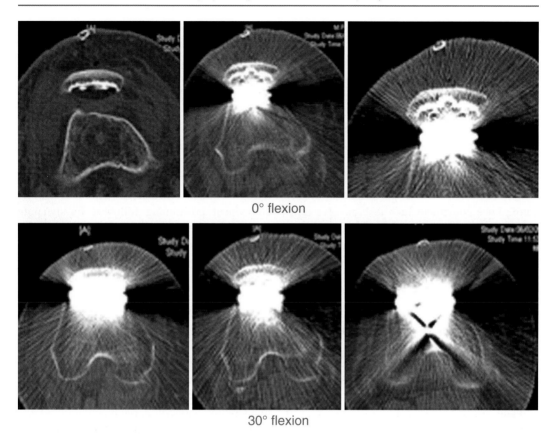

0° flexion

30° flexion

Fig. 15.17 Use of multiple flexion angle CT in PFJR

provide a pitfall for the unwary and inexperienced surgeon, and severe maltracking provides a challenge even for the experienced surgeon. Radiographic features, particularly patellar shift, can be easily assessed preoperatively to identify those cases at increased risk of requiring additional soft tissue work at the time of implantation [9]. Multiple flexion angle CT can also be used to measure shifts, tilts, contact and congruence in relation to the underlying tibiofemoral axes (Fig. 15.17). This type of examination can demonstrate how accurate the tracking has to be, particularly in the case of isolated PFJR, when using a femoral component with a narrow trochlear flange.

Perhaps one of the most important current concepts in total knee arthroplasty is the term 'synchronisation' used by Lee et al. [29]. The term implies the active coordination of

dynamic events in knee arthroplasty to create a well-functioning system. His group used connecting instruments to check that femur and tibia were lined up as well as possible. Perhaps of most relevance in the context of the PFJ was the finding that only 83 % of the 70 patellae studied tracked centrally and that some cases had high tilt angles.

Computer assistance to study patellar tracking in vitro in total knee arthroplasty was used by Belvedere et al. [6] to demonstrate the feasibility of monitoring patellofemoral kinematics intraoperatively. They felt that, by monitoring the situation in this way, the surgeon would have a more complete prediction of the performance of the final implant and thereby assist the making of critical surgical decisions. In vivo studies have been carried out by Anglin et al. [2], who also thought that enhanced intraoperative awareness could aid surgical decision-making.

It seems, therefore, that tibiofemoral and patellofemoral kinematics have to be measured intraoperatively in order to optimise all aspects of balancing and tracking. However, there seems little point in observing patellar motion in isolation from tibiofemoral motion. Therefore, stress testing into varus, valgus and tibial internal and external motion seems necessary to fully test the performance of the whole knee construct. Such tests involve temporary capsular closure followed by dropping and pushing the knee into flexion and extension while loading the knee into valgus, varus, tibial

external and tibial internal positions. In this way, one can observe a 'potential envelope of motion' for that particular combination of component positions and soft tissue balance. Navigation can then quantify the effects of any surgical adjustments. Therefore, in terms of optimisation of patellar motion in the axial dimension, a 'correction algorithm' seems necessary (Fig. 15.18).

Any procedure should therefore start with trying to obtain satisfactory femoral and tibial component positioning followed by dynamic checks upon their synchronised relative motions. This is then followed by any adjustments to component positions and gap balancing as required. If abnormal motions are noted in any compartment, then the process should be repeated as often as necessary. Even if all seems well in the tibiofemoral compartment, there may still be an indication of the need to perform some degree of controlled and limited soft tissue balancing of the extensor mechanism, particularly in the case of prior chronic patellar maltracking. Hopefully, such attention to the dynamics of each individual knee will not only provide satisfactory radiographs but also improve clinical results (Fig. 15.19). In conclusion, therefore, the goal must always be to make the patella track consistently well whatever the initial status of the knee.

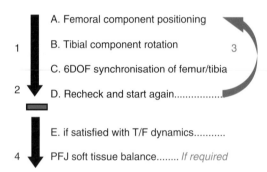

Fig. 15.18 Algorithm for optimisation of tibiofemoral and patellofemoral dynamics in TKA

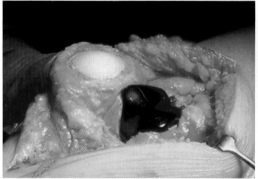
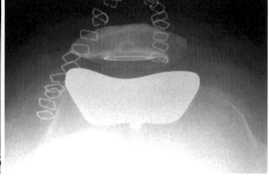

Fig. 15.19 The final result

References

1. Amis AA, Senavongse W, Bull AMJ (2006) Patellofemoral kinematics during knee flexion-extension – an in-vitro study. J Orthop Res 24: 2201–2211

2. Anglin C, Ho KC, Briard JL, de Lambilly C, Plaskos C, Nodwell E, Stindel E (2008) In vivo patellar kinematics during total knee arthroplasty. Comput Aided Surg 13:377–391

3. Archibeck MJ, Camarata D, Trauger J, Allman J, White RE Jr (2003) Indications for lateral retinacular release in total knee replacement. Clin Orthop Relat Res 414:157–161

4. Baldini A, Anderson JA, Cerulli-Mariani P, Kalyvas J, Pavlov H, Sculco TP (2007) Patellofemoral evaluation after total knee arthroplasty. Validation of a new weight-bearing axial radiographic view. J Bone Joint Surg Am 89(8):1810–1817

5. Baldwin JL (2009) The anatomy of the medial patellofemoral ligament. Am J Sports Med 37:2355–2361

6. Belvedere C, Catani F, Ensini A, Moctezuma de la Barrera JL, Leardini A (2007) Patellar tracking during total knee arthroplasty: an in vitro feasibility study. Knee Surg Sports Traumatol Arthrosc 15:985–993

7. Bicos J, Fulkerson JP, Amis A (2007) Current concepts review: the medial patellofemoral ligament. Am J Sports Med 35:484–492

8. Briard JL, Hungerford DS (1989) Patellofemoral instability in total knee arthroplasty. J Arthroplasty 4(Suppl):S87–S97

9. Chia SL, Merican AM, Devadasan B, Strachan RK, Amis AA (2009) Radiographic features predictive of patellar maltracking during total knee arthroplasty. Knee Surg Sports Traumatol Arthrosc 17:1217–1224

10. Cho WS, Woo JH, Park HY, Youm YS, Kim BK (2011) Should the 'no thumb technique' be the golden standard for evaluating patellar tracking in total knee arthroplasty? Knee 18:177–179

11. Christoforakis J, Bull AM, Strachan RK, Shymkiw R, Senavongse W, Amis AA (2006) Effects of lateral retinacular release on the lateral stability of the patella. Knee Surg Sports Traumatol Arthrosc 14(3):273–277

12. Conlan T, Garth WP Jr, Lemons JE (1993) Evaluation of the medial soft-tissue restraints of the extensor mechanism of the knee. J Bone Joint Surg Am 75: 682–693

13. Cook JL, Scuderi GR, Tenholder M (2006) Incidence of lateral release in total knee arthroplasty in standard and mini-incision approaches. Clin Orthop Relat Res 452:123–126

14. Desio SM, Burks RT, Bachus KN (1998) Soft tissue restraints to lateral patellar translation in the human knee. Am J Sports Med 26:59–65

15. Ghosh KM, Merican AM, Iranpour F, Deehan DJ, Amis AA (2009) The effect of overstuffing the patellofemoral joint on the extensor retinaculum of the knee. Knee Surg Sports Traumatol Arthrosc 17: 1211–1216

16. Ghosh KM, Merican AM, Iranpour-Boroujeni F, Deehan DJ, Amis AA (2009) Length change patterns of the extensor retinaculum and the effect of total knee replacement. J Orthop Res 27:865–870

17. Healy WL, Iorio R, Warren P (2004) Mesh expansion release of the lateral patellar retinaculum during total knee arthroplasty. J Bone Joint Surg Am 86-A(Suppl 1 (Pt 2)):193–200

18. Iranpour F, Merican AM, Amis AA, Cobb JP (2008) The width:thickness ratio of the patella: an aid in knee arthroplasty. Clin Orthop Relat Res 466:1198–1203

19. Iranpour F, Merican AM, Dandachli W, Amis AA, Cobb JP (2010) The geometry of the trochlear groove. Clin Orthop Relat Res 468:782–788

20. Iranpour F, Merican AM, Rodriguez-y-Baena F, Cobb JP, Amis AA (2010) Patellofemoral joint kinematics: the circular path of the patella. J Orthop Res 28:589–594

21. Jenny JY, Boeri C (2004) Low reproducibility of the intra-operative measurement of the transepicondylar axis during total knee replacement. Acta Orthop Scand 75:74–77

22. Jerosch J, Peuker E, Philipps B, Filler T (2002) Interindividual reproducibility in perioperative rotational alignment of femoral components in knee prosthesis surgery using the transepicondylar axis. Knee Surg Sports Traumatol Arthrosc 10:194–197

23. Katchburian MV, Bull AMJ, Shih YF, Heatley FW, Amis AA (2003) Measurement of patellar tracking: assessment and analysis of the literature. Clin Orthop Relat Res 412:241–259

24. Kessler O, Patil S, Colwell CW Jr, D'Lima DD (2008) The effect of femoral component malrotation on patellar biomechanics. J Biomech 41:3332–3339

25. Kusuma SK, Puri N, Lotke PA (2009) Lateral retinacular release during primary total knee arthroplasty: effect on outcomes and complications. J Arthroplasty 24:383–390

26. Lachiewicz PF, Soileau ES (2006) Patella maltracking in posterior-stabilized total knee arthroplasty. Clin Orthop Relat Res 452:155–158

27. Laskin RS (2001) Lateral release rates after total knee arthroplasty. Clin Orthop Relat Res 392:88–93

28. Lee GC, Cushner FD, Scuderi GR, Insall JN (2004) Optimizing patellofemoral tracking during total knee arthroplasty. J Knee Surg 17:144–149

29. Lee DH, Seo JG, Moon YW (2008) Synchronisation of tibial rotational alignment with femoral component in total knee arthroplasty. Int Orthop 32:223–227

30. Malo M, Vince KG (2003) The unstable patella after total knee arthroplasty: etiology, prevention, and management. J Am Acad Orthop Surg 11:364–371

31. Merican AM, Ghosh KM, Iranpour F, Deehan DJ, Amis AA (2011) The effect of femoral component

rotation on the kinematics of the tibiofemoral and patellofemoral joints after total knee arthroplasty. Knee Surg Sports Traumatol Arthrosc 19:1479–1487

32. Pagnano MW, Trousdale RT, Stuart MJ, Hanssen AD, Jacofsky DJ (2004) Rotating platform knees did not improve patellar tracking: a prospective, randomized study of 240 primary total knee arthroplasties. Clin Orthop Relat Res 428:221–227

33. Senavongse W, Amis AA (2005) The effects of articular, retinacular, or muscular deficiencies on patellofemoral joint stability: a biomechanical study in vitro. J Bone Joint Surg Br 87B:577–582

34. Shaw JA (2003) Patellar retinacular peel: an alternative to lateral retinacular release in total knee arthroplasty. Am J Orthop 32:189–192

35. Sodha S, Kim J, McGuire KJ, Lonner JH, Lotke PA (2004) Lateral retinacular release as a function of femoral component rotation in total knee arthroplasty. J Arthroplasty 19:459–463

36. Strachan RK, Merican AM, Devadasan B, Maheshwari R, Amis AA (2009) A technique of staged lateral release to correct patellar tracking in total knee arthroplasty. J Arthroplasty 24:735–742

37. Verlinden C, Uvin P, Labey L, Luyckx JP, Bellemans J, Vandenneucker H (2010) The influence of malrotation of the femoral component in total knee replacement on the mechanics of patellofemoral contact during gait: an in vitro biomechanical study. J Bone Joint Surg Br 92:737–742

38. Weber AB, Worland RL, Jessup DE, Van Bowen J, Keenan J (2003) The consequences of lateral release in total knee replacement: a review of over 1000 knees with follow up between 5 and 11 years. Knee 10:187–191

39. Yoshino N, Takai S, Ohtsuki Y, Hirasawa Y (2001) Computed tomography measurement of the surgical and clinical transepicondylar axis of the distal femur in osteoarthritic knees. J Arthroplasty 16:493–497

Revision Total Knee Arthroplasty

16

F. Iacono, Laura Nofrini, D. Bruni, G. Raspugli,
B. Sharma, I. Akkawi, M. Lo Presti, M. Nitri, Stefano
Zaffagnini, and Maurilio Marcacci

16.1 Introduction

Total knee arthroplasty (TKA) is one of the most successful orthopaedic procedures performed today. This is due to the substantial pain relief and restoration of function after TKA. As a result of its success [15, 21], indications for TKA have included younger and more active patients. Therefore, the number of revision TKAs is also rising with a projected increase of 601 % from 2005 to 2030 [14]. Although the results of primary TKAs are well documented with implant survivorship at 15 years greater than 95 % [29], the results of revision procedures are less

F. Iacono • D. Bruni • G. Raspugli • M.L. Presti
S. Zaffagnini • M. Marcacci
Laboratorio di Biomeccanica e Innovazione Tecnologica,
Istituto Ortopedico Rizzoli,via di Barbiano 1/10,
Bologna 40136, Italy
Clinica Ortopedica e Traumatologica III, Istituto
Ortopedico Rizzoli,
via di Barbiano 1/10, Bologna 40136, Italy

L. Nofrini (✉)
Laboratorio di Biomeccanica e Innovazione Tecnologica,
Istituto Ortopedico Rizzoli,
via di Barbiano 1/10, Bologna 40136, Italy

Orthokey LLC,
Lewes, DE, USA
e-mail: l.nofrini@biomec.ior.it

B. Sharma • I. Akkawi • M. Nitri
Clinica Ortopedica e Traumatologica III,
Istituto Ortopedico Rizzoli,
via di Barbiano 1/10, Bologna 40136, Italy

predictable and encouraging with an 82 % survivorship at 12 years. Predominant revision failure modes include infection (46 %), aseptic loosening (19 %) and instability (13 %) [28].

Revision TKA is a technically demanding procedure with many potential complications. Its successful performance requires preoperative planning, adherence to principles of revision knee arthroplasty, availability of diverse implant options and adequate bone graft. Before considering a revision TKA, the aetiology of failure should be defined so the same mistake is not made again in the revision surgery [32]. Revision TKA must address soft tissue integrity and bone stock that is often compromised. The implant choice must be based on these factors. Contemporary designs of revision knee prostheses have evolved to provide designs with increasing levels of constraint. Considering that long-term durability of the prosthetic components, as well as fixation, is inversely proportional to prosthetic constraint, it is preferable to select the least constrained prosthetic components to achieve these objectives [6, 25].

The modular posterior stabilised implants with their conforming articulation and post and cam mechanism provide adequate stability when the collateral ligaments are intact. In cases of varus–valgus instability or increased flexion gap laxity, the post-cam mechanism is not sufficient, and a nonlinked condylar constrained prosthesis is needed. In patients with complete loss of the medial collateral ligament or with massive bony defects with resulting extension and flexion gap mismatch or extensor mechanism insufficiency, a rotating

F. Catani, S. Zaffagnini (eds.), *Knee Surgery using Computer Assisted Surgery and Robotics*,
DOI 10.1007/978-3-642-31430-8_16, © ESSKA 2013

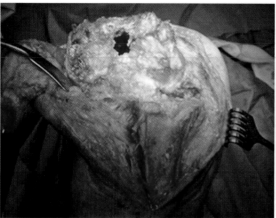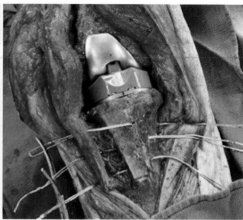

Fig. 16.1 After implant removal, tibial and distal and posterior femoral bone loss must be appreciated before cutting. May be difficult to identify relevant bone landmarks required for the joint reconstruction. In this case, osteotomy of the tibial tuberosity while maintaining intact muscle attachment laterally to preserve the vascularity was performed for exposure. Repair with wires was performed according to Whiteside technique

hinge implant may be indicated [2, 5, 30]. In our experience, in the majority of revision cases, a constrained prosthesis is used. Increasing constraint is not without problems, however, as forces across the knee may be transmitted to the stem-bone interface, resulting in radiographic loosening of stemmed components. Rotating hinge components have now gained wide acceptance in the salvage revision arthroplasties. In fact short-term survival rates are promising, and rotating hinge components are implanted in 10–30 % of RTKA [1, 8, 30, 31].

16.2 Revision with Constrained Prosthesis: Conventional Surgical Technique

The objective of revision arthroplasty is the same as primary surgery: to restore the limb alignment with proper implant positioning, to achieve an appropriate soft tissue balance and restoration of joint line with a good range of motion. Once the old implant and cement have been removed, the knee is ready for the new prosthesis. The proximal tibial and distal femoral cuts will determine the correct limb alignment. It is important to remember that adjustments on the femoral side can affect the knee in flexion or extension, whereas any adjustments on the tibial side will affect both. The proximal tibial cut should be perpendicular to the mechanical axis of the tibia in the coronal and sagittal planes. An intramedullary cutting guide is usually used for this cut. Minimal good bone sacrifice is the goal. In the case of a bone defect, this must be identified but not eliminated by an increased cut (Fig. 16.1). The defects will be subsequently treated by using bone graft or metal augmentations. The medullary canal is opened using hand reamers. A suitable trial rod with a good fit to the canal is selected and attached to a trial tibial component and put in place. The selected tibial implant should cover the cortical rim of the proximal tibia. Overhang of the tibial prosthesis on the medial side should be avoided to prevent impingement on the medial collateral ligament.

The distal femoral cut is made at 5–7° of valgus in reference to the shaft of the femur. An intramedullary cutting guide is usually used for this cut. As with the tibial cut, the objective is minimal bone removal with a flat femoral distal cut. Residual bone deficiencies will be treated at a subsequent time. Medial and lateral epicondyles will serve as reference for rotational position of the femoral component. The lateral femoral epicondyle lies slightly posterior to the medial femoral epicondyle. The next step is to choose the size of the femoral component. Its correct sizing is complex and very important, and it must be made simultaneously with soft tissue balance as the two issues are intimately related.

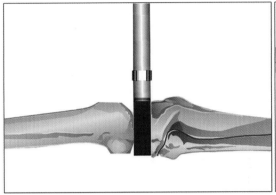 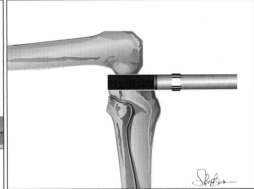

Fig. 16.2 The 'extension gap' is created by resection of the proximal tibia and distal femoral condyles, whereas the 'flexion gap' is created by resection of the proximal tibia and posterior femoral condyles. Therefore, while tibial cut will affect both gaps, distal and posterior femoral cuts can affect the knee in flexion or extension. Equal flexion and extension gaps are necessary to balance the knee (Design by Silvia Bassini)

The goals of femoral implant selection should be the creation of equal flexion and extension gaps (Fig. 16.2), correction of joint line level and fit of the implant to the remaining bone.

The final choice of revision femoral component size will be determined not by residual bone but by the soft tissue, specifically the collateral ligaments. Always after implant removal, there is distal and posterior femoral bone loss that must be appreciated. In fact, if a femoral component that simply fits the remaining bone is chosen, a smaller than normal size will be selected. The result will be the selection of a thicker polyethylene to achieve stability both in flexion and extension. This will lead to proximalisation of the joint line. Sometimes, a smaller femoral component may result in an arthroplasty that is unstable in flexion (flexion space larger than extension space), in which an excessive distal femoral cut must be performed to accommodate the thicker polyethylene selected to have flexion stability. Undue resection of the distal femur results in a proximally displaced joint line. For these reasons in revision TKA, the joint line is often proximalised [16, 20]. The size of the failed component, if it was sized appropriately, or lateral radiograph of the contralateral knee, if not replaced, may be used to estimate the size of the revision component. Stability in flexion is determined not only by the size but also by the anteroposterior location of the femoral component. It is good practice to position the

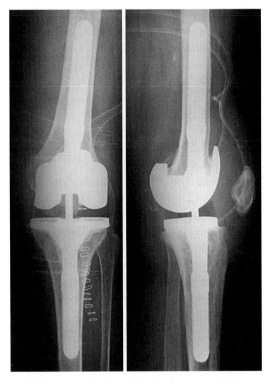

Fig. 16.3 AP and lateral radiographs of a total condylar III for revision arthroplasty. To balance the knee in flexion and extension, the femoral component is placed as posterior as possible, and a posterior augmentation is used to fill the space between the implant and the bone

femoral component as posterior as possible without notching. Augmentation can be added posteriorly to fit the implant to the bone (Fig. 16.3).

Augmentation can be used asymmetrically and in different amounts to achieve an appropriate rotation of the femoral component according to the epicondylar axis. Once the appropriate sized femoral component is set in the correct rotation, the objective is to restore the joint line level. Re-establishing the joint line to the true anatomic level is required for optimal stability and joint kinematics. When posterior cruciate substitution is selected, restoration of the joint line to within 8 mm is necessary to optimise function [3, 7, 20]. The femoral epicondyles again provide a valuable landmark. In fact, more detailed anatomic studies have determined the joint line to be positioned at a mean distance of 3.0 cm below the medial epicondyle and 2.5 cm below the lateral epicondyle [27]. The trial femoral component is then set to re-establish the distal joint line. With the provisional components in place, the knee is stabilised in flexion: the thickest polyethylene that fills the flexion space is inserted. The knee is brought into full extension. If the knee is stable (equal extension space), no adjustments are necessary. If there is a discrepancy between flexion and extension gaps, additional adjustments are required.

When the knee is balanced in flexion and loose in extension, if the size of femoral component is correct, distal femoral augmentation is added. It is important that the joint line is not displaced distally because this can produce patella maltracking.

The most common problem is a flexion gap larger than the extension gap: in this case a series of checks and adjustments are necessary.

The first step is to reduce the distal augmentation.

The second step is to check the sagittal position and the size of the femoral component:

(a) If it is set too anterior, then it is moved posteriorly by using an offset stem and a thicker posterior augmentation.

(b) If the size is too small, a larger size should be chosen, but caution should be taken not to oversize the femur because of the adverse effect on motion.

(c) In case of a stable knee in extension and persistent flexion laxity after joint line restoration, a compromise could be to seat more proximally

the femoral component and increase the thickness of polyethylene accepting an elevation of joint line that does not have a clinical adverse effects if it is less than 8 mm.

(d) If the knee cannot be stabilised because of deficiency of one or both collateral ligaments, then a rotating hinge prosthesis may be considered.

Once the appropriate alignment and stability have been achieved, the final components are assembled. With constrained implants extension stems are usually used to improve the fixation. It is our practice to cement the tibial and femoral component and insert press-fit stems. The integrity of the bone and the dimension of the intramedullary canal determine the length and the diameter of stems, respectively.

As described above, the primary challenge in revision TKA is the restoration of an adequate joint stability and joint line. This may be complicated by a loss of bone stock and difficulties in identifying relevant bone landmarks [9, 20].

16.3 Computer-Assisted Revision Total Knee Arthroplasty

Computer assistance can be extremely useful in revision situations. Navigation can be a helpful decision-making tool to overcome lack of anatomical and functional information due to loss of bone stock and ligamentous insufficiency often observed after the removal of the failed prosthesis. This chapter reports our experience in computer-assisted total knee revision.

16.3.1 Our First Experience: RTKANav System

Our experience started in 2005 with the development of an innovative computer-assisted surgical technique for total knee revision [17]. This technique was based on the use of a dedicated navigation system, RTKANav, a prototype developed by our group in collaboration with ORTHOKEY (Lewes, DE, USA). Even if first attempts of navigated revision total knee arthroplasty were already being performed using navigation system for primary TKA, we decided to develop a dedicated system for revision total knee arthroplasty because in our opinion anatomical landmarks available were not suitable to give correct indications using a primary TKA navigation system. In fact, since those systems require anatomical parameters detected on the failed metal component to be removed, proposed surgical planning is based on rough anatomical landmarks that do not reflect the patient's original anatomy. RTKANav was the first system specifically developed for revision total knee arthroplasty.

RTKANav allows one:

- To identify the best joint line position to be restored according to the indication reconstructed from the residual anatomical landmarks
- To identify the best component size combination restoring the joint line position and guaranteeing the best soft tissue balance possible and allow the surgeon to virtually test different solutions, controlling those two crucial factors
- To accurately reproduce on the patient the planned operative decisions

16.3.2 System Description

The main components of the navigation system RTKANav are a passive optical localiser (Polaris System NDI, Northern Digital Inc., Ontario, Canada) to determine the position and the orientation of the instruments in the scene, dedicated software specifically developed for this application and some sensorised surgical tools, part of which have been purposely developed for this application.

Sensorised surgical instrumentation designed to be used together with the conventional instrumentation consists of:

- Two reference arrays to be fixed to the femur and to the tibia, used to track the anatomy during the intervention
- A pointer used to acquire anatomical landmarks
- Two tools, called FemoralMod and TibialMod, developed to acquire the direction of the

medullary canal of the two bones and to provide indications for a correct rotational and anteroposterior prosthesis positioning

The last tool is a custom-made spacer, called key tensor, developed to measure the gap between the femur and the tibia in flexion and extension. During gap acquisition, key tensor features allow the femur and the tibia to assume a position depending exclusively on ligament constraints, enabling the surgeon, together with the information provided by the software, to perform a navigated ligament balancing.

The system does not require preoperative medical images. Moreover, landmarks useful to correctly plan and navigate the intervention are acquired on patient anatomy after prosthesis removal.

Joint line computation and gap measuring steps implemented on the system are independent from the surgical instrumentation used, while virtual planning phase and implant positioning navigation depend on the prosthesis model.

16.3.3 Surgical Technique

After performing the surgical access, the two reference arrays are fixed to the bones using two bicortical pins, being careful to avoid possible impingement between the bicortical pins and the cutting guides or femoral and tibial intramedullary rods. After prosthesis removal and medullary canal reaming, the surgeon by using the sensorised instruments detects several anatomical landmarks on patient anatomy, medullary canal direction and the tibial and distal femoral residual planes orientation (Fig. 16.4). Using those data, RTKANav reconstructs the 3D representation of the patient's lower limb and the references to plan the intervention.

Using the conventional surgical technique, tibial and distal femoral resection is executed to the level required to establish a viable surface and preserve bone stock. On the femoral side, in the final implant, augmentation will be employed to correct possible imbalance.

The last data required by RTKANav to define the surgical strategy are the gaps in extension and

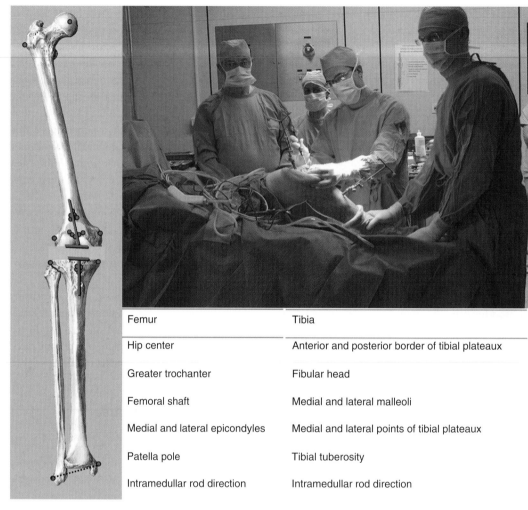

Femur	Tibia
Hip center	Anterior and posterior border of tibial plateaux
Greater trochanter	Fibular head
Femoral shaft	Medial and lateral malleoli
Medial and lateral epicondyles	Medial and lateral points of tibial plateaux
Patella pole	Tibial tuberosity
Intramedullar rod direction	Intramedullar rod direction

Fig. 16.4 Anatomical data required to build patient model and to plan the intervention. Even if during acquisition phase some specific points were missing due to the bone deficiencies (e.g. one or both the epicondyles), since for each prosthetic component several criteria to set each degree of freedom are considered and compared, the system is always able to suggest an intervention plan

in flexion: with the FemoralMod and the TibialMod positioned on the bones, with the relative planes tangent to the most protruding part of each bone, using the key tensor to obtain the desired ligament tension, joint space measuring in extension and in 90° flexion is performed, and the symmetry of each gap is evaluated (Fig. 16.5).

RTKANav shows on the interface the relative positions between medio-lateral axis of the two planes together with numerical information about their distance and the angle between them in the frontal plane, updated in real time.

During flexion space assessment, RTKANav helps the surgeon to establish correct femoral rotational positioning considering both anatomical references and soft tissue balancing: in addition to FemoralMod and TibialMod references, also the transepicondylar line reference is represented, together with the measure of the angle that it forms with the FemoralMod reference [10–12, 24, 27]. Gathered data are

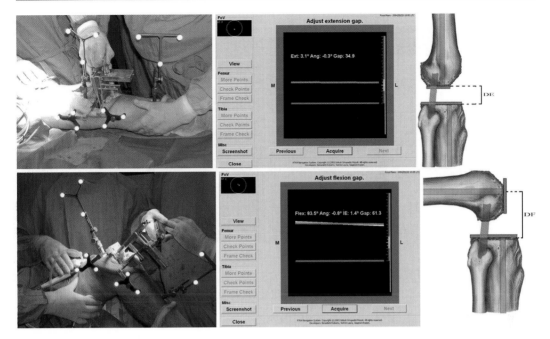

Fig. 16.5 Estimation of extension and flexion space using the key tensor. On the interface the TibialMod reference (*blue line*) and the FemoralMod reference (*orange line*) together with numerical data allow to assess the gap parallelism. During flexion space estimation, also the transepicondylar line reference is shown (*upper white line*) to determine proper femoral prosthesis rotational positioning

used by the system to automatically plan the intervention.

16.3.4 Planning Criteria

A range of acceptability for the joint line level is determined relative to the medial and lateral epicondyles' height, the patella pole position in extension and the fibular head, based on anatomical data reported in literature [3, 4, 11, 16, 19, 20]. The most appropriate joint line height is set considering the determined acceptability interval and the measured extension space, providing also indications about the required tibial polyethylene insert size and possible need of femoral augmentation. The tibial polyethylene insert size that is chosen is the one that best fits the space between the tibial cut and the joint line height determined at the previous step on the basis of measured extension space.

The femoral components size to be implanted in order to have a correct flexion-extension soft tissue balancing is determined considering the flexion space, the prosthesis features and the relationship between the canal position and the anterior femoral shaft [4, 11, 13, 22].

The system proposes a plan of the intervention and provides the surgeon with tools to analyse and modify the proposed plan monitoring the behaviour of the residual joint gap in flexion and in extension (Fig. 16.6).

It should be underlined that even if during acquisition phase, some specific points were missing due to the bone deficiencies (e.g. one or both the epicondyles), since for each prosthetic component several criteria to set each degree of freedom are considered and compared, the system is always able to suggest an intervention plan.

Once the intervention plan is refined, the system tools enable the surgeon to correctly position the cutting guides in order to reproduce on the patient the planned strategy.

The final position of the tibial and femoral implants can be checked by displaying the postoperative leg alignment and residual joint gap. If the check with the trials satisfies the surgeon's requirements, the definitive components are inserted with cement.

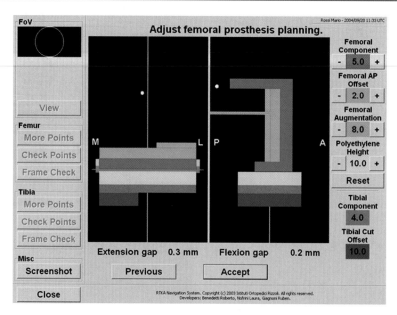

Fig. 16.6 System interface during planning phase. In this system prototype each implant component is represented by a simple geometrical model, which is drawn considering only the characteristics useful for planning purposes. The limb is represented by the femoral and tibial mechanical axis together with some reference points, useful for planning refinement. The joint line range of acceptability is represented as an area drawn with different shades of green (from *dark green* to *yellow*), depending on the amount of conditions fulfilled. A white line is drawn corresponding to the middle of the darkest green area, and it shows the best joint line height (BJLH) satisfying most of set conditions. Some buttons labelled '+' and '−' allow the surgeon to modify the size of components that can be replaced and to check different components combination. Measurements of the critical data resulting from the current configuration are reported

16.4 Our Second Experience: RHO System

Recently we started a new experience in computer-assisted revision total knee arthroplasty with the development of a software for hinged prosthesis implant. We developed this software in collaboration with ORTHOKEY, and now it is included in the set of applications available with the BLU-IGS platform (BLU-IGS, Orthokey, Lewes, DE, USA).

Hinged prostheses for revision TKA are used in cases of severe bone loss, high instability, insufficiency or absence of one or both collateral ligaments and chronic dysfunction of the extensor mechanism. Proper implant positioning and correct joint line position are crucial for a successful outcome.

RHO assists the surgeon to:

- Restore the joint line level based on the residual anatomical landmarks still available
- Recreate the correct rotational positioning of the component

16.4.1 System Description

RHO is based on the use of an optical localiser and of some sensorised instruments to be tracked during the surgery. In particular the sensorised instrumentation consists of:

- Two reference arrays to be fixed to the femur and to the tibia.
- A pointer used both for anatomical landmark acquisition and to enable the tracking of the conventional instrumentation in the most critical steps of prosthesis components positioning. Using the conventional

Femur
- Hip center
- Anterior shaft
- Medial and lateral
  epicondyles
- Medullary canal entry point
- Distal residual bone

Tibia
- Medullary canal entry point
- Fibular head
- Tibial tuberosity
- Proximal residual bone
- Tibial posterior condyle
  tangent
- Medial and lateral malleoli

Patella
Inferior patella pole

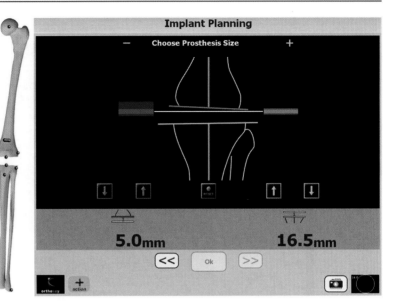

Fig. 16.7 RHO landmarks acquisition and joint line planning interface. After landmark acquisition, the system shows on the interface the optimal joint line position with respect to femoral and tibial residual planes and the areas where joint line anatomical constraint is satisfied. Even if during acquisition phase some specific points were missing due to the bone deficiencies (e.g. one or both the epicondyles), since several criteria are considered and compared, the system is always able to suggest a solution

instrumentation allows one to exploit all the instrument features for an optimal prosthesis implant.

As for RTKANav, as with RHO, preoperative medical images are not required, and all the computations are based on the anatomical acquisitions done after prosthesis removal.

16.4.2 Surgical Technique

After performing the surgical access, the femoral reference array is fixed to the bone medially on the distal femoral metaphysis, using two monocortical screws. Then, the tibial array is fixed as distally as possible on the shaft with two bicortical 3 mm diameter screws.

Anatomical landmark acquisition is performed after prosthesis removal, and starting from those points, RHO reconstructs the best joint line level for both the tibia and femur (Fig. 16.7). In this case, since a hinged prosthesis is implanted, the best joint line position is reconstructed using the anatomical data and not soft tissue information.

16.4.2.1 Planning Criteria

In RHO criteria used to determine the joint line position include more criteria in addition to those implemented in RTKANav, making joint line reconstruction even more reliable [10, 18, 23, 26].

Those criteria are considered and compared as described for RTKANav.

The system shows on the interface the position of the optimal joint line with respect to the distal femoral plane and the proximal tibial plane and together with the representation for each landmark of the areas where the associated constraints are satisfied. A set of buttons allows the surgeon to adapt the proposed solution to any patient-specific need.

Using the navigated pointer together with the conventional instrumentation, RHO assists the surgeon during cutting block positioning, trial prosthesis and definitive component implant, to correctly reproduce the planned rotational position and for joint line restoration: the current component position is shown on the frontal and axial view together with the reference (Figs. 16.8 and 16.9).

Moreover, it is always possible to assess limb alignment, measuring varus–valgus deformity

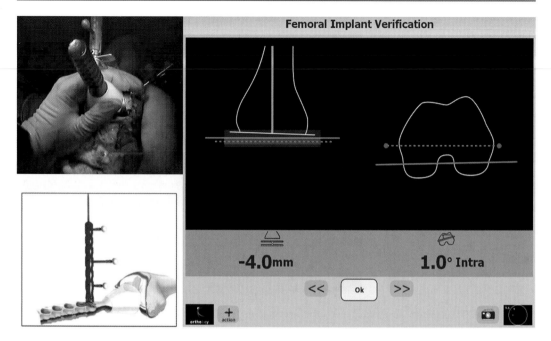

Fig. 16.8 Femoral implant positioning navigation. Using the navigated pointer together with the conventional instrumentation, during prosthesis positioning it is possible to monitor in real time resulting joint line position and rotational positioning with respect to the anatomical references

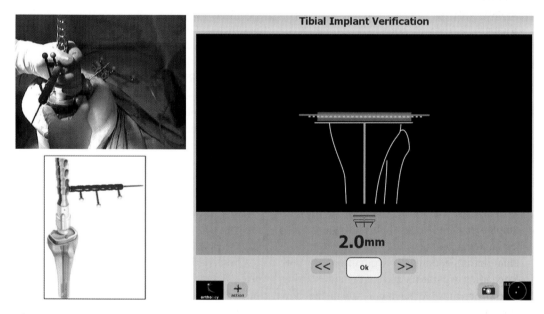

Fig. 16.9 Tibial implant positioning navigation. Using the navigated pointer together with the conventional instrumentation, during prosthesis positioning it is possible to monitor in real time resulting joint line position with respect to the anatomical references

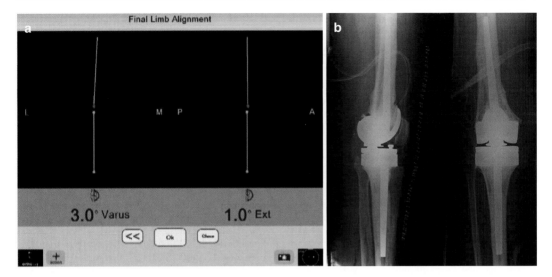

Fig. 16.10 (a) Intraoperative limb assessment. (b) Postoperative X-ray carried out immediatly after revision surgery with LINK Endo-Model

and range of motion obtained with the current solution (Fig. 16.10).

Conclusion

Revision total knee arthroplasty remains a challenging procedure, and computer-assisted surgery can be very useful to provide crucial indications to define the surgical strategy to adopt. Different from other navigated applications in which the navigation system allows one to detect in a more accurate way or in a less invasive manner information that can be retrieved with manual instrumentation, the most important aspect of computer-assisted revision is to provide the surgeon with fundamental information that cannot be retrieved with manual instruments.

The case of modular prosthesis, criteria implemented for flexion and extension spaces estimation using the key tensor, with the bones that during gap opening assume a position depending exclusively on ligament constraints, allows one to solve the main problems of inaccuracy in spaces assessment.

Another crucial aspect is that during planning phase the system allows the surgeon to define the best operative strategy that guarantees joint line restoration and soft tissue balancing, analysing the consequences of each decision he takes, including the opportunity to check different implant solutions.

Several authors report joint line elevation with conventional technique. Present computer-assisted techniques, allowing one to compute optimal joint line position, can help to determine the correct augment thickness to be implanted. Moreover, giving a permanent knowledge of the joint line position during the most crucial steps of the procedure, both techniques allow one to easily reproduce the planned surgical strategy on the patient.

Limb alignment restoration is one of the objectives of revision arthroplasty. Even if both systems allow limb alignment control, it should be considered that the longer the stem is, the more difficult it is to change the alignment of the component. So the component takes up the alignment of the medullary canal, which is not the same as the mechanical axis.

Finally, navigation can be a helpful decision-making tool for choosing more constrained implants in case joint line elevation exceeds 1 cm with respect to the ideal level.

In our experience, navigation contributed valuable information throughout the procedure with minimal extra time or expense, providing indications very useful for the surgeon both in simple revision cases, allowing control of joint line restoration, ligament balancing and limb alignment and in case of severe bone loss to calculate the height of bone to be reconstructed, in order to restore a satisfactory anatomy.

References

1. Barrack RL (2002) Rise of the rotating hinge in revision total knee arthroplasty. Orthopedics 25: 1020–1058
2. Barrack RL, Lyons TR, Ingraham RQ et al (2000) The use of a modular rotating hinge component in salvage revision total knee arthroplasty. J Arthroplasty 15: 858–866
3. Bellemans J (2004) Restoring the joint line in revision TKA: does it matter? Knee 11:3–5
4. Bourne RB, Crawford HA (1998) Principles of revision total knee arthroplasty. Orthop Clin North Am 29(2):331–337
5. Cameron HU, Hu C, Vyamont D (1997) Hinge total knee replacement revisited. Can J Surg 40: 278–283
6. Dennis DA (2007) A stepwise approach to revision total knee arthroplasty. J Arthroplasty 22:32–39
7. Figgie HE, Goldberg VM, Heipel KG, Miller HS, Gordon NH (1986) The influence of tibial patellofemoral location on function of the knee in patients with the posterior stabilized knee prosthesis. J Bone Joint Surg Am 68A:1035–1040
8. Fuchs S, Sandmann C, Gerdemann G et al (2004) Quality of life and clinical outcome in salvage revision total knee replacement: hinged vs. total condylar design. Knee Surg Sports Traumatol Arthrosc 12: 140–143
9. Gofton WT, Tsigaras H, Butler RA et al (2002) Revision total knee arthroplasty: fixation with modular stems. Clin Orthop 404:158–168
10. Griffin FM, Math K, Scuderi GR, Insall JN, Poilvache PL (2000) Anatomy of the epicondyles of the distal femur: MRI analysis of normal knees. J Arthroplasty 15(3):354–359
11. Hoeffel DP, Rubash HE (2000) Revision total knee arthroplasty: current rationale and techniques for femoral component revision. Clin Orthop Relat Res 380:116–132
12. Jerosch J, Peuker E, Philipps B, Filler T (2002) Interindividual reproducibility 27 in perioperative rotational alignment of femoral components in knee prosthetic surgery using the transepicondylar axis. Knee Surg Sports Traumatol Arthrosc 10(3): 194–197
13. Krackow KA (2002) Revision total knee replacement ligament balancing for deformity. Clin Orthop Relat Res 404:152–157
14. Kurtz S, Ong K, Lau E, Mowat F, Halpern M (2007) Projections of primary and revision hip and knee arthroplasty in the United States from 2005 to 2030. J Bone Joint Surg Am 89:780–785
15. Lachiewicz PF, Soileau ES (2006) Ten year survival and clinical results of constrained components in primary total knee arthroplasty. J Arthroplasty 21:803
16. Laskin R (2002) Joint line position restoration during revision total knee replacement. Clin Orthop 404: 169–171
17. Marcacci M, Nofrini L, Iacono F et al (2007) A novel computer-assisted surgical technique for revision total knee arthroplasty. Comput Biol Med 37(12): 1771–1779
18. Mountney J, Karamfiles R, Breidahl W, Farrugia M, Sikorski JM (2007) The position of the joint line in relation to the trans-epicondylar axis of the knee: complementary radiologic and computer-based studies. J Arthroplasty 22(8):1201–1207
19. Neyret P, Robinson AH, Le Coultre B, Lapra C, Chambat P (2002) Patellar tendon length – the factor in patellar instability? Knee 9(1):3–6
20. Partington PF, Sawhney J, Rorabeck CH, Barrack RL, Moore J (1999) Joint line restoration after revision total knee arthroplasty. Clin Orthop 367:165–171
21. Pradhan NR, Gambhir A, Porter ML (2006) Survivorship analysis of 3234 primary total knee arthroplasties implanted over a 26-year period: a study of eight different implant designs. Knee 13:7–11
22. Ries MD, Haas SB, Windsor RE (2004) Soft-tissue balance in revision total knee arthroplasty. Surgical technique. J Bone Joint Surg Am 86-A(Suppl 1): 81–86
23. Romero J, Seifert B, Reinhardt O, Ziegler O, Kessler O (2010) A useful radiologic method for preoperative joint-line determination in revision total knee arthroplasty. Clin Orthop Relat Res 468(5):1279–83
24. Schneider B, Laubenberger J, Jemlich S et al (1997) Measurement of femoral antetorsion and tibial torsion by magnetic resonance imaging. Br J Radiol 70(834): 575–579
25. Scuderi GR (2001) Revision total knee arthroplasty. How much constraint is enough? Clin Orthop 392: 300–305
26. Servien E, Viskontas D, Giuffrè BM, Coolican MR, Parker DA (2008) Reliability of bony landmarks for restoration of the joint line in revision knee arthroplasty. Knee Surg Sports Traumatol Arthrosc 16(3): 263–9
27. Stiehl JB, Abbott BD (1995) Morphology of the transepicondylar axis and its application in primary and revision total knee arthroplasty. J Arthroplasty 10: 785–789
28. Suarez J, Griffin W, Springer B et al (2008) Why do revision knee arthroplasties fail? J Arthroplasty 23:99–103

29. Vessely MB, Whaley AL, Harmsen WS et al (2006) Long-term survivorship and failure modes of 1000 cemented condylar total knee arthroplasties. Clin Orthop 452:28

30. Walker PS, Manktelow AR (2001) Comparison between a constrained condylar and a rotating hinge in revision knee surgery. Knee 8:269–279

31. Westrich GH, Mollano AV, Sculco TP et al (2000) Rotating hinge total knee arthroplasty in severely affected knee. Clin Orthop 379:195–208

32. Windsor RE, Scuderi GR, Moran MC et al (1989) Mechanisms of failure of the femoral and tibial components in total knee arthroplasty. Clin Orthop 248:15–20

Tibiofemoral Joint Kinematics

17

Nicola Lopomo, Simone Bignozzi, Cecilia Signorelli,
Francesca Colle, Giulio Maria Marcheggiani Muccioli,
Tommaso Bonanzinga, Alberto Grassi,
Stefano Zaffagnini, and Maurilio Marcacci

N. Lopomo (✉) • F. Colle
Laboratorio di Biomeccanica e Innovazione Tecnologica,
Istituto Ortopedico Rizzoli,
via di Barbiano 1/10, Bologna, 40136, Italy

Laboratorio di NanoBiotecnologie – NaBi,
Istituto Ortopedico Rizzoli, Bologna, Italy
e-mail: n.lopomo@biomec.ior.it; f.colle@biomec.ior.it

S. Bignozzi
Laboratorio di Biomeccanica e Innovazione Tecnologica,
Istituto Ortopedico Rizzoli,
via di Barbiano 1/10, Bologna, 40136, Italy

Orthokey LLC, Lewes, DE, USA
e-mail: s.bignozzi@biomec.ior.it

C. Signorelli
Laboratorio di Biomeccanica e Innovazione Tecnologica,
Istituto Ortopedico Rizzoli, via di Barbiano 1/10,
Bologna, 40136, Italy

Dipartimento di Bioingegneria,
Politecnico di Milano, Milan, Italy
e-mail: c.signorelli@biomec.ior.it

G.M.M. Muccioli • T. Bonanzinga • A. Grassi
Laboratorio di Biomeccanica e Innovazione Tecnologica,
Istituto Ortopedico Rizzoli, via di Barbiano 1/10,
Bologna, 40136, Italy
e-mail: marcheggianimuccioli@me.com;
t.bonanzinga@tiscali.it; alberto.grassi3@studio.unibo.it

S. Zaffagnini • M. Marcacci
Laboratorio di Biomeccanica e Innovazione Tecnologica,
Istituto Ortopedico Rizzoli, via di Barbiano 1/10,
Bologna, 40136, Italy

Clinica Ortopedica e Traumatologica III,
Istituto Ortopedico Rizzoli,
via di Barbiano 1/10, Bologna 40136, Italy
e-mail: s.zaffagnini@biomec.ior.it

17.1 Introduction

Computer-assisted surgery (CAS), as well as robotics, has been extensively used for tibiofemoral joint surgery over the course of the last few decades.

Ligament surgery – with great care to anterior cruciate ligament (ACL) injury treatment – and joint arthroplasty, including total knee arthroplasty (TKA) as well as unicompartmental knee arthroplasty (UKA), represent the major field of application.

The first step in using CAS technology for knee surgery was the improvement of the accuracy of the intervention (limb alignment or isometric graft) and to enhance surgical outcome [6, 37], using information collected preoperatively via computed tomography (CT) or magnetic resonance imaging (MRI) scans.

CAS for orthopedic purposes has entered the mainstream only in the last 10 years, providing in addition to surgical guidance for reconstructive surgery, the valuable feedback for kinematic analysis [16], above all for the tibiofemoral joint. In fact, with the aid of anatomical registration, CAS systems allow evaluation of the passive range of motion and laxity associated with each specific reconstruction, both ligamentous and prosthetic ones. A global and accurate kinematic evaluation should in fact be recommended for all reconstruction procedures, to reach parameters as close as possible to normal knee function, and for the development of a new generation of implants and surgical techniques.

F. Catani, S. Zaffagnini (eds.), *Knee Surgery using Computer Assisted Surgery and Robotics*,
DOI 10.1007/978-3-642-31430-8_17, © ESSKA 2013

In this chapter, we wanted to highlight our approach to the use of CAS systems in tibiofemoral kinematic analysis concerning:

- ACL-deficient knees before and after reconstruction with several different surgical procedures
- Osteoarthritic (OA) knees before and after the installation of implants, both TKA and UKA

Hereinafter we are going to describe in detail the technology we adopted and the approach we used to address the surgeons' specific requirements for tibiofemoral kinematic assessment. We report a set of successful clinical applications as well.

17.2 Navigation Methodology

17.2.1 Tracking Technology and Hardware Specifications

In our experience in intraoperative tibiofemoral kinematic analysis, we adopted a specific navigation system (BLU-IGS, Orthokey, Lewes, DE, USA) consisting of an optoelectronic localizer, combined with dedicated software (KLEE, Orthokey, Lewes, DE, USA), specifically developed for intraoperative acquisition and evaluation of tibiofemoral kinematics (Fig. 17.1). The platform allows one to measure limb and tool movement: translation and rotation of each wireless three-marker navigation tool is tracked by optically measuring the positions of the passive reflective spherical markers (10.5 mm Ø). A single marker position can be identified with a 3D root-mean-square (RMS) volumetric accuracy of 0.25 mm, with a 95 % confidence interval of 0.5 mm [4].

17.2.2 Intraoperative Protocol

Usually this kind of navigation system is placed about 2 m away from the operating table [21, 29–32, 40]. Tibial and femoral frames (formally the bone trackers, Fig. 17.1) are implanted on bones with two small surgical pins to achieve reduced patient morbidity just before the acquisition of

anatomical landmarks, and they are removed after the last kinematic test. They are required for tracking the limb movement.

Preparation and surgical approach are not modified by the use of the navigation system for kinematic analysis, and standard surgical equipment is used to perform the surgery. In general the used software provides only information about the limb kinematics; thus, it is not used for guiding the surgery, above all in ACL reconstructions. The operating area has to be optimized to minimize light reflexes and interference and to guarantee an unobstructed line of sight between the optical localizer and the markers on the tools.

ACL surgery and arthroplasty are similar in the anatomical registration phase. In particular, the identification of some specific anatomical and functional landmarks is required:

- Hip center: functionally defined by a pivoting motion
- Medial and lateral femoral epicondyles: identified with a tracked probe
- Medial and lateral tibial malleoli: identified with a tracked probe
- Medial and lateral extremities of tibial plateaus: identified with a tracked probe

Additionally, it is possible to arthroscopically acquire with the probe internal landmarks and/or surfaces in order to have a complete view of joint characteristics (e.g., joint line, tibial plateau centers, ACL insertion areas and tunnel in ligament reconstruction, condyles, and plateaus surface in arthroplasty).

The femoral anatomical reference system is defined by setting the Z-axis as the femoral mechanical axis, the X-axis as the transepicondylar line normalized with respect to the Z-axis, and the Y-axis as the cross product between the Z-axis and X-axis [21, 29–32, 40]. The origin lies at the midpoint between the epicondyles. Similarly, the tibial anatomical reference system was defined by setting the Z-axis as the tibial mechanical axis, the X-axis as the line joining the tibial plateau extremities normalized with respect to the Z-axis, and the Y-axis as the cross product between Z-axis and X-axis. The origin is fixed at the midpoint between the medial and lateral ends of the tibial plateau (Fig. 17.2).

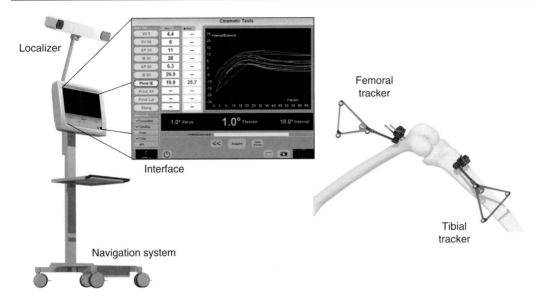

Fig. 17.1 Navigation system details: localizer, user interface, and positioned trackers (Courtesy of Orthokey LLC, Lewes, DE, USA)

Fig. 17.2 Anatomical reference systems defined for the femur and for the tibia. *ME* medial epicondyle, *LE* lateral epicondyle, *HJC* hip joint center, *MTP* medial tibial plateaux, *LTP* lateral tibial plateaux, *MM* medial malleolus, *LM* lateral malleolus

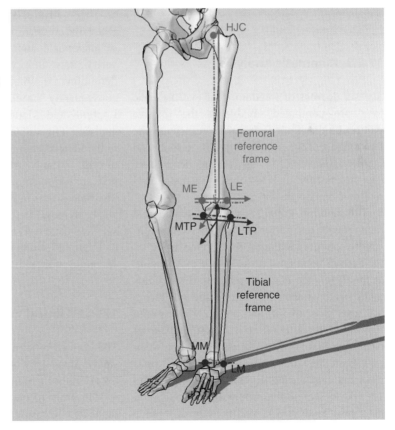

17.2.2.1 Landmark Identification Error

As described by Martelli et al. [29], the landmarks used in the definition of anatomical reference systems could be subject to identification errors.

Table 17.1 Average STD (mm) in landmark coordinate identification

MM	LM	MTP	LTP	ME	LE
2.55	2.46	1.35	2.75	2.75	2.92

MM medial malleolus, *LM* lateral malleolus, *MTP* medial tibial plateaux, *LTP* lateral tibial plateaux, *ME* medial epicondyle, *LE* lateral epicondyle

Table 17.1 reports an analysis of the possible error in the identification through palpation of anatomic landmarks due to the presence of the skin. The values, performed in ten cases, refer to the average standard deviation (STD) in the landmark coordinates. Each landmark was identified three times by the same surgeon on each patient. The average error in the identification on the whole set of specimen for each landmark was 2.53 mm.

As reported in Lopomo et al. [23], the error related to the functional definition of hip joint center is less than 25 mm in the worst case, tracking the pivoting motion of the femur around the acetabulum.

17.2.3 Kinematic Analysis

The six degrees of freedom (DoF) of the knee joint are computed, analyzing the relative motion of the tibial frame with respect to the femoral one [21, 29–32, 40]. The Grood and Suntay approach [11] was used to decompose the movements and to obtain instantaneous rotations and displacements.

Tibiofemoral kinematics are evaluated real time for each test performed both in ACL reconstructive surgery and arthroplasty. In particular, the system computes varus/valgus (VV) laxity as the difference between maximum and minimum instantaneous rotations achieved during VV tests at 0° (VV0) and 30° (VV30) around the anterior–posterior axis, internal/external (IE) rotational laxity as the difference between maximum and minimum instantaneous rotations achieved during IE tests at 30° (IE30) and 90° (IE90) around the proximo/distal axis, and the antero/posterior (AP) laxity as the difference between maximum and minimum instantaneous

displacements achieved during the Lachman's (AP30) and drawer (AP90) tests along the anterior–posterior axis. Since the pivot-shift (PS) test is a complex maneuver, the decomposition of the kinematics corresponding to this test involves the analysis of both IE rotations and AP displacement, specifically of the lateral compartment. For TKA and UKA analysis, the passive range of motion (PROM) is evaluated in its globality analyzing the corresponding flexion/extension, varus/valgus, and internal/external rotation angles.

17.2.3.1 Error Propagation in Kinematic Analysis

Due to the presence of the error in the identification of anatomical landmarks, it is fundamental to verify how this variability can modify the definition of the anatomical reference system and consequently the clinical quantitative outcome. Lopomo and Martelli [23, 29] reported that, applying a maximum of 40 mm of random error in the identification of the hip center and 10 mm of error in the position of the epicondyles, tibial plateau, and malleoli, the obtained variation was less than 2 mm in AP value, less than 2° in IE value, and less than 1.5° in VV value on an average kinematic test sample (Table 17.2).

Figure 17.3 reports an example of kinematic decomposition with superimposed errors.

17.2.4 Clinical Validation

The clinical reliability of the described system was evaluated by performing intra- and inter-tester trials in blinded conditions [21, 29–32, 40]. In order to measure intra-tester reliability, in the first 30 cases, an expert surgeon performed the kinematic tests at maximum force three times

Table 17.2 Simulated error analysis for Grood and Suntay motion decomposition

M/L	A/P	P/D	F/E	V/V	I/E
2.23	1.82	1.43	0.73	1.32	1.91

M/L medio/lateral, *A/P* anterior/posterior, *P/D* proximal/distal, *F/E* flexion/extension, *V/V* varus/valgus, *I/E* internal/external rotation

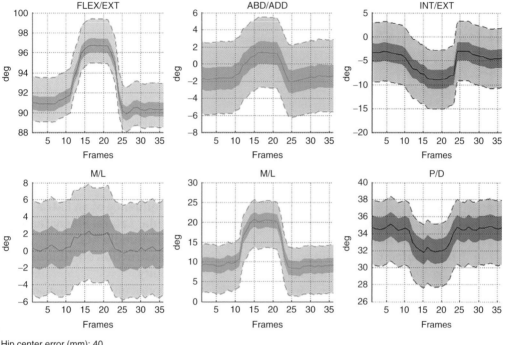

Hip center error (mm): 40
Femoral epicondyles error (mm): 10
Tibial plateaus error (mm): 10
Tibial malleoli error (mm): 10

Fig. 17.3 Example of distribution of random error propagation on kinematic analysis

consecutively in extension, 30° knee flexion and 90° knee flexion, both before and after ACL reconstruction. To measure inter-tester reliability, in 30 more cases, three different surgeons used the described system to measure knee laxity. According to the literature regarding in vivo kinematic measurements [10, 18, 35, 39], to estimate the measurement variability, the percentage standard error (SE%) and standard deviation of repeated trials have been reported. They also used the (item) interclass correlation (ICC) and the repeatability coefficient to estimate the intra-surgeon and the inter-surgeon reliability of laxity measurements.

Hereinafter (Tables 17.3 and 17.4) we summarize of the results of the clinical evaluation of navigated methodology.

17.3 Clinical Studies

17.3.1 Tibiofemoral Kinematics in ACL Surgery

The kinematic analysis in ACL surgery has a great impact in the evaluation of knee stability, related to ligament surgery. We report a set of analysis we performed on ACL surgery using an

Table 17.3 Analysis of variance in repeated measurements of laxity

Test	Intra-test SE%	Intra-test SD	Inter-test SE%	Inter-test SD
AP	4.9 %	0.7 mm	12.3 %	1.2 mm
VV	7.3 %	0.6°	18.9 %	0.9°
IE	4.6 %	1.3°	9.7 %	2.4°

AP anteroposterior displacement stress test, *VV* varus–valgus rotation stress test, *IE* internal–external rotation stress test; *SE%* average percentage standard error; *SD* average standard deviation

Table 17.4 Interclass correlation for repeated measurements

Test	Intra-test ICC A	Inter-test ICC AB	Inter-test ICC AC	Inter-test ICC BC
AP	0.95	0.71	0.6	0.88
VV	0.85	0.46	0.69	0.62
IE	0.89	0.77	0.72	0.82

ICC intraclass correlation between: *A* expert surgeon, *B* intermediate surgeon, *C* novice surgeon

intraoperative navigation system, highlighting the advantages given by the introduction of this technology and the obtained clinical outcomes.

17.3.1.1 The Influence of Combined Lesions in ACL Injury on Tibiofemoral Stability

In the study reported in 2007 by Zaffagnini et al. [41], they intraoperatively quantified, with the help of the developed navigation system, the knee laxity in AP and VV directions in isolated ACL injury compared with combined ACL and medial collateral ligament (MCL) grade II sprain. Fifty-seven patients who underwent arthroscopic over-the-top double-bundle ACL reconstruction performed with a hamstring tendon technique [27] were included in the study. The analysis prospectively classified patients in two groups: 37 patients with isolated ACL lesion (control group, group I) and 20 patients with grade II injury of the medial collateral ligament combined with ACL lesion study group (group II).

To verify the hypothesis that some residual laxities may remain in patients with combined ACL and MCL injuries even after ACL reconstruction, they compared the differences in knee stability between group I and group II. The results confirm the hypothesis in the patients with associated lesions. VV laxity at 30° of flexion was approximately 1° greater in group II with respect to group I. In extension no statistical difference was found. The AP laxity remained approximately 1.3 mm, greater ($p = 0.0024$) in group II at

90° of flexion with respect to group I. Table 17.5 reports the results.

17.3.1.2 The Influence of an Extra-articular Lateral Plasty During Single-Bundle ACL Reconstruction on Tibiofemoral Stability

In the study reported in 2009 by Bignozzi et al. [3], 28 consecutive patients who underwent an arthroscopic single-bundle ACL reconstruction performed with a hamstring tendon technique with additional extra-articular procedure [28] had laxity tests performed before the reconstruction, then the single-bundle (SB) graft was inserted, fixed with two staples on the over-the-top position to reconstruct the anterior-medial bundle of native ACL and laxity tests repeated. After this step, the remaining part of the graft was passed under the fascia lata to reach Gerdy's tubercle where it was fixed with another staple (extra-articular procedure), and the tests were repeated.

In order to quantify the effect of the SB graft and the extra-articular procedure in controlling knee stability, they compared knee laxities due to the stress tests performed with ACL-deficient knee, after SB graft fixation and after extra-articular procedure. To evaluate the effect of the reconstructive technique in controlling secondary rotatory laxities during AP test, they compared the reduction of AP displacement, after SB fixation and after extra-articular plasty

Table 17.5 Results of postoperative laxity test

Test	VV 0°(°)	VV 30° (°)	AP 30° (mm)	AP 90° (mm)
Group I	2.67 ± 0.98	2.39 ± 0.93	5.23 ± 1.83	4.42 ± 1.30
Group II	3.10 ± 0.71	3.42 ± 1.37	6.21 ± 1.61	5.73 ± 1.53
p	0.1022	0.0021*	0.545	0.0024*

Values are given as means ± SD. Group I: with pure ACL injury; Group II: with ACL injury and associated grade II MCL tear
ACL anterior cruciate ligament, *AP* anterior–posterior, *MCL* medial collateral ligament
*$p < 0.05$ is statistically significant

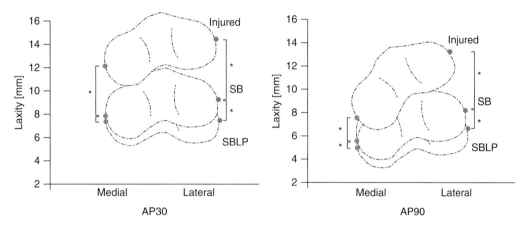

Fig. 17.4 Knee AP laxity decomposition. Medial and lateral plateaux displacement is highlighted during AP30 and AP90 test, and corresponding translations are reported. *$p < 0.05$

procedure, also on the medial and lateral tibial compartments.

As highlighted in Fig. 17.4, the analysis of the medial and lateral compartment during AP stress showed that at 30° of flexion, the SB graft causes a similar reduction of laxity in both compartments. The additional extra-articular procedure does not reduce the AP laxity in the medial compartment, while it controls the lateral compartment reducing AP displacement. On the contrary, at 90° of flexion, the SB graft reduces AP laxity more in the lateral compartment than in the medial one. The additional extra-articular procedure causes a further reduction of knee laxity in both compartments.

17.3.1.3 Knee Dynamic Stability in Anatomical Double-Bundle ACL Reconstruction

Lopomo et al. [24] evaluated 15 patients that consecutively underwent anatomical double-bundle ACL reconstruction; to evaluate the knee joint dynamic stability, the operating surgeon manually performed both clinical static tests at maximum force and a dynamic pivot-shift test before the reconstruction. Anatomical DB ACL reconstruction was then performed, and the same kinematic tests were reacquired (for what concerns specifically pivot-shift test the decomposition of AP translation, IE and VV rotations with respect to flexion/extension angle). For each decomposition, they evaluated the areas included by the curves (the "hysteresis" of the unstable joint) and the difference in the coupled peaks before and after the surgery at a specific flexion angle. Figure 17.5 shows a typical result.

As shown in Fig. 17.6, interesting results have been obtained with the analysis of the pivot-shift test: coupled peaks in AP translation, above all for what concerns the lateral compartment, and also in IE rotation are reduced after surgery. The analysis of the area highlighted a huge recovery of the dynamic stability of the joint.

Fig. 17.5 Example of pivot-shift decomposition. The limb is fully extended (*I*); applying a valgus force and maintaining the tibia in internal rotation, the limb is then flexed (path *A*); the surgeon maintains the force until 60/70° of flexion (*II*); the limb is the normally extended (path *B*). The reduction happens once reached the peak. Peak and area are the parameters used in the analysis

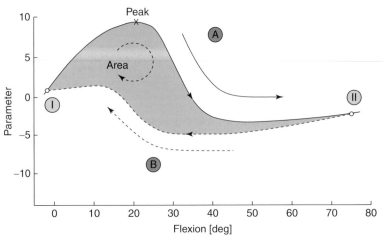

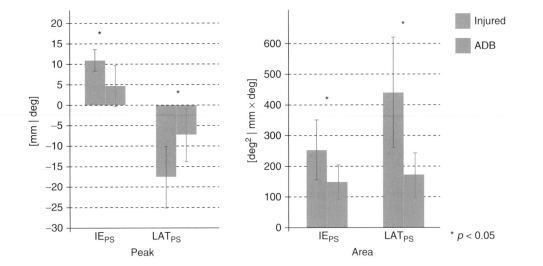

Fig. 17.6 Peaks and areas associated to internal rotation (IE_{PS}) [internal (+)/external (−)] and lateral compartment translation (LAT_{PS}) [anterior (−)/posterior (+)] during pivot-shift test

17.3.1.4 Anatomic Double-Bundle vs. Over-the-Top Single-Bundle with Additional Extra-articular Tenodesis: Different Reconstruction Behaviors on Tibiofemoral Stability

In the study reported by Zaffagnini et al. [42], included 35 consecutive patients, with an isolated anterior cruciate ligament injury, underwent both anatomic double-bundle (ADB group – 15 patients) and over-the-top single-bundle with additional lateral plasty (SBLP group – 20 patients) ACL reconstruction. After performing the anatomic registration, the operating

surgeon manually performed at maximum force the kinematic tests. After fixing the graft as described by the specific surgical procedure, the previously described clinical tests were repeated and acquired by the navigation system.

In order to highlight the possible specific contribution of the extra-articular tenodesis, they also analyzed the antero/posterior displacement of both the lateral and medial compartment during AP30, AP90, IE30, and IE90 and maximal medial and maximal lateral joint opening during VV0 and VV30. Lopomo et al. [24] analyzed the maximal anterior displacement of the lateral tibial compartment and the area included by the translation during PS phenomenon with respect to flexion/extension angle. The posterior acceleration reached by the lateral compartment during tibial reduction [17] was evaluated as well.

Focusing on the behavior of each compartment, they found that SBLP presented more reduction with respect to ADB, concerning the lateral compartment displacement during AP90, the maximal lateral joint opening during VV0 and VV30, and concerning both medial and lateral AP displacement during IE90 (Fig. 17.7).

In the ADB group, the post-reconstruction values of dynamic laxity were lower if compared with the corresponding pre-surgery values for all the parameters describing the lateral tibial plateau. Moreover, the ADB group reported a lower peak in anterior displacement and a lower value of acceleration during the reconstruction relative to the SBLP group (Fig. 17.8).

17.3.2 Tibiofemoral Kinematics in Knee Arthroplasty

The outcome of knee replacement depends on various factors; in particular, the accuracy of implantation and the recovery of normal knee kinematics are both well-known factors for the long-term survival of knee replacement [33, 34, 36]. Computer-assisted systems have been developed for total knee arthroplasty (TKA) and recently for unicompartmental knee arthroplasty (UKA) and should allow a higher precision of implantation than conventional instruments as they offer a complete guide for the correct alignment of the prosthesis [14, 15].

Navigation systems have the potential to bring into the operating room all the computational methodologies adopted in in vitro and postoperative studies on knee behavior. Most of the knowledge about osteoarthritic (OA) and reconstructed knees comes from anatomical investigations, gait analysis, and postoperative radiographic analysis [8, 20]. However, such information is difficult to correlate to the intraoperative assessment after knee replacement or

to the surgical actions. It is still not clear which are the most important parameters to evaluate and how to use kinematics information to improve knee replacement outcome.

Hereinafter we report the use of navigation system in intraoperative kinematic evaluations of minimally invasive unicompartmental knee arthroplasty (UKA) and total knee arthroplasty (TKA).

17.3.2.1 Intraoperative Evaluation of Tibiofemoral Kinematic Behavior in UKA and TKA

As reported by Casino et al. [5], this study was conducted on 20 consecutively selected patients who were undergoing UKA (Preservation Uni, DePuy, Warsaw, IN, USA) and posterior-substituting, rotating-platform TKA (PFC Sigma RP-F, DePuy, Warsaw, IN, USA). Ten patients met the inclusion criteria for UKA surgery, whereas ten other met TKA surgery indications. Standard equipment was used to perform surgery. Since the system was used only to evaluate implant performance and to obtain further kinematic data on OA and reconstructed knees, preparation of the patient and surgical approach were not modified by the use of the navigation system.

The kinematic acquisitions were executed before and after the standard surgical procedures. The kinematic elaboration proposed in this study was focused on the analysis of PROM. The pattern of internal–external (IE) rotation as a function of flexion and the amount of rotation during flexion were computed. For comparison, instantaneous values of IE were plotted by a polynomial fit of fifth degree and $2°$ resampling from $10°$ to $110°$ of flexion. Mean curves obtained during the PROM test in the UKA and TKA groups were calculated underlying differences in pattern and amount of IE rotation before and after the implants.

The amount of IE rotation during the PROM was similar in OA knees and knees after UKA. Similar patterns of tibial rotation were in fact seen before and after UKA (Fig. 17.9). In the TKA group, IE rotation during flexion was not significantly different before and after TKA. On

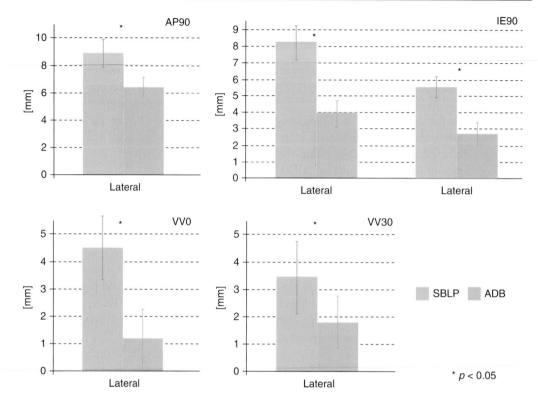

Fig. 17.7 Laxity reduction of the lateral (*lateral*) and medial (*medial*) compartment: differences in AP displacements for AP90 and IE90 tests were analyzed, whereas differences in maximal joint opening were reported for VV0/VV30 tests. *$p < 0.05$

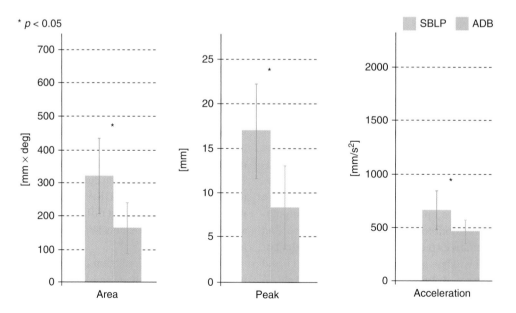

Fig. 17.8 Absolute values of areas, peaks, and accelerations reached by the lateral tibial compartment during PS test after ACL reconstruction, classified according to reconstruction techniques. *$p < 0.05$

Fig. 17.9 Tibial internal (+)/external (−) rotation during knee flexion in OA knees before (*red circles*) and following (*green circle*) TKA and UKA (mean values with shaded standard deviations)

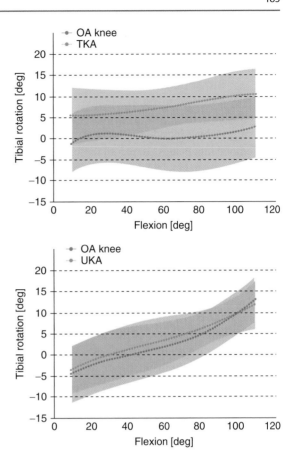

the other hand, the trend of IE rotation during knee flexion lost its original path, related to screw-home mechanism. TKA improved internal rotation during flexion (Fig. 17.9).

Conclusions

The navigation system (BLU-IGS, Orthokey, Lewes, DE, USA), based on an optoelectronic localizer and combining a dedicated acquisition software (KLEE, Orthokey, Lewes, DE, USA), allowed us to perform a set of very different analysis on tibiofemoral kinematics. The system was characterized and its clinical reliability in kinematic analysis verified. The kinematic knee model defined on these landmarks was validated in order to correctly evaluate joint kinematics, static, and dynamic laxities: in particular the general clinical evaluation implies varus/valgus (VV), internal/external rotation (IE), anterior/posterior (AP) stress tests, normal passive range of motion (PROM), and pivot-shift test.

Since 2005, the navigation system has been used on more than 150 ACL reconstructions with different techniques and more than 100 arthroplasties.

The CAS approach, with the combination of measuring knee kinematic properties and standard clinical tests, helped to distinguish between healthy and pathological knees in in vivo conditions.

The development of the kinematic approach has shown its huge potential and has been contributing in a significant manner to several research works in different clinical fields; specifically the kinematic methodology was successfully used in the analysis of the comparison between the outcome of different ACL reconstructions and tibiofemoral replacement.

17.3.3 Future Developments

17.3.3.1 Forces Measurements During Intraoperative Clinical Examinations

At present most navigation systems, above all for ACL surgery, have introduced the ability to record tibiofemoral kinematics. To record these data, the surgeon has to manipulate the limb into varus and valgus, and the navigation system records the varus/valgus angle between the tibial and femoral mechanical axes and calculates the magnitude of the bicompartmental gaps between femur and tibia with the knee in full extension and in flexion [16]. As reported in this chapter, while several studies have presented data on knee laxity recorded with navigation, detailed characterizations of joint laxity require an accurate means of recording both the forces applied to the limb and the resultant displacements. As navigation systems do not have instrumentation to record forces, this remains the next step in intraoperative analysis and an open challenge for system developers, even if some researchers are working on it [4].

17.3.3.2 Noninvasive Assessment of Knee Stability

A pivot-shift test seems to be the most relevant test in the analysis of tibiofemoral knee dynamic laxity. To quantify a pivot-shift test, quite complex systems which need markers [7], footplates [1], and robotic technology [9], magnetic resonance imaging [38] has been proposed; nevertheless, when intraoperatively required, PS quantification needed the support of a navigation system [24]. Less invasive methodologies based on electromagnetic sensors were dedicated to quantitatively evaluate PS test [2, 13, 19], even if they present quite complicated equipment (wires, specific surgical instrumentation, and setup) and costs incompatible with office practice. In the last few years, several efforts have been made to use noninvasive systems based on inertial [22, 25, 26] or image analysis [12] in quantifying the pivot-shift test, thus allowing a quantitative assessment also in an ambulatory setup, where CAS technology still has a lot to give.

References

1. Amis A, Bull A, Lie D (2005) Biomechanics of rotational instability and anatomic anterior cruciate ligament reconstruction. Operat Tech Orthop 15:29–35. doi:10.1053/j.oto.2004.10.009
2. Amis AA, Cuomo P, Rama RBS et al (2008) Measurement of knee laxity and pivot-shift kinematics with magnetic sensors. Operat Tech Orthop 18:196–203. doi:10.1053/j.oto.2008.12.010
3. Bignozzi S, Zaffagnini S, Lopomo N et al (2009) Does a lateral plasty control coupled translation during antero-posterior stress in single-bundle ACL reconstruction? An in vivo study. Knee Surg Sports Traumatol Arthrosc 17:65–70. doi:10.1007/s00167-008-0651-6
4. Cammarata M, Lopomo N, Cerveri P et al (2009) Accuracy characterization of an integrated optical-based system for loads measurements in computer aided surgery. J Mech Med Biol 10(4):577. doi:10.1142/S0219519410003575
5. Casino D, Martelli S, Zaffagnini S et al (2009) Knee stability before and after total and unicondylar knee replacement: in vivo kinematic evaluation utilizing navigation. J Orthop Res 27:202–207. doi:10.1002/jor.20746
6. Chauhan SK, Scott RG, Breidahl W, Beaver RJ (2004) Computer-assisted knee arthroplasty versus a conventional jig-based technique. A randomised, prospective trial. J Bone Joint Surg Br 86:372–377
7. Csintalan RP, Ehsan A, McGarry MH et al (2006) Biomechanical and anatomical effects of an external rotational torque applied to the knee: a cadaveric study. Am J Sports Med 34:1623–1629. doi:10.1177/0363546506288013
8. Dennis DA, Komistek RD, Hoff WA, Gabriel SM (1996) In vivo knee kinematics derived using an inverse perspective technique. Clin Orthop Relat Res (331):107–117
9. Diermann N, Schumacher T, Schanz S et al (2009) Rotational instability of the knee: internal tibial rotation under a simulated pivot shift test. Arch Orthop Trauma Surg 129:353–358. doi:10.1007/s00402-008-0681-z
10. Fleming BC, Brattbakk B, Peura GD et al (2002) Measurement of anterior-posterior knee laxity: a comparison of three techniques. J Orthop Res 20:421–426. doi:10.1016/S0736-0266(01)00134-6
11. Grood ES, Suntay WJ (1983) A joint coordinate system for the clinical description of three-dimensional motions: application to the knee. J Biomech Eng 105:136–144
12. Hoshino Y, Araujo P, Irrgang JJ et al (2011) An image analysis method to quantify the lateral pivot shift test. Knee Surg Sports Traumatol Arthrosc 20(4):703–707. doi:10.1007/s00167-011-1845-x
13. Hoshino Y, Kuroda R, Nagamune K et al (2007) In vivo measurement of the pivot-shift test in the anterior

cruciate ligament-deficient knee using an electromagnetic device. Am J Sports Med 35:1098–1104. doi:10.1177/0363546507299447

14. Jenny J-Y, Boeri C (2004) Low reproducibility of the intra-operative measurement of the transepicondylar axis during total knee replacement. Acta Orthop Scand 75:74–77. doi:10.1080/00016470410 001708150

15. Jenny J-Y, Boeri C, Picard F, Leitner F (2004) Reproducibility of intra-operative measurement of the mechanical axes of the lower limb during total knee replacement with a non-image-based navigation system. Comput Aided Surg 9:161–165. doi:10.3109/10929080500095517

16. Klein GR, Parvizi J, Rapuri VR et al (2004) The effect of tibial polyethylene insert design on range of motion: evaluation of in vivo knee kinematics by a computerized navigation system during total knee arthroplasty. J Arthroplasty 19:986–991

17. Kuroda R, Hoshino Y, Nagamune K et al (2008) Intraoperative measurement of pivot shift by electromagnetic sensors. Operat Tech Orthop 18:190–195. doi:10.1053/j.oto.2008.12.011

18. Kärrholm J, Selvik G, Elmqvist LG et al (1988) Three-dimensional instability of the anterior cruciate deficient knee. J Bone Joint Surg Br 70:777–783

19. Labbe DR, de Guise JA, Mezghani N et al (2010) Feature selection using a principal component analysis of the kinematics of the pivot shift phenomenon. J Biomech 43:3080–3084. doi:10.1016/j.jbiomech.2010.08.011

20. Li G, Moses JM, Papannagari R et al (2006) Anterior cruciate ligament deficiency alters the in vivo motion of the tibiofemoral cartilage contact points in both the anteroposterior and mediolateral directions. J Bone Joint Surg Am 88:1826–1834. doi:10.2106/ JBJS.E.00539

21. Lopomo N, Bignozzi S, Martelli S et al (2009) Reliability of a navigation system for intra-operative evaluation of antero-posterior knee joint laxity. Comput Biol Med 39:280–285. doi:10.1016/j. compbiomed.2009.01.001

22. Lopomo N, Signorelli C, Bonanzinga T et al (2012) Quantitative assessment of pivot-shift using inertial sensors. Knee Surg Sports Traumatol Arthrosc 20(4):713–717. doi:10.1007/s00167-011-1865-6

23. Lopomo N, Sun L, Zaffagnini S et al (2010) Evaluation of formal methods in hip joint center assessment: an in vitro analysis. Clin Biomech (Bristol, Avon) 25:206–212. doi:10.1016/j.clinbiomech.2009.11.008

24. Lopomo N, Zaffagnini S, Bignozzi S et al (2010) Pivot-shift test: analysis and quantification of knee laxity parameters using a navigation system. J Orthop Res 28:164–169. doi:10.1002/jor.20966

25. Lopomo N, Zaffagnini S, Signorelli C et al (2011) An original clinical methodology for non-invasive assessment of pivot-shift test. Comput Methods Biomech Biomed Engin. doi:10.1080/10255842.2011.591788

26. Maeyama A, Hoshino Y, Debandi A et al (2011) Evaluation of rotational instability in the anterior cruciate ligament deficient knee using triaxial accelerometer: a biomechanical model in porcine knees. Knee Surg Sports Traumatol Arthrosc 19(8):1233–1238. doi:10.1007/s00167-010-1382-z

27. Marcacci M, Molgora AP, Zaffagnini S et al (2003) Anatomic double-bundle anterior cruciate ligament reconstruction with hamstrings. Arthroscopy 19:540–546. doi:10.1053/jars.2003.50129

28. Marcacci M, Zaffagnini S, Iacono F et al (1998) Arthroscopic intra- and extra-articular anterior cruciate ligament reconstruction with gracilis and semitendinosus tendons. Knee Surg Sports Traumatol Arthrosc 6:68–75

29. Martelli S, Lopomo N, Bignozzi S et al (2007) Validation of a new protocol for navigated intraoperative assessment of knee kinematics. Comput Biol Med 37:872–878. doi:10.1016/j.compbiomed.2006.09.004

30. Martelli S, Zaffagnini S, Bignozzi S et al (2006) Validation of a new protocol for computer-assisted evaluation of kinematics of double-bundle ACL reconstruction. Clin Biomech (Bristol, Avon) 21:279–287. doi:10.1016/j.clinbiomech.2005.10.009

31. Martelli S, Zaffagnini S, Bignozzi S et al (2007) Description and validation of a navigation system for intra-operative evaluation of knee laxity. Comput Aided Surg 12:181–188

32. Martelli S, Zaffagnini S, Bignozzi S et al (2007) KIN-Nav navigation system for kinematic assessment in anterior cruciate ligament reconstruction: features, use, and perspectives. Proc Inst Mech Eng H 221:725–737. doi:10.1243/09544119JEIM262

33. Pandit H, Van Duren BH, Gallagher JA et al (2008) Combined anterior cruciate reconstruction and Oxford unicompartmental knee arthroplasty: in vivo kinematics. Knee 15:101–106. doi:10.1016/j.knee.2007.11.008

34. Patil S, Colwell CW, Ezzet KA, D'Lima DD (2005) Can normal knee kinematics be restored with unicompartmental knee replacement? J Bone Joint Surg Am 87:332–338. doi:10.2106/JBJS.C.01467

35. Shoemaker SC, Markolf KL (1982) In vivo rotatory knee stability. Ligamentous and muscular contributions. J Bone Joint Surg Am 64:208–216

36. Siston RA, Giori NJ, Goodman SB, Delp SL (2006) Intraoperative passive kinematics of osteoarthritic knees before and after total knee arthroplasty. J Orthop Res 24:1607–1614. doi:10.1002/jor.20163

37. Sparmann M, Wolke B, Czupalla H et al (2003) Positioning of total knee arthroplasty with and without navigation support. A prospective, randomised study. J Bone Joint Surg Br 85:830–835

38. Tashiro Y, Okazaki K, Miura H et al (2009) Quantitative assessment of rotatory instability after anterior cruciate ligament reconstruction. Am J Sports Med 37:909–916. doi:10.1177/0363546508330134

39. Wroble RR, Van Ginkel LA, Grood ES et al (1990) Repeatability of the KT-1000 arthrometer in a normal population. Am J Sports Med 18:396–399

40. Zaffagnini S, Bignozzi S, Martelli S et al (2006) New intraoperative protocol for kinematic evaluation of ACL reconstruction: preliminary results. Knee Surg

Sports Traumatol Arthrosc 14:811–816. doi:10.1007/s00167-006-0057-2

41. Zaffagnini S, Bignozzi S, Martelli S et al (2007) Does ACL reconstruction restore knee stability in combined lesions?: An in vivo study. Clin Orthop Relat Res 454:95–99. doi:10.1097/BLO.0b013e31802b4a86

42. Zaffagnini S, Signorelli C, Lopomo N et al (2011) Anatomic double-bundle and over-the-top single-bundle with additional extra-articular tenodesis: an in vivo quantitative assessment of knee laxity in two different ACL reconstructions. Knee Surg Sports Traumatol Arthrosc 20(1):153–159. doi:10.1007/s00167-011-1589-7

Patellar Tracking in Computer-Assisted Surgery

18

Claudio Belvedere, Andrea Ensini, Alberto Leardini,
Alessandro Feliciangeli, and Sandro Giannini

18.1 Why Is It Important to Track Patellar Motion?

18.1.1 Basics on Patellar Tracking

It is well known that the human knee is a complex structure that joins the thigh with the shank and, because of the presence of three bones that articulate within this anatomical plexus, it consists of two joints, the tibio-femoral (TFJ) and the patello-femoral joint (PFJ), the latter being the smaller of the two. Regardless of its size and sesamoid development, the patella plays two crucial roles within the knee: the transmission of tensile forces generated by all heads of the quadriceps to the patellar tendon and the tibia, and the increase

of the lever arm of the extensor muscles during TFJ flexion-extension, i.e. ultimately the increase of the efficacy of the whole extensor mechanism of the knee [18, 25, 50, 53, 55]. The motion of the patella relative to the distal femur is generally called either PFJ kinematics or patellar tracking, and the important biomechanical functions cited above are successfully achieved only when this motion occurs correctly [18, 50, 53]. Patellar tracking is a full six-degree-of-freedom motion, i.e. the patellar bone is not constrained in its motion. This motion can be described as translations and rotations along and about, respectively, predefined axes [15, 18, 26, 60]. Among all kinematic variables, only a few are generally considered of clinical importance, and these are PFJ flexion, rotation and tilt, these being assessed on the knee sagittal, coronal and transverse plane, respectively, and patella translation along the medio-lateral axis of the distal femur. All references, both on the patella and the femur, have variable definitions [60].

Patellar tracking has been extensively investigated in clinics, for diagnosis and conservative or surgical treatments [42, 43, 77, 88, 99], and in biomechanics for the development of more accurate and realistic knee models [11, 20, 44, 78, 81]. No univocal consensus exists on what is normality for patellar motion [18, 26, 60]. It is still debated, and thus the source of misunderstanding, which nomenclature is most appropriate to describe and/or define patellar rotation and translation [48] and which methodology is most appropriate to study PFJ kinematics, i.e. by tracking all six degrees of

C. Belvedere, Ph.D. (✉) • A. Leardini, Ph.D.
Movement Analysis Laboratory,
Istituto Ortopedico Rizzoli,
via di Barbiano 1/10, Bologna 40136, Italy
e-mail: belvedere@ior.it; leardini@ior.it

A. Ensini, M.D. • A. Feliciangeli, M.D.
Department of Orthopaedic Surgery,
Istituto Ortopedico Rizzoli, University of Bologna,
via di Barbiano 1/10, Bologna 40136, Italy
e-mail: andrea.ensini@ior.it

S. Giannini, M.D.
Movement Analysis Laboratory,
Istituto Ortopedico Rizzoli,
via di Barbiano 1/10, Bologna 40136, Italy

Department of Orthopaedic Surgery,
Istituto Ortopedico Rizzoli, University of Bologna,
via di Barbiano 1/10, Bologna 40136, Italy

F. Catani, S. Zaffagnini (eds.), *Knee Surgery using Computer Assisted Surgery and Robotics*,
DOI 10.1007/978-3-642-31430-8_18, © ESSKA 2013

Fig. 18.1 Computed-tomography scan showing patellar dislocation in the natural knee

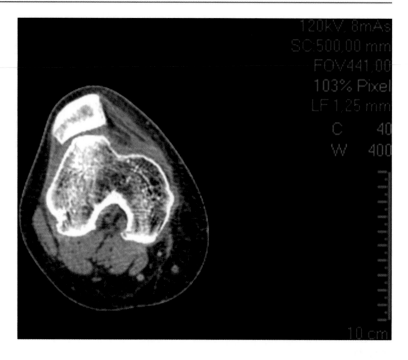

freedom of PFJ during TFJ flexion-extension [4, 15, 18, 26, 60], or, according to a more bi-dimensional graphical approach based on x-ray images, by assessing the location of the patella with respect to the geometry of the femoral groove on the Merchant's view [23, 60, 79]. Abnormal patellar tracking or patella maltracking refers to several different conditions in which the patella does not slide properly within the trochlear groove of the distal femur throughout the knee flexion arc. In the natural knee, this maltracking can be due to idiopathic factors; a relevant small overview is reported for completeness in the next section. Conversely, after total knee replacement (TKR), abnormal patellar tracking can derive from a number of complex factors, and this will be discussed more extensively.

18.1.2 Patella Maltracking in the Natural Knee

The literature reports how abnormal PFJ kinematics in the natural knee can frequently result in a number of joint disorders, which are usually the source of anterior knee pain [37, 42, 45, 47]. Idiopathic patellar maltracking is generally due to anatomical abnormalities in the articular interface between the patellar posterior aspect and the femoral groove, such as trochlear dysplasia and deficit of patellar posterior crest (Fig. 18.1).

Other factors can be the excessive tightening of surrounding soft tissue structures, in particular the two retinacula and the patellar tendon, and general lower limb malrotations, such as abnormal internal-external knee rotation, and misalignment, as in the case of excessive Q-angle [37, 42, 43, 49, 88] and unnatural patellar height [22, 34, 86], or to muscle-related problems [81, 82]. More specifically, the shape of the patellar articular crest and the distal femur and the percentage of PFJ contact area during patellar engagement into the femoral sulcus affect largely PFJ kinematics. Generally, anatomical abnormalities on the femoral side are associated with patellar sub- or complete luxation [3, 21], whereas when the percentage of patellar articular crest overlapping the trochlea is less than 30 %, the patella tends to sublux [70]. Ultimately, patella maltracking resulting in repetitive abnormal loading on the cartilage of the PFJ complex can evolve towards PFJ osteoarthritis [97].

18.1.3 Patella Maltracking in Total Knee Replacement

The literature reports how patellar maltracking can occur after TKR, frequently resulting in anterior knee pain and ultimately leading to the failure of the arthroplasty [15, 52, 80, 84]. This surgical procedure continues to be an efficient treatment, as evidenced both by the survivorship rate and long-term results [59, 73, 74], and by the satisfactory functional performances assessed at follow-up, and, ultimately, it seems to allow the restoration of normal knee motion after joint replacement [13, 14, 71, 72]. It is worth remembering that post-implant problems still persist, these being accounted for mainly by polyethylene wear, aseptic loosening, instability, infection, arthrofibrosis, prosthesis component malalignment or malposition, deficient extensor mechanism, avascular necrosis in the patella, periprosthetic fracture and isolated patellar resurfacing [27, 46, 87]. Generally, TKR provides significant pain relief and general patient satisfaction, but its success is unequivocally considered as dependent on a number of factors, the geometry of the prosthetic articular surfaces, posterior condylar offset, cruciate ligament retaining/sacrificing, soft tissue balancing and final lower limb alignment achieved at surgery [29, 30, 85]. All these aspects involve only the TFJ complex, almost completely neglecting the PFJ one. During TKR, patellar management and PFJ kinematics assessment, both with and without resurfacing, represent only one step within the whole surgical procedure, and these are often relegated to secondary importance and dealt with summarily [69]. In the case of patellar resurfacing, the most frequent scenario is a quick estimation of the relevant bone thickness followed by equally quick bone cutting, drilling and component cementing and visual/manual inspection of patellar motion for eventual soft tissue release; without resurfacing, just the latter step is executed. To

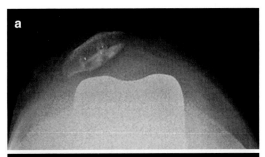
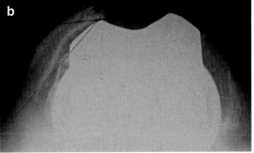

Fig. 18.2 X-ray images showing patellar dislocation after TKR with (**a**) and without (**b**) patellar resurfacing

intraoperatively assess the real status of patellar tracking during TKR, a number of methods have been proposed [32, 92], the lateral release being performed according to relevant results. The so-called no-thumb technique is most frequently applied to evaluate PFJ kinematics [32] by means of manually imposed knee flexion-extension without any external pressure on the patella; a high number of false positives resulting in a high incidence of lateral retinacular releases are reported [9, 32, 92].

The surgeon must pay particular attention to the patella since complications at the PFJ complex after TKR results in abnormal patellar tracking. The literature reports that this is mainly accounted for by a number of critical factors that inadvertently occur during surgery. The most important are [15, 57, 58, 61, 69, 76, 80, 84, 95]: (1) the misalignment of the lower limb mechanical axis altering the normal Q-angle; (2) inappropriate femoral/tibial bone cut execution and relevant prosthesis component malpositioning, resulting in improper joint line restoration at both the TFJ and the PFJ complex; and (3) inappropriate patellar resurfacing (Fig. 18.2), resulting in under- or overstuffed implanted bone with subsequent alteration of the physiological lever arm length and in the tightened state of the surrounding soft tissues.

The latter factor, alone or in concomitance with the inappropriate joint line restoration at both articular complexes, can alter normal patellar height with respect to the distal femur with likely invalidation of the efficacy of the whole extensor apparatus with post-operative recurrence of anterior knee pain [5, 35, 69, 83].

18.1.4 Patellar Tracking in Computer-Assisted Total Knee Replacement: State-of-the-Art

Within computer-assisted techniques, knee surgical navigation systems have been developed for TKR to optimise femoral and tibial prosthesis component implantation via intraoperative tracking of the femur and the tibia before, i.e. at the original arthritic knee joint, and after trial and final prosthesis components implantation [15, 64, 90, 91]. Generally, these systems, in addition to offering greater visibility of the areas of intervention, prediction of the effect of surgical actions and higher accuracy in component positioning, allow preoperative planning of the surgical goal, the intraoperative monitoring and prediction of the final functional result of the replaced joint. These systems can also be used to check for surgeon-specific technique performance and instrumental accuracy [63, 93]. Navigated TKR is revealed to be far more accurate than those performed by means of the standard surgical procedures [17, 38, 39, 90], since intraoperative monitoring allows the surgeon to check and correct a number of surgical actions intraoperatively. There is still a margin of error which is constantly narrowing thanks to novel hardware and software solutions. Besides some inescapable incorrect surgical actions, limited in number but still to be considered, there are a limited number of kinematic pieces of information provided by the current knee navigation systems. This limitation does not allow complete support during all the surgical steps and to achieve a thorough kinematics assessment of the joint under replacement. These systems would benefit from the introduc-

tion of additional navigated steps dedicated to patellar tracking assessment and/or soft tissue monitoring [15, 19, 33, 36, 67, 89, 96].

Even by means of navigated procedures, the techniques in TKR used to assess patellar motion and to collect patellar morphological data are the same as those illustrated in the previous section, i.e. based only on visual inspections of the patellar articular aspect and manual manoeuvres and by means of a simple calliper reading to check for patellar thickness [7, 19, 40, 41]. All these actions are ultimately achieved without any computer assistance, this being essential for more accurate measurements and three-dimensional representations [15, 16, 19]. Even though the inclusion of a procedure for tracking the PFJ kinematics based on patient-specific bone references seems fundamental in in vivo navigated TKR, this has been completely disregarded so far within current knee surgical navigation systems. Recent findings have revealed the intraoperative feasibility of patellar tracking and data collection for patellar resurfacing in the context of the most modern operative techniques in in vitro experiments [15, 19, 41] and recently also in in vivo initial experiences [16]. The next section will be dedicated to illustrating a number of experiences recently performed for the purpose of patellar tracking assessment under different aspects.

18.2 Patellar Tracking in Computer-Assisted Total Knee Replacement: Recent Development

18.2.1 Three-Dimensional Anatomy-Based Patellar Tracking in In Vitro Navigated Total Knee Replacement

Abnormal patellar tracking may result in many PFJ disorders. In the intact knee, this is generally due to abnormalities in the PFJ interface and lower limb rotations, whereas after TKR, even with navigated procedures, this can be attributed to prosthesis component misalignment in both the TFJ and the PFJ complex, erroneous soft tissue balancing and incorrect patellar resurfacing. All these might lead to pain and, ultimately, to replacement failure [15, 52, 80, 84]. It is therefore necessary to develop computer-assisted surgery techniques that allow the acquisition of patellar motion data and the assessment of the PFJ kinematics according to which the identification of patellar maltracking could be feasible [1, 15, 18, 26]. This is of primary importance during TKR since all involved bones, including the patella in case of resurfacing, can be properly prepared for relevant implant positioning by taking into account the kinematic behaviour of both the TFJ and PFJ [15, 18].

Patellar tracking has been studied using several methodological approaches and measuring devices [1, 2, 6, 8, 10, 15, 18, 24, 31, 45, 54, 58, 62, 65, 66, 94, 98]. Only a few studies dealt with the comparison of this tracking before and after TKR [6, 8, 15, 18, 56]. Among these, two in vitro studies reported the feasibility of tracking intra-operatively patella motion before, during and after the standard TKR procedures using a current knee surgical navigation system adapted for the purpose of bony landmarks digitization and bone position measurements [15, 56].

In one study [15], patellar tracking was assessed during TKR (cruciate-retaining Scorpio, Stryker®-Orthopaedics, Mahwah, NJ, USA.) with patellar resurfacing in 0–140° TFJ flexion arc and with 100 N force vertically applied on the quadriceps using the Stryker® knee surgical navigation system (Stryker®-Leibinger, Freiburg im Breisgau, Germany) in six fresh-frozen specimens from inter-iliac abdominal amputation. In this study, a novel tracking tool for patellar-dedicated acquisition was manufactured, much lighter and smaller than the standard ones fixed onto the femur and tibia in order to introduce small inertial effect during acquisitions (Fig. 18.3).

Particularly, in this original study [15], an anatomy-based convention for assessing the PFJ kinematics (Fig. 18.4), in addition to the TFJ kinematics, was derived from a relevant proposal [26] recommending a three-cylinder open chain representation of the PFJ, which closely corresponds to a standard mechanical convention for describing human joint motion [51]. Furthermore,

in the same study, an original anatomical-based convention (Fig. 18.4) for defining a patellar-embedded reference frame was proposed; this closely corresponds to previous recommendations for defining bone-embedded reference frames from lower limb anatomical landmarks [28]. Corresponding repeatability tests were also performed, and relevant results reported, to check for the robustness of this convention by assessing the corresponding variability in orientation about and position along the three anatomical planes, less than 6.5° and 1.3 mm, on average, on all anatomical planes and along all anatomical axes, respectively. A repeatable path of motion over repetitions was observed in the six intact knees, in both the TFJ and PFJ, the mean standard deviation being less than 1.5° and 1.3 mm over TFJ flexion for all rotation and translation, respectively. Restoration of the original patellar tracking in the intact knees was generally not fully accomplished in the replaced knees (Fig. 18.5).

Belvedere et al. [15] reported that patellar flexion was very similar over the specimens before and after TKR, whereas the original patellar tilt was well replicated after TKR in only two specimens and with a discrepancy varying from 5° to 10° in the other knees, although a similar pattern was observed over the specimens. The original patellar shift, i.e. the medio-lateral patellar translations along the femoral medio-lateral axes, was well replicated in three specimens, whereas an opposite pattern with a difference as large as 12 mm was observed in the other specimen.

Heinert et al. [56] compared the PFJ kinematics in nine specimens in normal knees and after the sequential implantation of two different prosthesis components for TKR. A fixed-bearing TKR was initially implanted on these knees and relevant measurements acquired; afterwards, a mobile-bearing prosthesis was implanted by changing only the components on the tibial side, and relevant measurements were acquired. Both TKR designs (DePuy®-Orthopaedics, Warsaw, IN, USA) shared the same femoral prosthesis component. In this study, a knee surgical navigation system was used to assess patellar movements in addition to standard TFJ kinematics (Unlimited Knee Patella Tracking software,

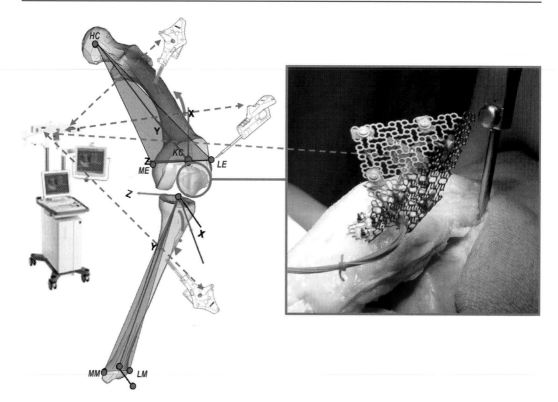

Fig. 18.3 Experimental setup for in vitro tests: the standard trackers are pinned onto the femur and tibia. The special patellar tracker, shown in the close-up, is fixed onto the cortical anterior surface of the patella by means of four metal screws and is powered and controlled by a small external unit. Three light-emitting diodes are attached to each of the two orthogonal planes in known relative positions and are alternatively seen by the localizer. Depending on the typology of data acquisition, one of the two diode planes is visible when the patella is in place over the femoral trochlea for standard knee joint motion or the patella is partially everted to access the inner articular surface for the original landmark calibration procedure. The localizer must be oriented in order to see all light-emitting diodes on each cluster. The anatomical landmarks, directly digitised or estimated, used in the definition of the femur and tibial anatomical reference frame are also indicated: on the thigh, the medial (*ME*) and lateral (*LE*) epicondyle, the centre of the femur head (*HC*), and the knee centre (*KC*); on the shank, the medial (*MM*) and lateral (*LM*) malleolus, the ankle centre (*AC*) and the centre of the tibial plateau (*CT*)

Brainlab, Munich) in 0–90° TFJ flexion arc, and the form and the position of the trochlea in the natural knee and the patellar groove of the TKR femoral component were also analysed. No differences in TFJ and PFJ kinematics were observed between the fixed-bearing and mobile-bearing prosthesis. After TKR, independent of the adopted design, the patellar tilt was larger than that in the natural knee from 50° to 90° of TFJ flexion, whereas no significant differences were observed in the absolute medio-lateral translation and in the translation relative to the patellar groove. The patella after TKR lost contact with the femoral groove earlier than in the intact knee.

The results from these two studies [15, 56] demonstrated the feasibility and necessity of patellar tracking during TKR. Measurements of PFJ flexion tilt and shift of the intact knee, together with the other standard TFJ kinematics variables, may assist the surgeon in the choice of the best alignment for the femoral, tibia and, in case of resurfacing, patellar prosthesis components because of the more comprehensive assessment of the original knee kinematics. Standard surgical navigation recommends assessment of the TFJ kinematics after implantation of the prosthetic trial components to be compared with the original or with target kinematics, and this

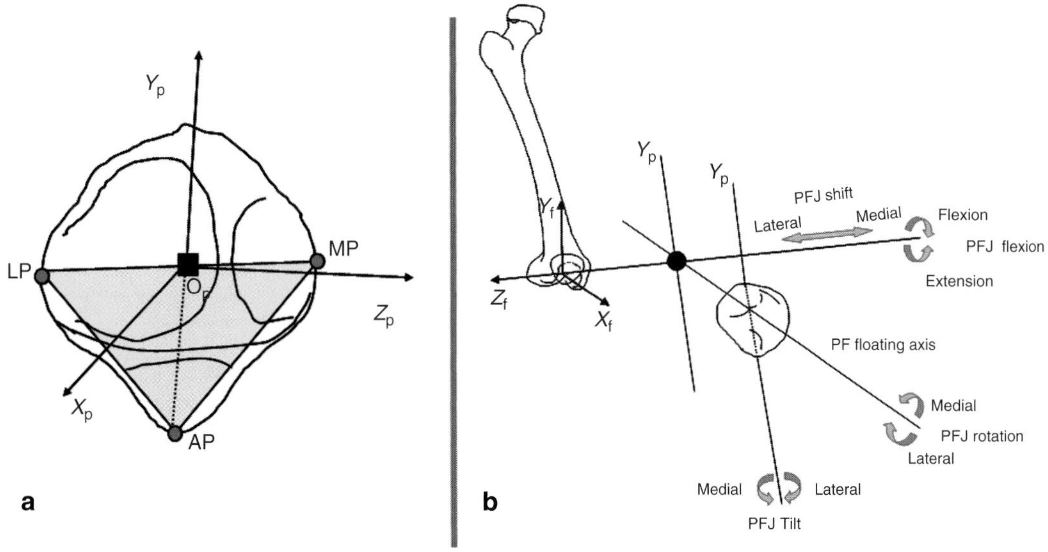

Fig. 18.4 Anatomical reference frame for the patella (**a**) and mechanical convention (**b**) used to assess PFJ kinematics. On the patella, the medial (*MP*) and lateral (*LP*) prominences and the patellar distal apex (*AP*) are digitised in the internal aspect of the bone in order to define the patellar anteroposterior, proximo-distal and medio-lateral axis (X_p, Y_p and Z_p, respectively). Particularly,

X_p is defined as the axis orthogonal to the plane through *MP*, *LP* and *AP*, Y_p as the axis between *AP* and *Op*, the latter being the midpoint between *MP* and *LP*, and Z_p as perpendicular to both X_p and Y_p. PFJ flexion and shift are about and along Z_f, this being the femur medio-lateral axis tilt; PFJ tilt and rotation are respectively about Y_p, and the floating axis perpendicular to both Z_f and Y_p.

seems feasible for the assessment of the PFJ kinematics. As observed in these two studies, the intraoperative analysis of relevant kinematics can reveal possible patella maltracking, and this could be corrected, intraoperatively, by adjusting the preliminary patellar bone cut and selecting a more appropriate size of patellar component. Ultimately, by intraoperatively monitoring PFJ kinematics, the surgeon has a more complete view and prediction of the final knee implant. Preliminary experiences achieved in vitro will be reported in the next section.

18.2.2 Computer-Assisted Patellar Resurfacing in In Vitro Navigated Total Knee Replacement

In TKR with patellar resurfacing, patellar resection has received little attention compared to the tibia and femur bone preparation for relevant prosthesis component implantation. Although a

variety of devices and techniques have been developed for the purpose of optimising the patellar cut, surgeons still cut the patella freehand. Incorrect patellar resection can introduce an additional offset in PFJ tilting and may result in over- or understuffed after final component implantation. This has been associated with a number of patellar disorders resulting in anterior knee pain [6, 12, 19, 41, 75]. Even by means of computer-assisted TKR, the techniques utilised to assess patellar motion and to collect patellar morphological data are still based only on visual inspections, manual manoeuvres and by means of a simple calliper reading to check for patellar thickness [7, 19, 40, 41]. It is fundamental to assess PFJ kinematics intraoperatively in order to allow the surgeon to comprehend the effect in advance of every relevant surgical action on the PFJ, and it is also helpful to monitor bone preparation and component positioning for the patella in case of resurfacing [8, 15, 36, 89].

As reported above, knee surgical navigation systems support the surgeon in the execution of

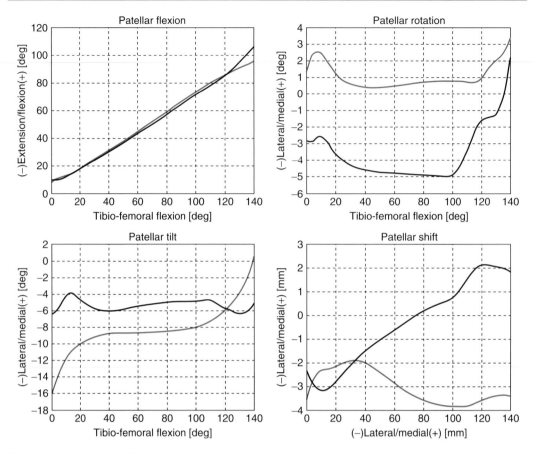

Fig. 18.5 Patterns of patellar motion from a well-representative specimen: comparison between intact (*red line*) and replaced (*black line*) knees during flexion

more accurate femoral and tibial cuts [68, 90], but none of the systems on the market provide computer assistance for patellar resection during navigated TKR [19]. Recently, in vitro experiences were performed for this purpose reporting encouraging results about the feasibility and relevance of the introduction of computer-based support for patellar resurfacing [19, 41].

In a preliminary study [19], a procedure for the navigation of the patella in TKR with patellar resurfacing was reported (Fig. 18.6) and assessed on a single specimen implanted with a posterior-stabilised TKR and domed patellar component (Scorpio®, Stryker Orthopaedics, Mahwah, NJ, USA). In this study, bone tracking was performed according to recent methodology [15]. Patellar flexion, tilt, rotation and shift were measured according to recent anatomical and mechanical proposals [15, 18, 26] in the

intact knee and after navigated TKR, before and after conventional, i.e. not navigated, patellar resurfacing. Orientation of the patellar osteotomy and position of the most posterior point of the patellar component were identified in the patellar anatomical reference frame by digitization with the pointer. After the comparison of the PFJ kinematic variables with a predefined reference for normality [18] and the posterior patellar crest location after freehand resurfacing and the corresponding values in the intact patella, the patella was cut again and the patellar component repositioned in such a way that the patellar resection plane was parallel to the predefined patellar coronal plane, the amount of removed bone was as thick as the thickness of the patellar component selected for the implant, and the latter was positioned close to the location of the original, i.e. bony, patellar crest.

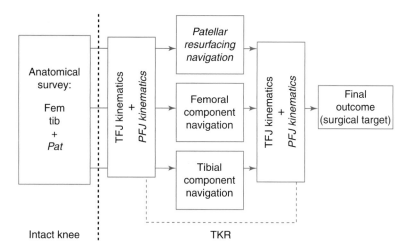

Fig. 18.6 Flow chart for the conceptual sequence of the knee surgical navigation steps including also the navigation of the patellar resurfacing. Standard and new procedures (in normal and in italics, respectively) are indicated. In addition to the standard anatomical survey for the femur and the tibia, required by the standard knee navigation, it is necessary to perform the anatomical survey also for the patella in order to define an anatomy-based patellar frame used as reference for a more proper alignment of cutting jig during patellar cut execution and in patellar component positioning. All procedures can be iteratively performed until the surgical goal is reached, this being now based on assessments on both TFJ and PFJ kinematics

Afterwards, additional kinematics measurements were taken, and further adjustments were performed if necessary. The results showed that after resurfacing with the conventional technique, all PFJ variables were altered. Particularly, an abnormal lateral tilt, about 15° more than normality, and a medial translation (on average, 8 mm more than normality) were observed. Freehand patellar osteotomy resulted in a 22° lateral tilt with respect to the relevant anatomical frontal plane (i.e. less than necessary bone removed laterally), whereas the most posterior patellar component point was 5 mm more lateral with respect to the intact patella. After again cutting the patella and relevant component repositioning, both performed according to piece of information provided by the system in real time, patellar osteotomy resulted in a perfect realignment and the original patellar crest restored. The final results demonstrated full restoration of the normal kinematics both for the TFJ and PFJ, i.e. within the reference for normality.

In a recent study [41], a similar procedure was applied on six pairs of cadaveric knee specimens by two experienced surgeons using a knee surgical navigation system suitably adapted for this purpose and preliminarily validated on artificial bones [40]. The patellae of right knees were resurfaced according to the conventional technique, whereas the left knee according to the novel computer-assisted technique. The tracking system utilised in this study consisted of a custom-written software, an optoelectronic localizer (Spectra; Northern Digital Inc., Waterloo, Canada; 0.25 mm RMS accuracy), a custom-modified patellar marker array, instrument marker array, a digitising pointer and cut-plane digitising block (Praxim; Grenoble, France). In the novel procedure for navigated patellar resurfacing, the surgeon positioned the saw guide based on a real-time display that compared the current saw guide plane to the ideal resection, the same as that in the previous study [19]. The achievement of this goal was also confirmed on computed-tomography scans. The results showed better resection repeatability in terms of orientation on the patellar sagittal plane than that performed with the conventional technique. Also this study demonstrated that computer-assisted patellar resection is feasible and better results can derive from its adoption.

18.2.3 Three-Dimensional Anatomy-Based Patellar Tracking in In Vivo Navigated Total Knee Replacement

A number of factors can affect PFJ kinematics during TKR including component position, implant design, joint alignment and soft tissue tension. The impact of this arthroplasty on patellar tracking has been reported in depth in in vitro studies, as illustrated in Sect. 18.2.1. This has also been assessed in vivo [8, 16]. From a technical point of view, recent knee surgical navigation systems offer great potential for tracking PFJ motion in vivo during TKA surgery. The enhancement of these current systems plus the possible development of novel ad hoc algorithms can be derived from related in vitro experiences reported in the past.

In one study [8], a computer-assisted system for navigated TKR (Praxim®, Grenoble, France) was suitably adapted to measure the preoperative PFJ kinematics, to display the patellar motion path onto the surface of the planned femoral component and to compare the post-operative PFJ kinematics to the preoperative one. These measurements were performed on 18 patients during the implantation of posterior-stabilised TKR (DePuy®-Orthopaedics, Warsaw, IN, USA). Relevant results revealed a small, but consistent, proximal translation of the tibial joint lines that could result in pseudo patella-baja, i.e. a more distal contact of the patella on the femoral component. Significant changes between pre- and postoperative PFJ kinematics were generally observed, but the greatest magnitude of change was observed in patellar medio-lateral translation and tilt. Generally, female patients had more lateral tilt on average than male patients throughout flexion.

In a recent study [16], a novel procedure has been developed, together with relevant software and surgical instrumentation, as an extension of the current standard knee surgical navigation system (Stryker®-Leibinger, Freiburg, Germany), for measuring in vivo and intraoperatively in six patients during TKR with domed patellar resurfacing (NRG, Stryker®-Orthopaedics, Mahwah,

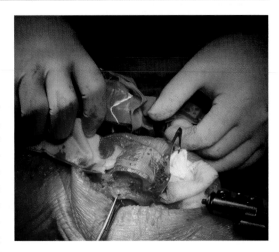

Fig. 18.7 Patellar tracker used intraoperatively during in vivo TKR

NJ, USA) the effects of every surgical action on both TFJ and PFJ kinematics. In the first series of experimental application, a second surgical navigation system for patellar-dedicated acquisition was added to the standard, with which TFJ data were shared. In the operating room, before surgery, both systems were initialized; the patellar tracker was assembled by shaping a titanium mesh equipped with three markers to be tracked by the second navigation system only (Fig. 18.7) and mounted onto the patellar anterior aspect by four mono-cortical screws.

In this original study [16], the additional patellar-resection-plane and patellar-cut-verification probes were instrumented with a standard tracker, and a relevant reference frame was defined on these by digitization using the second navigation system. Afterwards, the procedures for standard navigation were performed to calculate preoperative joint deformities and TFJ kinematics. The patellar anatomical reference frame was defined with the second navigation system, and PFJ kinematics were according to a recent proposal [15]. Standard procedures for femoral and tibial component implantation and TFJ kinematics assessment were then performed by using relevant trial components. Once the surgeon had arranged and fixed the patellar cutting jig at the desired position, the patellar-resection-plane probe was inserted into the slot for the saw

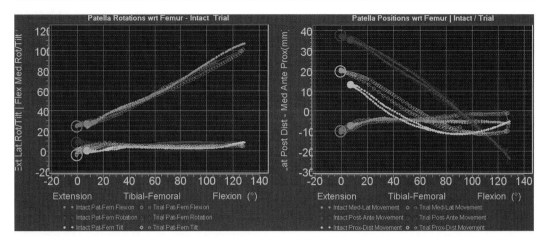

Fig. 18.8 Screen snapshot of the navigation system used for patellar-dedicated acquisitions showing PFJ rotations (*left*) and translation (*right*) from a well-representative TKR case. In order to allow a comparison between two different situations, data are reported both at the intact knee and after the implantation with the femoral, tibial and patellar trial components

blade. With this in place, the second navigation system captured tracker data to calculate the planned level of patellar bone cut and the patellar cut orientation. Then the cut was executed, and the accuracy of this actual bone cut was assessed by means of the patellar-cut-verification probe. The trial patellar component was positioned, and, with all three trial components in place, TFJ and PFJ kinematics were assessed (Fig. 18.8).

Using this novel technique [16], possible adjustments in component positioning could still be performed, and final TFJ and PFJ kinematics were acquired after final component cementing. A sterile calliper and pre- and post-implantation lower limb x-rays were used to check for patellar thickness and final lower limb alignment. The novel surgical technique was performed in vivo successfully, resulting in a 30-min longer TKR. Relevant data, including the patella related ones, were all acquired intraoperatively and finally stored after surgery. On average, the final lower limb alignment was within 0.5°, the discrepancy between intact and resurfaced patellar thickness was 0.4 mm and the patellar cut was 1.5° laterally tilted. Generally, PFJ kinematics was taken within the reference for normality [18]. The patella implantation parameters were confirmed by x-ray inspection; discrepancies in thickness up to 5 mm were observed between SNS- and calliper-based measurements.

18.3   Concluding Remarks

This chapter analysed different aspects related to the patella. The overview on patellar tracking, from basics to recent experimental tests, reveals the relevance, the feasibility and the efficacy of tracking patellar motion in computer-assisted TKR. The encouraging results derived from in vivo applications may lay the ground work for the design of a clinical navigation system that the surgeon can utilise to execute a more comprehensive assessment of the original whole knee anatomy and kinematics, including the patella and related PFJ kinematics. Within the same results, patellar bone preparation in case of TKR with patellar resurfacing, patellar component positioning results in a more suitably performed surgery. Conceptually, computer-assisted patellar tracking may be useful in not resurfacing if patellar anatomy and tracking assessment by surgical navigation system reveals no abnormality. By intraoperatively analysing PFJ kinematics of the intact knee, no resurfacing could be preferred by the surgeon if the original patellar tracking is nearly physiological. From this perspective, resurfacing could be performed more selectively, as in the case of severe deforming arthritis causing patellar maltracking.

In the future, if this procedure is routinely applied during navigated TKR, abnormalities at both the TFJ and PFJ complex and related kinematics can be corrected intraoperatively by more cautious bone cut preparation on the femur, tibia and patella, in case of resurfacing, and by correct prosthetic component positioning.

References

1. Ahmed AM, Duncan NA, Tanzer M (1999) In vitro measurement of the tracking pattern of the human patella. J Biomech Eng 121:222–228
2. Ahmed AM, Shih HN, Hyder A, Chan KH (1988) The effect of the quadriceps tension characteristics on the patellar tracking pattern. Trans Orthop Res Soc 13:280
3. Amis AA, Oguz C, Bull AM, Senavongse W, Dejour D (2008) The effect of trochleoplasty on patellar stability and kinematics: a biomechanical study in vitro. J Bone Joint Surg Br 90:864–869
4. Amis AA, Senavongse W, Bull AM (2006) Patellofemoral kinematics during knee flexion-extension: an in vitro study. J Orthop Res 24:2201–2211
5. Anagnostakos K, Lorbach O, Kohn D (2011) Patella baja after unicompartmental knee arthroplasty. Knee Surg Sports Traumatol Arthrosc 20(8):1456–1462
6. Anglin C, Brimacombe JM, Hodgson AJ, Masri BA, Greidanus NV, Tonetti J, Wilson DR (2008) Determinants of patellar tracking in total knee arthroplasty. Clin Biomech (Bristol, Avon) 23:900–910
7. Anglin C, Fu C, Hodgson AJ, Helmy N, Greidanus NV, Masri BA (2009) Finding and defining the ideal patellar resection plane in total knee arthroplasty. J Biomech 42:2307–2312
8. Anglin C, Ho KC, Briard JL, de Lambilly C, Plaskos C, Nodwell E, Stindel E (2008) In vivo patellar kinematics during total knee arthroplasty. Comput Aided Surg 13:377–391
9. Archibeck MJ, Camarata D, Trauger J, Allman J, White RE Jr (2003) Indications for lateral retinacular release in total knee replacement. Clin Orthop Relat Res 414:157–161
10. Asano T, Akagi M, Koike K, Nakamura T (2003) In vivo three-dimensional patellar tracking on the femur. Clin Orthop Relat Res 413:222–232
11. Ateshian GA, Hung CT (2005) Patellofemoral joint biomechanics and tissue engineering. Clin Orthop Relat Res 436:81–90
12. Baldini A, Anderson JA, Zampetti P, Pavlov H, Sculco TP (2006) A new patellofemoral scoring system for total knee arthroplasty. Clin Orthop Relat Res 452:150–154
13. Banks SA, Hodge WA (2004) Implant design affects knee arthroplasty kinematics during stair-stepping. Clin Orthop Relat Res 426:187–193
14. Banks SA, Markovich GD, Hodge WA (1997) The mechanics of knee replacements during gait. In vivo fluoroscopic analysis of two designs. Am J Knee Surg 10:261–267
15. Belvedere C, Catani F, Ensini A, Moctezuma de la Barrera JL, Leardini A (2007) Patellar tracking during total knee arthroplasty: an in vitro feasibility study. Knee Surg Sports Traumatol Arthrosc 15:985–993
16. Belvedere C, Ensini A, Moctezuma de la Barrera JL, Feliciangeli A, Leardini A, Catani F (2011) Patellar tracking assessment in surgical navigation for total knee replacement: initial experience in patient. In: 11th Annual meeting of computer assisted orthopaedic surgery – international proceedings, CAOS, London
17. Belvedere C, Ensini A, Leardini A, Bianchi L, Catani F, Giannini S (2007) Alignment of resection planes in total knee replacement obtained with the conventional technique, as assessed by a modern computer-based navigation system. Int J Med Robot 3:117–124
18. Belvedere C, Leardini A, Ensini A, Bianchi L, Catani F, Giannini S (2009) Three-dimensional patellar motion at the natural knee during passive flexion/extension. An in vitro study. J Orthop Res 27:1426–1431
19. Belvedere C, Leardini A, Ensini A, Feliciangeli A, Catani F, Giannini S (2008) Preliminary patello-femoral joint navigation in computer assisted total knee arthroplasty. An in-vitro study. In; 8th Annual meeting of computer assisted orthopaedic surgery – international proceedings, CAOS, Hong Kong, pp 205–208
20. Besier TF, Gold GE, Beaupre GS, Delp SL (2005) A modeling framework to estimate patellofemoral joint cartilage stress in vivo. Med Sci Sports Exerc 37: 1924–1930
21. Biedert RM, Netzer P, Gal I, Sigg A, Tscholl PM (2011) The lateral condyle index: a new index for assessing the length of the lateral articular trochlea as predisposing factor for patellar instability. Int Orthop 35:1327–1331
22. Bollier M, Fulkerson JP (2011) The role of trochlear dysplasia in patellofemoral instability. J Am Acad Orthop Surg 19:8–16
23. Brossmann J, Muhle C, Schroder C, Melchert UH, Bull CC, Spielmann RP, Heller M (1993) Patellar tracking patterns during active and passive knee extension: evaluation with motion-triggered cine MR imaging. Radiology 187:205–212
24. Brunet ME, Brinker MR, Cook SD, Christakis P, Fong B, Patron L, O'Connor DP (2003) Patellar tracking during simulated quadriceps contraction. Clin Orthop Relat Res 414:266–275
25. Buff HU, Jones LC, Hungerford DS (1988) Experimental determination of forces transmitted through the patello-femoral joint. J Biomech 21:17–23
26. Bull AM, Katchburian MV, Shih YF, Amis AA (2002) Standardisation of the description of patellofemoral motion and comparison between different techniques. Knee Surg Sports Traumatol Arthrosc 10:184–193
27. Callaghan JJ, O'rourke MR, Saleh KJ (2004) Why knees fail: lessons learned. J Arthroplasty 19:31–34
28. Cappozzo A, Catani F, Croce UD, Leardini A (1995) Position and orientation in space of bones during movement: anatomical frame definition and determination. Clin Biomech (Bristol, Avon) 10:171–178

29. Catani F, Belvedere C, Ensini A, Feliciangeli A, Giannini S, Leardini A (2011) In-vivo knee kinematics in rotationally unconstrained total knee arthroplasty. J Orthop Res 29:1484–1490

30. Catani F, Ensini A, Belvedere C, Feliciangeli A, Benedetti MG, Leardini A, Giannini S (2009) In vivo kinematics and kinetics of a bi-cruciate substituting total knee arthroplasty: a combined fluoroscopic and gait analysis study. J Orthop Res 27:1569–1575

31. Chew JT, Stewart NJ, Hanssen AD, Luo ZP, Rand JA, An KN (1997) Differences in patellar tracking and knee kinematics among three different total knee designs. Clin Orthop Relat Res 345:87–98

32. Cho WS, Woo JH, Park HY, Youm YS, Kim BK (2011) Should the 'no thumb technique' be the golden standard for evaluating patellar tracking in total knee arthroplasty? Knee 18:177–179

33. Clemens U, Miehlke RK (2005) Advanced navigation planning including soft tissue management. Orthopedics 28:s1259–s1262

34. Colvin AC, West RV (2008) Patellar instability. J Bone Joint Surg Am 90:2751–2762

35. Eisenhart-Rothe R, Vogl T, Englmeier KH, Graichen H (2007) A new in vivo technique for determination of femoro-tibial and femoro-patellar 3D kinematics in total knee arthroplasty. J Biomech 40:3079–3088

36. Eisenhuth SA, Saleh KJ, Cui Q, Clark CR, Brown TE (2006) Patellofemoral instability after total knee arthroplasty. Clin Orthop Relat Res 446:149–160

37. Elias DA, White LM (2004) Imaging of patellofemoral disorders. Clin Radiol 59:543–557

38. Ensini A, Catani F, Biasca N, Belvedere C, Giannini S, Leardini A (2011) Joint line is well restored when navigation surgery is performed for total knee arthroplasty. Knee Surg Sports Traumatol Arthrosc 20(3): 495–502

39. Ensini A, Catani F, Leardini A, Romagnoli M, Giannini S (2007) Alignments and clinical results in conventional and navigated total knee arthroplasty. Clin Orthop Relat Res 457:156–162

40. Fu CK, Wai J, Lee E, Hutchison C, Myden C, Batuyong E, Anglin C (2012) Computer-assisted patellar resection system: development and insights. J Orthop Res 30:535–540

41. Fu C, Wai J, Lee E, Myden C, Batuyong E, Hutchison CR, Anglin C (2012) Computer-assisted patellar resection for total knee arthroplasty. Comput Aided Surg 17:21–28

42. Fulkerson JP (2002) Diagnosis and treatment of patients with patellofemoral pain. Am J Sports Med 30:447–456

43. Fulkerson JP, Shea KP (1990) Disorders of patellofemoral alignment. J Bone Joint Surg Am 72: 1424–1429

44. Gill HS, O'Connor JJ (1996) Biarticulating two-dimensional computer model of the human patellofemoral joint. Clin Biomech (Bristol, Avon) 11:81–89

45. Goh JC, Lee PY, Bose K (1995) A cadaver study of the function of the oblique part of vastus medialis. J Bone Joint Surg Br 77:225–231

46. Gonzales AG (1976) On the insanity defense. J Fla Med Assoc 63:436–437

47. Grelsamer RP (2000) Patellar malalignment. J Bone Joint Surg Am 82-A:1639–1650

48. Grelsamer RP (2005) Patellar nomenclature: the Tower of Babel revisited. Clin Orthop Relat Res 436:60–65

49. Grelsamer RP, Dejour D, Gould J (2008) The pathophysiology of patellofemoral arthritis. Orthop Clin North Am 39(3):269–274, v

50. Grelsamer RP, Weinstein CH (2001) Applied biomechanics of the patella. Clin Orthop Relat Res 389:9–14

51. Grood ES, Suntay WJ (1983) A joint coordinate system for the clinical description of three-dimensional motions: application to the knee. J Biomech Eng 105:136–144

52. Harwin SF (1998) Patellofemoral complications in symmetrical total knee arthroplasty. J Arthroplasty 13:753–762

53. Heegaard J, Leyvraz PF, Curnier A, Rakotomanana L, Huiskes R (1995) The biomechanics of the human patella during passive knee flexion. J Biomech 28:1265–1279

54. Hefzy MS, Jackson WT, Saddemi SR, Hsieh YF (1992) Effects of tibial rotations on patellar tracking and patello-femoral contact areas. J Biomed Eng 14:329–343

55. Hehne HJ (1990) Biomechanics of the patellofemoral joint and its clinical relevance. Clin Orthop Relat Res 258:73–85

56. Heinert G, Kendoff D, Preiss S, Gehrke T, Sussmann P (2011) Patellofemoral kinematics in mobile-bearing and fixed-bearing posterior stabilised total knee replacements: a cadaveric study. Knee Surg Sports Traumatol Arthrosc 19:967–972

57. Hsu RW (2006) The management of the patella in total knee arthroplasty. Chang Gung Med J 29: 448–457

58. Hsu HC, Luo ZP, Rand JA, An KN (1997) Influence of lateral release on patellar tracking and patellofemoral contact characteristics after total knee arthroplasty. J Arthroplasty 12:74–83

59. Jones CA, Beaupre LA, Johnston DW, Suarez-Almazor ME (2007) Total joint arthroplasties: current concepts of patient outcomes after surgery. Rheum Dis Clin North Am 33:71–86

60. Katchburian MV, Bull AM, Shih YF, Heatley FW, Amis AA (2003) Measurement of patellar tracking: assessment and analysis of the literature. Clin Orthop Relat Res 412:241–259

61. Kelly MA (2001) Patellofemoral complications following total knee arthroplasty. Instr Course Lect 50:403–407

62. Koh TJ, Grabiner MD, De Swart RJ (1992) In vivo tracking of the human patella. J Biomech 25: 637–643

63. Koyonos L, Stulberg SD, Moen TC, Bart G, Granieri M (2009) Sources of error in total knee arthroplasty. Orthopedics 32:317

64. Krackow KA, Phillips MJ, Bayers-Thering M, Serpe L, Mihalko WM (2003) Computer-assisted total knee arthroplasty: navigation in TKA. Orthopedics 26:1017–1023

65. Lafortune MA, Cavanagh PR, Sommer HJ III, Kalenak A (1992) Three-dimensional kinematics of the human knee during walking. J Biomech 25:347–357

66. Laprade J, Lee R (2005) Real-time measurement of patellofemoral kinematics in asymptomatic subjects. Knee 12:63–72

67. Laskin RS, Beksac B (2006) Computer-assisted navigation in TKA: where we are and where we are going. Clin Orthop Relat Res 452:127–131

68. Mason JB, Fehring TK, Estok R, Banel D, Fahrbach K (2007) Meta-analysis of alignment outcomes in computer-assisted total knee arthroplasty surgery. J Arthroplasty 22:1097–1106

69. McPherson EJ (2006) Patellar tracking in primary total knee arthroplasty. Instr Course Lect 55:439–448

70. Monk AP, Doll HA, Gibbons CL, Ostlere S, Beard DJ, Gill HS, Murray DW (2011) The patho-anatomy of patellofemoral subluxation. J Bone Joint Surg Br 93:1341–1347

71. Moro-oka TA, Hamai S, Miura H, Shimoto T, Higaki H, Fregly BJ, Iwamoto Y, Banks SA (2008) Dynamic activity dependence of in vivo normal knee kinematics. J Orthop Res 26:428–434

72. Moro-oka TA, Muenchinger M, Canciani JP, Banks SA (2007) Comparing in vivo kinematics of anterior cruciate-retaining and posterior cruciate-retaining total knee arthroplasty. Knee Surg Sports Traumatol Arthrosc 15:93–99

73. Noble PC, Conditt MA, Cook KF, Mathis KB (2006) The John Insall Award: patient expectations affect satisfaction with total knee arthroplasty. Clin Orthop Relat Res 452:35–43

74. Noble PC, Gordon MJ, Weiss JM, Reddix RN, Conditt MA, Mathis KB (2005) Does total knee replacement restore normal knee function? Clin Orthop Relat Res 431:157–165

75. Pagnano MW, Trousdale RT (2000) Asymmetric patella resurfacing in total knee arthroplasty. Am J Knee Surg 13:228–233

76. Parker DA, Dunbar MJ, Rorabeck CH (2003) Extensor mechanism failure associated with total knee arthroplasty: prevention and management. J Am Acad Orthop Surg 11:238–247

77. Post WR (2005) Patellofemoral pain: results of nonoperative treatment. Clin Orthop Relat Res 436:55–59

78. Powers CM, Chen YJ, Scher I, Lee TQ (2006) The influence of patellofemoral joint contact geometry on the modeling of three dimensional patellofemoral joint forces. J Biomech 39:2783–2791

79. Powers CM, Shellock FG, Pfaff M (1998) Quantification of patellar tracking using kinematic MRI. J Magn Reson Imaging 8:724–732

80. Ritter MA, Pierce MJ, Zhou H, Meding JB, Faris PM, Keating EM (1999) Patellar complications (total knee arthroplasty). Effect of lateral release and thickness. Clin Orthop Relat Res 367:149–157

81. Sakai N, Luo ZP, Rand JA, An KN (1996) Quadriceps forces and patellar motion in the anatomical model of the patellofemoral joint. Knee 3:1–7

82. Sakai N, Luo ZP, Rand JA, An KN (2000) The influence of weakness in the vastus medialis oblique muscle on the patellofemoral joint: an in vitro biomechanical study. Clin Biomech (Bristol, Avon) 15:335–339

83. Sasaki H, Kubo S, Matsumoto T, Muratsu H, Matsushita T, Ishida K, Takayama K, Oka S, Kurosaka M, Kuroda R (2011) The influence of patella height on intra-operative soft tissue balance in posterior-stabilized total knee arthroplasty. Knee Surg Sports Traumatol Arthrosc. [Epub ahead of print]. doi:10.1007/s00167-011-1797-1

84. Scuderi GR, Insall JN, Scott NW (1994) Patellofemoral pain after total knee arthroplasty. J Am Acad Orthop Surg 2:239–246

85. Seil R, Pape D (2011) Causes of failure and etiology of painful primary total knee arthroplasty. Knee Surg Sports Traumatol Arthrosc 19:1418–1432

86. Shabshin N, Schweitzer ME, Morrison WB, Parker L (2004) MRI criteria for patella alta and baja. Skeletal Radiol 33:445–450

87. Sharkey PF, Hozack WJ, Rothman RH, Shastri S, Jacoby SM (2002) Insall Award paper. Why are total knee arthroplasties failing today? Clin Orthop Relat Res 404:7–13

88. Sheehan FT, Derasari A, Fine KM, Brindle TJ, Alter KE (2010) Q-angle and J-sign: indicative of maltracking subgroups in patellofemoral pain. Clin Orthop Relat Res 468:266–275

89. Siston RA, Giori NJ, Goodman SB, Delp SL (2007) Surgical navigation for total knee arthroplasty: a perspective. J Biomech 40:728–735

90. Sparmann M, Wolke B, Czupalla H, Banzer D, Zink A (2003) Positioning of total knee arthroplasty with and without navigation support. A prospective, randomised study. J Bone Joint Surg Br 85: 830–835

91. Stiehl JB (2007) Computer navigation in primary total knee arthroplasty. J Knee Surg 20:158–164

92. Strachan RK, Merican AM, Devadasan B, Maheshwari R, Amis AA (2009) A technique of staged lateral release to correct patellar tracking in total knee arthroplasty. J Arthroplasty 24:735–742

93. Stulberg SD (2003) How accurate is current TKR instrumentation? Clin Orthop Relat Res 416:177–184

94. Tang TS, MacIntyre NJ, Gill HS, Fellows RA, Hill NA, Wilson DR, Ellis RE (2004) Accurate assessment of patellar tracking using fiducial and intensity-based fluoroscopic techniques. Med Image Anal 8: 343–351

95. Theiss SM, Kitziger KJ, Lotke PS, Lotke PA (1996) Component design affecting patellofemoral complications after total knee arthroplasty. Clin Orthop Relat Res 326:183–187

96. Tria AJ Jr (2006) The evolving role of navigation in minimally invasive total knee arthroplasty. Am J Orthop (Belle Mead NJ) 35:18–22
97. Utting MR, Davies G, Newman JH (2005) Is anterior knee pain a predisposing factor to patellofemoral osteoarthritis? Knee 12:362–365
98. Van Kampen A, Huiskes R (1990) The three-dimensional tracking pattern of the human patella. J Orthop Res 8:372–382
99. Waters TS, Bentley G (2003) Patellar resurfacing in total knee arthroplasty. A prospective, randomized study. J Bone Joint Surg Am 85-A:212–217

How to Teach Total Knee Reconstruction Using Computer-Assisted Navigation

19

S. David Stulberg

19.1 Introduction

The original goals of applying computer-assisted surgical techniques to knee reconstructive procedures were to (1) increase the accuracy with which implants and limbs were aligned and soft tissues balanced and (2) improve the reliability with which the procedures were performed (i.e., reduce the incidence of alignment and soft-tissue balancing "outliers") [18, 80]. These goals were based upon the well-established observations that the clinical and functional outcomes of knee reconstructive procedures and the durability of these procedures were correlated with the accuracy of implant and limb alignment and the quality of soft-tissue balancing [1, 3, 4, 20, 21, 26, 30, 38–40, 49, 50, 59, 61, 62, 68, 69, 75, 78, 84–86, 89].

When surgeons experienced in the manual performance of the knee reconstruction procedures use computer-assisted surgical techniques, numerous reports have confirmed that average implant and limb alignment is improved and the incidence of "outliers" is reduced [2, 5–8, 10–13, 16, 17, 22, 23, 33, 36, 37, 41–46, 53–55, 57, 58, 60, 70, 72, 73, 76, 77, 79, 86, 88]. Moreover, recent reports indicate that when experienced surgeons use computer-assisted surgical techniques to perform knee reconstructive procedures, their ability to perform these procedures *manually* improves [81].

It had been anticipated by the developers of computer-assisted technologies for knee surgery that the goals of increased alignment accuracy and reproducibility would also be realized by surgeons who were less experienced with or performed relatively few major knee reconstruction procedures. It was hoped that computer technology could narrow or eliminate the differences in outcomes that have been reported based upon operative volumes.

However, current computer-assisted systems for knee reconstruction have proven relatively inaccessible to and inappropriate for surgeons who perform relatively few of these procedures or who have relatively little experience with these procedures. Computer navigation techniques require the use of new and different instrumentations. The procedures appear cumbersome and awkward in comparison to those of routine, manual primary knee reconstructions. Consequently, there is, in general, a relatively long learning curve associated with the use of computer-assisted techniques for knee reconstruction. Moreover, these techniques, even in the hands of experienced surgeons, prolong surgical procedures by 15–30 min, making their use by less-experienced surgeons daunting. Finally, computer-assisted surgical systems are expensive. It is often not possible or realistic for hospitals performing relatively few knee reconstruction procedures to invest in this technology at this time.

S.D. Stulberg, M.D.
Division of Joint Reconstruction and Implant Service,
Northwestern University, 680 N Lake Shore Dr,
Ste 1028, Chicago, IL 60611, USA
e-mail: jointsurg@northwestern.edu

F. Catani, S. Zaffagnini (eds.), *Knee Surgery using Computer Assisted Surgery and Robotics*,
DOI 10.1007/978-3-642-31430-8_19, © ESSKA 2013

There continues to exist, therefore, the need to develop technologies that can help surgeons who are less experienced with or who perform relatively few major knee reconstruction procedures achieve accurate and reproducible results. It is now beginning to be appreciated that computer-assisted technologies can be used in both teaching laboratories and the operating room as training tools for these surgeons. This application of computer technology could have a profound impact on the way in which surgeons are taught knee surgery.

19.2 The Evolution of the Teaching Model for Knee Surgery

Surgical training has always relied significantly on the importance of adequate operating room experience and sufficient exposure to actual surgical procedures [35]. However, a number of factors have emerged in the past few years that make actual operating room experience and volume less reliable and appropriate as the basis for acquiring and maintaining surgical expertise [65]. The shorter workweek for residents reduces this group of inexperienced surgeons' opportunities for learning in the operating room. Increased emphasis on operating room efficiencies reduces the time that surgeons feel willing to take to acquire new surgical skills. Concerns about the legal impact of using new technologies in the operating room make the use of this location increasingly less appropriate for learning new surgical techniques. As a result, surgical skills laboratories are rapidly becoming sites essential for teaching surgical residents basic surgical procedures and for training experienced surgeons in new techniques [9, 51, 64, 71]. These laboratories are stimulating a reexamination of the way surgeons learn and can be taught.

The theoretical foundation of surgical training most widely accepted and applied is based on the three stages of motor skill acquisition described by Fitts and Posner [27, 47] (Table 19.1). In the first stage, cognition, the procedure to be learned is explained and demonstrated to the surgical trainee. In the second stage, integration, the trainee practices the procedure and receives feedback from an experienced instructor. In the third phase, automation, the trainee becomes so adept at the procedure that he or she is no longer consciously aware of how the task is being performed. Surgical skills laboratories, rather than operating rooms, are increasingly becoming the sites at which the first two stages of training occur. This theoretical model of skill acquisition is particularly helpful in understanding how surgeons learn basic surgical techniques, e.g., suture tying.

An important advance in the understanding of how surgeons acquire skills has come from Ericsson's work on the nature of expert performance [24, 25]. Drawing on extensive study of superior athletes, chess players, and musicians, he evolved the concept of *deliberate practice* as the basis for the development of mastery or expertise of a particular skill. Ericsson's observations suggested that true experts not only practiced their skills frequently but did so in a specific, *deliberate* way. That is, experts engage in the practice of their skills with the primary goal of improving some aspect of their performance. An essential aspect of deliberate practice is the importance of repeated and accurate feedback on performance.

The practice of surgery, like the piloting of an airplane, allows for virtually no error in performance. Surgical skills, therefore, must not only be acquired but mastered. Computer technology is ideally suited to provide the essential requirements of both the Fitts and Posner concept of skill acquisition and the Ericsson model of expert performance. Computer technology, if properly applied in both the skills laboratory and operating room, offers the possibility that an expert's level of skill acquisition can be attained and practiced even by those who use the skill relatively infrequently.

19.3 The Use of Computer Technology in the Skills Laboratory

The first stage of the Fitts–Posner theory of motor skill acquisition is cognition, understanding the skill that is to be performed. This skill may be a simple task, e.g., tying a surgical knot, or may be

Table 19.1 The Fitts–Posner theory of motor skill acquisition

Stage	Goal	Activity
Cognition	Understand task	Explanation, demonstration
Integration	Translate knowledge of skill into conscious motor activity	Practice, receive feedback
Automation	Perform motor activity without thinking about it	Motor activity, a routine part of full procedure

Adapted from Fitts and Posner [27]

a complex one, requiring the performance of a number of simple physical tasks in a given sequence and in accordance with specific guidelines, e.g., a total knee replacement. The description and demonstration of the skill, whether simple or complex, has been traditionally performed in the laboratory by an instructor with the aid of written and visual materials. The computer dramatically extends the ability of an instructor to provide this description and carry out the demonstration. DVD productions illustrating a variety of simple and complex surgical skills are now available. Interactive computer programs make it possible for the student to confirm his or her understanding of the skill, even before attempting to perform it. A wide variety of simulations, from schematic body models to lifelike three-dimensional anatomic reproductions, can be presented in these interactive productions. These programs provide the learner with a wide range of visual and tactile prospectives of a motor skill. The programs can also be used by an instructor to demonstrate in an efficient and clear way both the proper and improper ways of performing a motor skill. Computer programs can also be used to demonstrate the consequences of performing a skill incorrectly, e.g., simulations of the impact of changing femoral implant rotation or size on the flexion gap in a TKA can be carried out by students learning to perform this step of the procedure. Moreover, a substantial amount of active cognition can take place even before the student comes to the laboratory to practice.

The second stage of the Fitts–Posner theory is integration, the translation of an understanding of the skill into appropriate motor behavior. In this stage, the skill is practiced by the learner in the laboratory while being supervised. Computers greatly enhance, and in some situations may make superfluous, the instructor's ability to provide the student with feedback (Fig. 19.1). Current computer-assisted knee reconstruction applications (e.g., TKA, ACL, HTO, UKA) can be used in conjunction with the performance of a specific surgical procedure to guide the student through steps of the operation and to measure the accuracy with which each step of the procedure is performed. This is a particularly useful method for teaching open surgical procedures. The computer is a very powerful tool for providing feedback to learners of surgical skills. However, there is virtually no data currently available [15] to support the use of computers in surgical laboratories in this way. Once such data are available, it is likely that computers will have a prominent presence in all knee reconstruction hands-on courses.

Computers linked to surgical simulators can also play a critical and powerful role in the integration stage of motor skill acquisition. Advances in virtual reality technology are occurring rapidly and are now the basis for a number of commercially available surgical simulators. These systems make it possible for the student to perform a surgical procedure in a virtual environment with tools that look, feel, and perform much like real instruments [35]. The student can receive accurate and instantaneous feedback about innumerable aspects of his or her performance of the surgical task. The student can monitor very accurately his or her progress in acquiring the surgical skill [14, 56]. Surgical simulators have been successfully used in a variety of general surgical, urologic, and vascular [29] training programs for the teaching of minimally invasive endoscopic and laparoscopic procedures [28, 31, 67, 72, 83]. These simulators can be used on a variety of models, including inanimate fabricated anatomical replications, cadavers, and live animals [32]. They can also be self-contained virtual reality

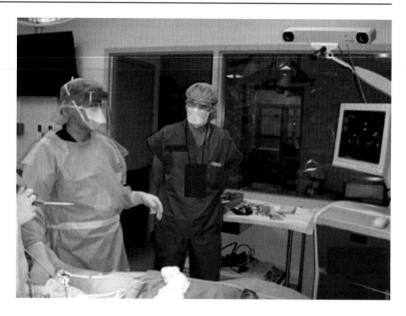

Fig. 19.1 Student carrying out a step of knee reconstruction procedure in laboratory while receiving visual feedback from computer-assisted program and guidance from instructor

units whose use can closely replicate the feel and look of live surgery. The use of computer-based surgical simulators for the teaching of knee surgery is just beginning to emerge. Simulators are particularly appropriate for the teaching of arthroscopic skills (personal communication: Howard J. Sweeney, M.D., Northwestern-Evanston Healthcare System). If the use of simulators for the teaching of arthroscopic knee surgery parallels their use in urologic, vascular, endoscopic, and laparoscopic surgery, it is likely that most orthopedic surgical training programs and many orthopedic surgical courses will devote a substantial amount of time to simulator-based training.

Perhaps the most significant impact of computer technology on the training of knee surgical procedures will be on the measurement of the efficacy of various educational techniques in teaching these surgical skills. Many efforts in the past few years have focused on establishing standard and reliable methods for evaluating the surgical performance of trainees. Objectively evaluating surgical performance in the operating room is difficult [83, 90]). Therefore, a substantial effort has been made to establish and validate objective measures of operative skills in the surgical laboratory. The Objective Structured Assessment of Technical Skills

(OSATS) requires students to perform a series of standardized surgical tasks on inanimate models under the direct observation of an expert [52, 66]. The examiners use a task-specific checklist consisting of 10–30 specific surgical maneuvers considered essential for the procedure and a global rating form consisting of 5–8 surgical behaviors (e.g., respect for soft tissue, appropriate use of assistants) important for the successful performance of the procedure to grade the student's performance. The OSATS validity and reliability have been well established [63, 66, 82]. The McGill Inanimate System for Training and Evaluation of Laparoscopic Skills (MISTELS) uses an inanimate box to simulate the basic skills needed to perform laparoscopic surgery [83]. Its validity and reliability for evaluating these skills have been confirmed. The Imperial College Surgical Assessment Device (ICSAD) tracks hand motion using sensors placed on the student's hands during the performance of the surgical skill [15, 83]. The sensors translate movement into computerized tracings of hand motion. This tracing is an index of the technical skill with which various laparoscopic and open procedures are performed. The ICSAD has been shown to have good concordance with OSATS scores [14]. Virtual simulators of surgical procedures will augment and, in some cases, replace the tools for measuring the efficacy of various surgical skill training techniques. As computing power expands and the cost of simulation equipment falls, the ability to use simulators to train and evaluate surgeons will increase. In the future, surgeons (residents and practicing orthopedists) will probably need to demonstrate proficiency in basic and complex techniques in the laboratory, measured by computer-based assessment tools, before performing new procedures in the operating room.

The evolution of a competence-based system of surgical education and evaluation will require the establishment of standards for the performance of technical skills [65]. This difficult task will become more urgent as advances in orthopedic technology are demonstrated to be clinically effective. Computer-based evaluation tools will undoubtedly play an important role in the establishment of unbiased, objective, and meaningful tools for measuring appropriate surgical skill acquisition.

The establishment of these evaluation tools will have to be based upon the demonstration that training programs in surgical skills laboratories result in both initial and sustained improvements in surgical performance in the operating room [65, 74]. Such evidence is now emerging for a number of general surgical and vascular minimally invasive procedures. Training in the laboratory on both physical laparoscopic and virtual reality laparoscopic simulators has led to measurable benefits for learners in the clinical setting. There is also some information that suggests that the improvement in surgical skills resulting from simulated training in the laboratory may eliminate, or reduce, the learning curve for a new procedure in the operating room.

19.4 The Role of the Computer as a Teaching Tool in the Operating Room

There exists extensive evidence from many surgical fields, including orthopedics, that there is a relationship between operative volume and clinical outcomes [34]. However, most knee reconstructive procedures are performed by surgeons who perform relatively few of these procedures. Thus, the third stage of Fitts and Posner's theory of motor skill acquisition, automation (the automatic performance of a skill requiring little or no cognitive input), will be difficult for many surgeons performing complex knee procedures to achieve. It is likely that, for the foreseeable future, a significant portion of these procedures will continue to be performed by a large number of surgeons doing relatively few. It is critical that efforts be made to assure that these surgeons perform the procedures accurately and reproducibly.

There is beginning to emerge information that indicates that the exposure to computer-assisted techniques for knee reconstruction during the actual performance of the procedures increases the understanding of these procedures by both experienced and novice surgeons and improves the accuracy and reliability with which these procedures are performed using conventional, non-navigated surgical techniques [81]. Although the exact mechanisms by which this learning takes place in the operating room are not yet well understood, a number of observations that might relate to these mechanisms have been made.

It is well recognized by experienced knee surgeons who have learned and extensively used computer-assisted systems that they are, as a result, "better surgeons" when performing the procedures using conventional surgical techniques. Although this information is anecdotal, it is remarkably consistent. The exact reasons given by these surgeons vary but usually include comments related to giving more attention to surgical detail, as a consequence of exposure to computer-assisted techniques, or to performing more intraoperative measurements at each step of the surgical procedure. Studies with computer-assisted techniques have clearly demonstrated the frequency with which errors occur at each step of knee procedures and have indicated the potential magnitude of these errors [48]. Surgeons experienced with computer navigation techniques are very aware of these issues and incorporate methods for addressing them (e.g., performing frequent measurements at each step of the procedure) when using conventional, non-navigated techniques.

Fig. 19.2 Example of a TKA computer screen present in the operating room to illustrate to the surgeon or surgical trainee the relationships between femoral rotation, femoral implant size, and the flexion and extension gaps

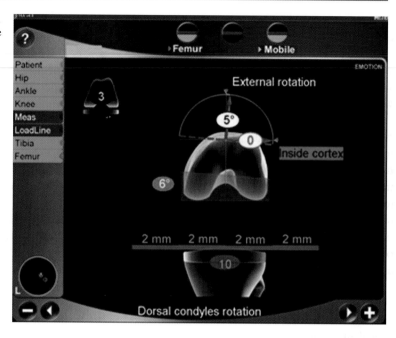

A recent study by a surgeon very familiar with navigation techniques indicated that after extensive exposure to these computer techniques, it was possible for him to perform a TKA with the same degree of accuracy and reproducibility using manual techniques as it was using navigation techniques [81]. In a previous study by the same surgeon carried out at the beginning of his navigation experience, he was able to perform TKA more accurately using navigation. It was suggested that the "real-time feedback" provided by computer-assisted techniques led, over time, to an increased appreciation of the factors related to accurately performing a TKA and to an increased ability to assess the accuracy with which each step of the procedure was performed. Moreover, many of the studies demonstrating an equivalency between computer-assisted and manual techniques have been carried out by surgeons very experienced with navigation. This finding of equivalency may, in fact, reflect a learning effect acquired by the surgeons as they become facile with computer navigation techniques.

Recently, a study from Scotland [19] revealed that trainees exposed to computer navigation techniques during the performance of TKA procedures were much more likely to understand the fundamental anatomical reference points and axes in TKA than trainees who had not had this exposure. The authors postulated that this increased understanding may be due to the visual information given by the navigation software during the performance of a TKA and to the real-time kinematic feedback provided by the software that made it possible to better understand the relationship between each part of the surgical procedure and the final alignment and soft-tissue balance outcome (Fig. 19.2).

The implication of all of these studies and observations is that there is a measurable and substantial benefit to both experienced and inexperienced surgeons to receiving real-time feedback during the performance of a knee reconstruction procedure. This feedback may allow surgeons who are relatively unfamiliar with the procedure or who perform relatively few procedures to carry out relatively complex knee reconstructions (e.g., TKA) as accurately and reproducibly as experienced, high-volume surgeons. Computer-assisted techniques are one type of technology capable of providing very accurate real-time feedback. However, current navigation systems have a number of design characteristics which make them inappropriate for widespread use as universal intraoperative measurement tools. The current systems are generally cumbersome. The learning curve for the use of the systems is often prolonged and awkward. The use of the current systems adds a significant amount of time to the procedure, even when used by experienced surgeons. The current systems do not interact easily with conventional, manual instrumentation. The current systems are too expensive to use as intraoperative measurement tools. Nevertheless, a number of developments are now occurring (e.g., pinless registration techniques that allow navigation equipment to be attached directly to manual-based instrumentation) that may make the widespread availability of this technology in the operating room feasible and desirable.

Conclusion

Surgical education is in the midst of a major and important transformation. This transformation is being driven by a number of factors. The operating room as the primary focus of learning for surgeons-in-training and for surgeons seeking refreshment of their surgical skills and knowledge is becoming less feasible. Residents have shorter workweeks, making them less available to assist in the operating room. There is an increased emphasis on the need for operating room efficiency which makes more difficult the allotment of time during the procedure for teaching of all types. The increased use of new technologies and the increased complexity of surgical procedures make it more difficult to use these surgical procedures for hands-on teaching. Concerns about the legal impact of using new technologies in the operating room make the use of this location increasingly less appropriate for teaching new surgical techniques.

The surgical skills laboratory and surgical learning centers are becoming increasingly accepted as desirable sites for teaching new skills and techniques. The number and sophistication of the teaching modalities available in these laboratories are growing. Orthopedic surgery was one of the first surgical fields to introduce computer-assisted surgical techniques in the operating room. Therefore, the incorporation of this technology as a teaching tool, especially for open surgical procedures, e.g., TKA, is conceptually relatively easy and accessible. Moreover, the computer-based simulation technologies being developed and successfully used in other fields of surgery to train surgeons to perform endoscopic and laparoscopic procedures have been validated as safe and effective. These technologies will become increasingly used to train and update surgeons in a wide range of arthroscopic-based knee procedures. The computer is likely to become the basic tool upon which a wide variety of teaching and skills assessment techniques will be based in the surgical learning centers of the future.

Surgical educators are increasingly recognizing the limits of the motor skill acquisition theories of Fitts and Posner when applied to current highly technical and complex surgical procedures, especially when these are performed by surgeons who do relatively few. The deliberate practice model of Ericsson, with its focus on expert performance, is much more consistent with the requirements of surgeons that they be highly accurate and consistent. Computer-based teaching modalities have the potential for providing one of the most essential aspects of the Ericsson model, accurate, unbiased, real-time performance feedback to the surgical trainee. The deliberate practice model is based upon the assumption that the trainee will acquire motor skills by "practicing" in an environment other than that in which the skill will ultimately be demonstrated (e.g., the concert violinist will practice in a studio not on the concert stage). However, the organization of surgeons' schedules does not permit the type of prolonged, intense practice of surgical procedures, even by those who specialize in a limited number of procedures, envisioned by Ericsson. In order to reap the benefits of the deliberate practice model, it will be necessary to incorporate its principles in the operating room environment. The computer may emerge as an ideal tool for providing the type of accurate, unbiased, real-time feedback that not only increases the accuracy of the surgical procedure but also improves the understanding and judgment of surgical trainees and experienced surgeons. The computer is likely to be the basis for the evolution of the concept that the operating room is both the primary performance stage and essential training location of the surgeon.

References

1. Aglietti P, Buzzi R (1988) Posteriorly stabilized total-condylar knee replacement. J Bone Joint Surg Br 70(2):211–216
2. Anderson KC, Buehler KC, Markel DC (2005) Computer assisted navigation in total knee arthroplasty: comparison with conventional methods. J Arthroplasty 20(7 Suppl 3):132–138
3. Ayers DC, Dennis DA, Johanson NA et al (1997) Common complications of total knee arthroplasty. J Bone J Surg Am 2(79A):278–311
4. Bargren JH, Blaha JD, Freeman MAR (1983) Alignment in total knee arthroplasty: correlated biomechanical and clinical observations. Clin Orthop 173:178–183
5. Bathis H, Perlick L, Tingart M et al (2004) Alignment in total knee arthroplasty. A comparison of computer-assisted surgery with conventional technique. J Bone Joint Surg Br 86:682–687
6. Bauwens K, Matthes G, Wich M et al (2007) Navigated total knee replacement. A meta-analysis. J Bone Joint Surg Am 89:261–269
7. Bohling U, Schamberger H, Grittner U et al (2005) Computerised and technical navigation in total knee arthroplasty. J Orthop Traumatol 6:69–75
8. Bolognesi M, Hofmann A (2005) Computer navigation versus standard instrumentation for TKA: a single-surgeon experience. Clin Orthop Relat Res 440:162–169
9. Cauraugh JH, Martin M, Martin KK (1999) Modeling surgical expertise for motor sill acquisition. Am J Surg 177:331–336
10. Chauhan SK, Scott RG, Breidahl W et al (2004) Computer-assisted knee arthroplasty versus a conventional jig-based technique. A randomized, prospective trial. J Bone Joint Surg Br 86:372–377
11. Chin PL, Yang KY, Yeo SJ et al (2005) Randomized control trial comparing radiographic total knee arthroplasty implant placement using computer navigation versus conventional technique. J Arthroplasty 20:618–626
12. Confalonieri N, Manzotti A, Pullen C et al (2005) Computer-assisted technique versus intramedullary and extramedullary alignment systems in total knee replacement: a radiological comparison. Acta Orthop Belg 71:L703–L709
13. Cossey AJ, Spriggins AJ (2005) The use of computer-assisted surgical navigation to prevent malalignment in unicompartmental knee arthroplasty. J Arthroplasty 20:29–34
14. Darzi A, Mackay S (2001) Assessment of surgical competence. Qual Health Care 10(Suppl 2):ii64–ii69
15. Datta V, Mackay SD, Mandalia M et al (2001) The use of electromagnetic motion tracking analysis to objectively measure open surgical skill in the laboratory-based model. J Am Coll Surg 193:479–485
16. Daubresse F, Vajeu C, Loquet J (2005) Total knee arthroplasty with conventional or navigated technique: comparison of the learning curves in a community hospital. Acta Orthop Belg 71:710–713
17. Decking R, Markmann Y, Fuchs J et al (2005) Leg axis after computer navigated total knee arthroplasty: a prospective randomized trial comparing computer-navigated and manual implantation. J Arthroplasty 20:282–288
18. Delp SL, Stulberg SD, Davies B, et al. (1998) Computer assisted knee replacement. Clin Orthop (354):49–56
19. Dillon JM, Clarke JV, Picard F et al (2007) Computer assisted navigation systems have a valuable teaching role in total knee arthroplasty. Poster. AAOS, San Diego
20. Dorr LD, Boiardo RA (1997) Technical considerations in total knee arthroplasty. Clin Orthop 205:5–11
21. Ecker ML, Lotke PA, Windsor RE et al (1987) Long-term results after total condylar knee arthroplasty. Significance of radiolucent lines. Clin Orthop 216:151–158
22. Eichorn H-J (2004) Image-free navigation in ACL replacement with the OrthoPilot System. In: Steihl JB, Konermann WH, Haaker RG (eds) Navigation and robotics in total joint and spine surgery. Springer, Berlin, pp 387–396
23. Ellis RE, Rudan JF, Harrison MM (2004) Computer-assisted high tibial osteotomies. In: DiGioia AM, Jaramaz B, Picard R, Nolte PL (eds) Computer and robotic assisted knee and hip surgery. Oxford University Press, Oxford, pp 197–212
24. Ericsson KA (1996) The acquisition of expert performance: an introduction to some of the issues. In: Ericsson KA (ed) The road to excellence: the acquisition of expert performance in the arts and sciences, sports, and games. Lawrence Erlbaum Associates, Mahwah, pp 1–50
25. Ericsson KA (2004) Deliberate practice and the acquisition and maintenance of expert performance in medicine and related domains. Acad Med 79(Suppl 10):S70–S81
26. Fehring TK, Odum S, Wl G et al (2001) Early failures in total knee arthroplasty. Clin Orthop 392:315–318
27. Fitts PM, Posner MI (1967) Human performance. Brooks/Cole, Belmont
28. Fried GM, Feldman LS, Vassiliou MC et al (2004) Proving the value of simulation in laparoscopic surgery. Ann Surg 240:518–528
29. Gallagher AG, Cates CU (2004) Approval of virtual reality training for carotid stenting: what this means for procedural-based medicine. JAMA 292:3024–3026

30. Gonzalez MH, Mekhail AO (2005) The failed total knee arthroplasty: evaluation and etiology. J Am Acad Orthop Surg 12:436–446
31. Grantcharov TP, Kristiansen VBG, Bendix J et al (2004) Randomized clinical trial of virtual reality simulation for laparoscopic skills training. Br J Surg 91:146–150
32. Grober ED, Hamstra SJ, Wanzel KR et al (2004) The educational impact of bench model fidelity on the acquisition of technical skill: the use of clinically relevant outcome measures. Ann Surg 240: 374–381
33. Haaker RG, Stockhelm M, Kamp M et al (2005) Computer-assisted navigation increases precision of component placement in total knee arthroplasty. Clin Orthop Relat Res 433:152–159
34. Halm EA, Lee C, Chassin MR (2002) Is volume related to outcome in health care? A systematic review and methodologic critique of the literature. Ann Intern Med 137:511–520
35. Haluck RS, Krummel TM (2000) Computers and virtual reality for surgical education in the 21st century. Arch Surg 135:786–792
36. Harnandez-Vaquero D, Suarez-Vazquez A, Garcia-Sandoval MA (2004) Computer-assisted implant in knee endoprosthesis with a wireless system. Prospective comparative study with conventional technique (abstract). J Bone Joint Surg Br 86(Suppl 3): 227. Abstract nr 01026
37. Hart R, Janecek M, Chaker A (2003) Total knee arthroplasty implanted with and without kinematic navigation. Int Orthop 27:366–369
38. Hsu HP, Garg A, Walker PS (1989) Effect on knee component alignment on tibial load distribution with clinical correlation. Clin Orthop 248: 135–144
39. Jeffcote B, Shakespeare D (2003) Varus/valgus alignment of the tibial component in total knee arthroplasty. Knee 10(3):243–247
40. Jeffery RS, Morris RW, Denham RA (1991) Coronal alignment after total knee replacement. J Bone Joint Surg Br 73B:709–714
41. Jenny JY, Boeri C (2002) Unicompartmental knee prosthesis. A case-control comparative study of two types of instrumentation with a five year follow-up. J Arthroplasty 17:1016020
42. Jenny JY, Clemens U, Kohler S et al (2005) Consistency of implantation of a total knee arthroplasty with a non-image-based navigation system: a case-control study of 235 cases compared with 235 conventionally implanted prostheses. J Arthroplasty 20:832–839
43. Keen G, Simpson D, Kalirajah Y et al (2006) Limb alignment in computer-assisted minimally invasive unicompartmental knee replacement. J Bone Joint Surg Br 88:44–48
44. Kim SJ, MacDonald M, Hernandez J et al (2005) Computer assisted navigation in total knee arthroplasty: improved coronal alignment. J Arthoplasty 20(7 Suppl 3):123–131
45. Kinzel V, Scaddan M, Bradley B et al (2004) Varus/valgus alignment of the femur in total knee arthroplasty. Can accuracy be improved by pre-operative CT scanning? Knee 11(3):197–201
46. Klein GR, Austn MS, Smith EB et al (2006) Total knee arthroplasty using computer-assisted navigation in patients with deformities of the femur and tibia. J Arthroplasty 21:284–288
47. Kopta JA (1971) The development of motor skills in orthopaedic education. Clin Orthop 75:80–85
48. Koyonos L, Granieri M, Stulberg SD (2005) At what steps in performance of a TKA do errors occur when manual instrumentation is used. Presented at the annual meeting of American Academy of Orthopaedic Surgeons, Washington, DC
49. Laskin RS (1984) Alignment of the total knee components. Orthopedics 7:62
50. Laskin RS (1990) Total condylar knee replacement in patients who have rheumatoid arthritis. A ten year follow-up study. J Bone Joint Surg Am 72A:529–535
51. Lossing AG, Hatswell EM, Gilas T et al (1992) A technical-skills course for 1st year residents in general surgery: a descriptive study. Can J Surg 35: 536–540
52. Martin JA, Regehr G, Reznick R et al (1997) Objective structured assessment of technical skill (OSATS) for surgical residents. Br J Surg 84:273–278
53. Matsumoto T, Tsumura N, Kurosaka M et al (2004) Prosthetic alignment and sizing in computer assisted total knee arthroplasty. Int Orthop 28:282–285
54. Matziolis G, Krocker D, Weiss U et al (2007) A prospective, randomized study of computer-assisted and conventional total knee arthroplasty. Three-dimensional evaluation of implant alignment and rotation. J Bone Joint Surg Am 89:236–243
55. Miehlke RK, Clemens U, Jens J-H et al (2001) Navigation in knee arthroplasty: preliminary clinical experience and prospective comparative study in comparison with conventional technique. Z Orthop Ihre Grenzgeb 139:109–129
56. Noble PC, Sugano N, Johnston JD et al (2003) Computer simulation: how can it help the surgeon optimize implant position? Clin Orthop (417):242-252. Review
57. Oberst M, Bertsch C, Wurstlin S et al (2003) CT analysis of leg alignment after conventional vs. navigated knee prosthesis implantation. Initial results of a controlled, prospective, and randomized study. Unfallchirurg 106:941–948. (German)
58. Perlick L, Bathis H, Tingart M et al (2004) Minimally invasive unicompartmental knee replacement with a nonimage-based navigation system. Int Orthop 28:193–197
59. Petersen TL, Engh GA (1988) Radiographic assessment of knee alignment after total knee arthroplasty. J Arthroplasty 3:67–72
60. Plaweski S, Cazal J, Roseli P et al (2006) Anterior cruciate ligament reconstruction using navigation: a comparative study on 60 patients. Am J Sports Med 34:542–552

61. Ranawat CS, Boachie-Adjei O (1988) Survivorship analysis and results of total condylar knee arthroplasty. Clin Orthop 226:6–13
62. Rand JA, Coventry MB (1988) Ten-year evaluation of geometric total knee arthroplasty. Clin Orthop 232: 168–173
63. Regehr G, MacRae H, Reznick RK et al (1998) Comparing the psychometric properties of checklists and global rating scales for assessing performance on an OSCE-format examination. Acad Med 73: 993–997
64. Reznick RK (1993) Teaching and testing technical skills. Am J Surg 165:358–361
65. Reznick RK, MacRae H (2006) Teaching surgical skills-changes in the wind. N Engl J Med 355: 2664–2669
66. Reznick R, Regehr G, MacRae H, Martin J et al (1997) Testing technical skill via an innovative "bench station" examination. Am J Surg 173:226–230
67. Risucci D, Cohen JA, Garbus JE et al (2001) The effects of practice and instruction on speed and accuracy during resident acquisition of simulated laparoscopic skills. Curr Surg 58:230–235
68. Ritter MA, Faris PM, Keating EM et al (1994) Postoperative alignment of total knee replacement. Its effect on survival. Clin Orthop 299:153–156
69. Ritter M, Merbst WA, Keating EM et al (1991) Radiolucency at the bone-cement interface in total knee replacement. J Bone Joint Surg Am 76A: 60–65
70. Saragaglia D, Picard F, Chaussard C et al (2001) Computer-assisted knee arthroplasty: comparison with a conventional procedure: results of 50 cases in a prospective randomized study. Rev Chir Orthop Reparatrice Appar Mot 87:18–28
71. Scallon SE, Fairholm DJ, Cochrane DD et al (1992) Evaluation of the operating room as a surgical teaching venue. Can J Surg 35:173–176
72. Scott DJ, Bergen PC, Rege RV et al (2004) Laparoscopic training on bench model simulators: a randomized controlled trial evaluating the durability of technical skill. J Urol 99:33–37
73. Seon JK, Song EK (2005) Functional impact of navigation-assisted minimally invasive total knee arthroplasty. Orthopedics 28(10 Suppl):s1251–s1254
74. Seymour NE, Gallagher AG, Roman SA et al (2002) Virtual reality training improves operating room performance: results of a randomized, double-blinded study. Ann Surg 236:458–463
75. Sharkey PF, Hozack WJ, Rothman RH et al (2002) Why are total knee arthroplasties failing today? Clin Orthop 404:7–13
76. Skowronski J, Bielecki M, Hermanowicz K et al (2005) The radiological outcomes of total knee arthroplasty

using computer assisted navigation ORTHOPILOT. Chir Narzadow Ruchu Ortop Pol 70:5–8
77. Sparmann M, Wolke B, Czupalla H et al (2003) Positioning of total knee arthroplasty with and without navigation support. A prospective, randomised study. J Bone Joint Surg Br 85:830–835
78. Stern SH, Insall JN (1992) Posterior stabilized prosthesis: results after follow-up of 9-12 years. J Bone Joint Surg Am 74A:980–986
79. Stulberg SD (2005) CAS-TKA reduces the occurrence of functional outliers. Presented at the annual meeting of Mid-America Orthopaedic Association, Amelia Island
80. Stulberg SD, Eichorn J, Saragaglia D et al (2003) The rationale for and initial experience with a knee suite of computer assisted surgical applications. In: Third International CAOS Meeting, Marbella
81. Stulberg SD, Yaffe MA, Koo SS (2006) Computer-assisted surgery versus manual total knee arthroplasty: a case-controlled study. J Bone Joint Surg Am 88:47–54
82. Szalay D, MacRae H, Regehr G et al (2000) Using operative outcome to assess technical skill. Am J Surg 180:234–237
83. Taffinder N, Sutton C, Fishwick RJ et al. (1998) Validation of virtual reality to teach and assess psychomotor skills in laparoscopic surgery: results from randomised controlled studies using the MIST VR laparoscopic simulator. Stud Health Technol Inform 50:124–130
84. Tew M, Waugh W (1985) Tibiofemoral alignment and the results of knee replacement. J Bone Joint Surg Br 67B:551–556
85. Townley CD. (1985) The anatomic total knee: instrumentation and alignment technique. The knee: papers of the first scientific meeting of the knee society. University Park Press, Baltimore, pp 39–54
86. Victor J, Hoste D (2004) Image-based computer-assisted total knee arthroplasty leads to lower variability in coronal alignment. Clin Orthop Relat Res 428:131–139
87. Vince KIG, Insall JN, Kelly MA (1989) The total condylar prosthesis. 10 to 12 year results of a cemented knee replacement. J Bone Joint Surg Br 71B:93–797
88. Werner FW, Ayers DC, Maletsky LP et al (2005) The effect of valgus/varus malalignment on load distribution in total knee replacements. J Biomech 38: 349–355
89. Winckel CP, Reznick RK, Cohen R et al (1994) Reliability and construct validity of a structured technical skills assessment form. Am J Surg 167: 423–427
90. Zorman D, Etuin P, Jennart H et al (2005) Computer-assisted total knee arthroplasty: comparative results in a preliminary series of 72 cases. Acta Orthop Belg 71:696–702

Index